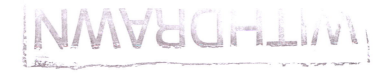

Complex Systems in Sport

Complex systems in nature are those with many interacting parts, all capable of influencing global system outcomes. There is a growing body of research that has modelled sport performance from a complexity sciences perspective, studying the behaviour of individual athletes and sports teams as emergent phenomena which self-organize under interacting constraints.

This book is the first to bring together experts studying complex systems in the context of sport from across the world to collate core theoretical ideas, current methodologies and existing data into one comprehensive resource. It offers new methods of analysis for investigating representative complex sport movements and actions at an individual and team level, exploring the application of methodologies from the complexity sciences in the context of sports performance and the organization of sport practice.

Complex Systems in Sport is important reading for any advanced student or researcher working in sport and exercise science, sports coaching, kinesiology or human movement.

Keith Davids is Professor of Motor Control at the Centre for Sports Engineering Research, Sheffield Hallam University, UK.

Robert Hristovski is Professor in the Faculty of Physical Education at the University of Ss. Cyril and Methodius, Republic of Macedonia.

Duarte Araújo is Associate Professor in the Faculty of Human Kinetics at University of Lisbon, Portugal.

Natàlia Balagué Serre is Professor of Exercise Physiology in the INEFC at the University of Barcelona, Spain.

Chris Button is Associate Professor of Motor Learning at the School of Physical Education, Sport and Exercise Sciences, University of Otago, Dunedin, New Zealand.

Pedro Passos is Assistant Professor of Motor Control in the Faculty of Human Kinetics at the University of Lisbon, Portugal.

Routledge Research in Sport and Exercise Science

The *Routledge Research in Sport and Exercise Science* series is a showcase for cutting-edge research from across sport and exercise sciences, including physiology, psychology, biomechanics, motor control, physical activity and health, and every core subdiscipline. Featuring the work of established and emerging scientists and practitioners from around the world, and covering the theoretical, investigative and applied dimensions of sport and exercise, this series is an important channel for new and groundbreaking research in the human movement sciences.

Also available in this series:

1. **Mental Toughness in Sport**
   Developments in Theory and Research
   Daniel Gucciardi and Sandy Gordon

2. **Paediatric Biomechanics and Motor Control**
   Theory and Application
   Mark De Ste Croix and Thomas Korff

3. **Attachment in Sport, Exercise and Wellness**
   Sam Carr

4. **Psychoneuroendocrinology of Sport and Exercise**
   Foundations, Markers, Trends
   Felix Ehrlenspiel and Katharina Strahler

5. **Mixed Methods Research in the Movement Sciences**
   Case Studies in Sport, Physical Education and Dance
   Oleguer Camerino, Marta Castaner and Teresa M. Anguera

6. **Complexity and Control in Team Sports**
   Dialectics in Contesting Human Systems
   Felix Lebed and Michael Bar-Eli

7. **Complex Systems in Sport**
   *Edited by Keith Davids, Robert Hristovski, Duarte Araújo,
   Natàlia Balagué Serre, Chris Button and Pedro Passos*

Complex Systems in Sport

Edited by
**Keith Davids, Robert Hristovski,
Duarte Araújo, Natàlia Balagué Serre,
Chris Button and Pedro Passos**

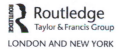
Routledge
Taylor & Francis Group

LONDON AND NEW YORK

First published 2014
by Routledge
2 Park Square, Milton Park, Abingdon, Oxon OX14 4RN

and by Routledge
711 Third Avenue, New York, NY 10017

Routledge is an imprint of the Taylor and Francis Group, an informa business

British Library Cataloguing in Publication Data
A catalogue record for this book is available from the British Library

Library of Congress Cataloging-in-Publication Data
Complex systems in sport / edited by Keith Davids, Robert Hristovski, Duarte
Araújo, Natàlia Balagué Serre, Chris Button and Pedro Passos. – First edition.
pages cm. – (Routledge research in sports and exercise science)
1. Sports sciences. 2. Exercise. 3. Human mechanics. 4. Complexity
(Philosophy) I. Davids, K. (Keith), 1953-
GV558.C65 2014
796.01'5–dc23
2013014582

ISBN: 978-0-415-80970-2 (hbk)
ISBN: 978-0-203-13461-0 (ebk)

Typeset in Times New Roman
by FiSH Books Ltd, Enfield

Contents

List of illustrations   *viii*

Contributors   *xv*

Acknowledgements   *xxiii*

Preface   *xxiv*
KEITH DAVIDS, ROBERT HRISTOVSKI, DUARTE ARAÚJO AND
NATÀLIA BALAGUÉ SERRE

PART 1
Theoretical bases for understanding complex systems in sport   **1**

1   Basic notions in the science of complex systems and nonlinear dynamics 3
     ROBERT HRISTOVSKI, NATÀLIA BALAGUÉ SERRE AND WOLFGANG SCHÖLLHORN

2   Coordination dynamics and cognition   18
     J. A. SCOTT KELSO

3   Why coordination dynamics is relevant for studying sport performance 44
     CHRIS BUTTON, JON WHEAT AND PETER LAMB

4   Psychobiological integration during exercise   62
     NATÀLIA BALAGUÉ SERRE, ROBERT HRISTOVSKI, ALFONSAS VAINORAS,
     PABLO VÁZQUEZ AND DANIEL ARAGONÉS

PART 2
Methodologies and techniques for data analyses in investigating
complex systems in sport   **83**

5   Nonlinear time series methods for analyzing behavioural sequences   85
     NIKITA KUZNETSOV, SCOTT BONNETTE AND MICHAEL A. RILEY

6 Interpersonal coordination tendencies induce functional synergies through co-adaptation processes in team sports 105
PEDRO PASSOS, DUARTE ARAÚJO, BRUNO TRAVASSOS, LUIS VILAR AND RICARDO DUARTE

7 The measurement of space and time in evolving sport phenomena 125
SOFIA FONSECA, ANA DINIZ AND DUARTE ARAÚJO

8 Self-organizing maps and cluster analysis in elite and sub-elite athletic performance 145
WOLFGANG SCHÖLLHORN, JIA YI CHOW, PAUL GLAZIER AND CHRIS BUTTON

9 Single camera analyses in studying pattern-forming dynamics of player interactions in team sports 160
RICARDO DUARTE, ORLANDO FERNANDES, HUGO FOLGADO AND DUARTE ARAÚJO

10 Using virtual environments to study interactions in sport performance 175
VANDA CORREIA, DUARTE ARAÚJO, GARETH WATSON AND CATHY CRAIG

11 Methods of measurement in studying team sports as dynamical systems 190
DANIEL MEMMERT AND JÜRGEN PERL

12 Team sports as dynamical systems 208
TIM MCGARRY, JÜRGEN PERL AND MARTIN LAMES

PART 3
Complexity sciences and sport performance **227**

13 Ecological dynamics as an alternative framework to notational performance analysis 229
LUIS VILAR, CARLOTA TORRENTS, DUARTE ARAÚJO AND KEITH DAVIDS

14 Talent development and expertise in sport 241
ELISSA PHILLIPS, KEITH DAVIDS, DUARTE ARAÚJO AND IAN RENSHAW

15 Creativity in sport and dance: ecological dynamics on a hierarchically soft-assembled perception–action landscape 261
ROBERT HRISTOVSKI, KEITH DAVIDS, DUARTE ARAÚJO, PEDRO PASSOS, CARLOTA TORRENTS, ALEXANDAR ACESKI AND ALEXANDAR TUFEKCIEVSKI

PART 4
Complexity sciences and training for sport 275

16 Variability in neurobiological systems and training 277
CHRIS BUTTON, LUDOVIC SEIFERT, DAVID O'DONOVAN AND KEITH DAVIDS

17 Individual pathways of change in motor learning and development 293
YEOU-TEH LIU AND KARL M. NEWELL

18 A constraints-based approach to the acquisition of expertise in outdoor
adventure sports 306
KEITH DAVIDS, ERIC BRYMER, LUDOVIC SEIFERT AND DOMINIC ORTH

19 Skill acquisition and representative task design 319
ROSS A. PINDER, IAN RENSHAW, JONATHON HEADRICK AND KEITH DAVIDS

Index *334*

Illustrations

Figures

1.1 Top: a stable linear system with one attractor and one basin of attraction (see converging arrows). Bottom: unstable linear system with one repeller and diverging flows toward infinity. There are no alternative stable states (attractors) for the behavioural variable Y   6

1.2 Nonlinear systems can possess repeller(s), but also two or more stable states of the behavioural variable Y and associated basins of attraction shown by converging arrows toward the attractors   7

1.3 Left panel: the increase of the inter-strike time interval for increasing of D control parameter (right-to-left direction). The whole cycle of leaning forward to strike – upright posture restoration – leaning forward to strike, increases, showing increase in the relaxation time toward the upright parallel-foot stance. For $D_0 - D < 0.05$, the relaxation time towards parallel stance tends to become infinite; that is, no relaxation toward the parallel stance exists anymore. The parallel stance loses its stability and transits to a more stable diagonal stance; see right panel   9

3.1 The interpretation of coupling angles; arrows represent the direction of a vector connecting data points on an angle-angle diagram   50

4.1 Feedback (A) and feed-forward (B) control of voluntary movement. A sign of correction is created in both mechanisms to change the action of the muscles according to the difference between the desired and achieved states   63

4.2 Quasi-static arm-curl exercise holding an Olympic bar with an elbow flexion of 90° at 80% of the one-repetition maximum until the fatigue-induced spontaneous termination point   68

4.3 A) Time series of the elbow-angle data for participant 1; B) A typical difference in the power spectral density values for the online fluctuations of the elbow angle in the first (a) and the last (b) third of the quasi-static exercise. The difference of the elbow angle variability between the first and the third phase spans over sub-second and seconds time scale. This signifies a correlated instability of the system under fatigue   69

4.4   Differences in means for the spectral degrees of freedom; horizontal axis: the first and third part of exercise; vertical axis: spectral degrees of freedom   70

4.5   Volition-state dynamics in six participants during the quasi-static elbow angle exercise   72

4.6   Cycle ergometer exercise   73

4.7   (Upper panel): standardized fluctuations from the data on revolutions per minute; (middle panel): power spectrum for the first half of the exercise with its slope of –1.5 showing anti-persistent fractional Brownian motion (fBm); (lower panel): power spectrum for the second half of the exercise with a slope of –2.2 showing persistent fBm   74

4.8   A: Treadmill exercise with a participant reporting through signs; B: sample of 11 individual time series of task-unrelated–task-related thought dynamics. Starting with the task-unrelated thoughts (TUT) state, one can observe the switches between TUT and task-related thoughts (TRT). Eventually, the TRT state becomes the one that precedes the exhaustion point. Numbers on the left signify participants   76

5.1   Simulated time series to illustrate the distinction between measures of central tendency and measures sensitive to the sequential properties of the time series. Panel A depicts random uncorrelated noise, while Panel B shows 'pink' or $1/f$ noise where each successive observation is positively correlated with the others   86

5.2   The phase space plot of the Lorenz attractor; we used the parameters $\rho = 10$, $\sigma = 28$ and $\beta = 8/3$ and initial conditions of $x = 1$, $y = 1$, $z = 1$ 88

5.3   Panel A shows the simulated time series used in the tutorial calculation of SampEn; panel B shows the same time series with added patterns of [1, 2, 3] values (shown in squares) to increase the regularity of the time series   95

5.4   Illustration of the digitization (quantization) effect on the SampEn calculation   100

6.1   The calculation of the coordinative variable   108

6.2   Angle between geometrical centre of each team and the goal position   116

6.3   Exemplar data of a network in water polo   118

7.1   Exemplar data of the distance from a sailing boat to a fixed starting position before the start of the regatta; the length of this time series is 579 data points   126

7.2   Simulated time series of length $n = 200$ of a stationary process (top), a non-stationary process with non-constant mean (middle) and a non-stationary process with non-constant variance (bottom)   127

7.3   Simulated time series of length $n = 200$ of a white noise (top) and respective sample autocorrelation function at lags $k = 0, \ldots, 50$ (bottom) with critical bounds (dashed lines)   129

7.4   Exemplar data of length $n = 579$ of the distance from a sailing boat to a fixed starting position before the regatta starting (top) and respective sample autocorrelation function at lags $k = 0, \ldots, 350$ (bottom) with critical bounds (dashed lines)   130

7.5   Simulated time series of length $n = 200$ of a white noise (top) and respective normalized periodogram at frequencies $\lambda_r = 2\pi r$ with $r = 0, \ldots, 0.5$ (bottom)   131

7.6   Exemplar data of length $n = 579$ of the distance from a sailing boat to a fixed starting position before the regatta starting (top) and respective normalized periodogram at frequencies $\lambda_r = 2\pi r$ with $r = 0$, ..., 0.5 (bottom)   132

7.7   Simulated time series of length $n = 200$ of a short-range correlation process (top), its sample autocorrelation function at lags $k = 0, \ldots, 50$ (middle) and normalized periodogram at frequencies $\lambda_r = 2\pi r$ with $r = 0, \ldots, 0.5$ (bottom)   133

7.8   Simulated times series of length $n = 400$ of a long-range correlation process (top), its sample autocorrelation function at lags $k = 0, \ldots, 50$ (middle) and normalized periodogram at frequencies $\lambda_r = 2\pi r$ with $r = 0, \ldots, 0.5$ (bottom)   135

7.9   Example of a set of points in a plane (A) and corresponding Voronoi diagram (B)   136

7.10 Spatial configurations: (A) attacker (grey areas) and defender (white areas) teams and; (B) attacker player breaking defence organization; the arrow indicates the direction of the attack   137

7.11 Example (one play) of the mean Voronoi area (VA) across time for each team; error bars represent the standard deviation   138

7.12 Comparison of the mean entropy of Voronoi area (VA) between teams in the same trial; error bars represent the standard deviation   139

7.13 Construction of the superimposed Voronoi diagram (bottom) from considering, separately, the Voronoi diagrams for team A (black dots) and team B (white dots)   139

7.14 Construction of the superimposed Voronoi diagram for (A) exclusively paired opponents and (B) randomly located individuals   140

7.15 Measures from the superimposed Voronoi diagram: (A) maximum percentage of overlapped area for each individual of the group marked with black dots; and (B) percentage of free area (in black)   140

7.16 Example (one play) of the observed percentage of free area (%FA) across time (solid line) and the 95% confidence interval for spatial random distribution (dashed lines)   142

8.1   Clustering dendrogram resulting from an average linkage algorithm; horizontal lines indicate the level of the rescaled distance at which the respective movements are grouped into one cluster   148

8.2   Linear versus nonlinear separation   152

8.3   Variations of data processing by means of self-organizing maps   153

9.1   Schematic representation of single-camera video motion capture   162

9.2   The TACTO 8.0 device window; manual tracking of a selected working point with a computer mouse allows virtual coordinates of the tracked player/object to be obtained   163

9.3   The direct linear transformation (2D-DLT) method for camera calibration and bi-dimensional reconstruction   164

9.4   Converted pitch coordinates (metres) allow the reproduction of movement displacement trajectories of players in the space of action   165

9.5   The two behavioural states of the order parameter; top panel shows the distance of the single centroid to the defensive boundary line of all the analyzed trials, synchronized by the assistance pass instant; bottom panel shows the order parameter subtracted by the own mean to highlight the qualitative changes associated with perturbations of the initial stability of teams   168

9.6   Identification of the nonlinear qualitative changes between the two behavioural states; top panel displays an exemplar play with increased slope in the transition between the two system states (down-sampled to 1 Hz); bottom panel shows the average and standard deviation bands of the first derivative of the order parameter in all plays, highlighting with an ellipse the high rate of change of the order parameter; the slope or high rate of change indicates the order–order transition   169

9.7   Moving average and standard deviation values of the inter-centroid distances (top panel) and relative stretch index (bottom panel); vertical dashed lines highlight the instant of the instabilities corresponding to the zero crossing of the order parameter previously identified in Figure 9.5   170

10.1   Illustrative immersive interactive virtual reality apparatus in the Movement Innovation Laboratory at Queen's University, Belfast. It shows a participant wearing a pair of gloves with attached hand trackers, a head-mounted display with attached head tracker and a back-pack housing the control unit   177

10.2   A schematic representation of what the ball-carrying participant could see in front of him/her (i.e. the defensive line) in a virtual environment simulated three-versus-three rugby task   183

11.1   (left) Self-organizing map (SOM: neurons are grouped to clusters which form the output; (right) feed-forward network (FFN): comparison of expected output O_{exp} and computed output O_{comp} is feedback and so changes the neuron connections to minimize the difference between expected and computed output   190

11.2   Network with a process trajectory and the corresponding type profile   193

11.3   (left): TeSSy input interface with video control (bottom), animation interface (left), attribute selection and input panel (top); (right): examples of a stroke frequency matrix and a stroke success matrix representing tactical concepts and technical skills, respectively   194

11.4   Squash court with game process BR–FR–BL (left); trained net representing the most frequent 4-position-sequences (right); BL = backhand left side, BR = backhand right side, FR = forehand right side   196

11.5   Tactical patterns of players depending on their opponents; A, B and D
       are the players. The squares represent the corresponding networks,
       where the circles represent the players' tactical concepts.
       Each circle corresponds to a stroke sequence, the frequency of
       which is encoded by the diameter of the circle   196
11.6   The network was trained with game processes from volleyball,
       presenting the most important sequences as circles, whose diameters
       represent the frequencies of the corresponding sequences, three of
       them being explained in more detail   197
11.7   (left): Trained net with a trajectory representing a sequence of player
       formations starting at the 'O' and ending at the 'X'; (right): scheme
       of a configuration prototype of a team formation, which could, for
       example, correspond to the marked cluster   198
11.8   Trajectories showing the preparation of the defence against the
       opponent's service   199
11.9   A two-dimensional replication of a match situation by means of
       position data   200
11.10 Net-based recognition of formation types and the recombination with
       position and time information   200
11.11 Example of the user interface of a tool for the combined quantitative
       and qualitative analysis of formations in football   202
11.12 Trained neural network with grey shaded areas that illustrate different
       quality levels (top left) and a representation of the trajectories of
       hockey training. The learning process begins in the dark grey square
       and ends in the light grey square; the colours of the neurons
       correspond to those in the large net graphic (top left)   203
12.1   Illustration of football as a complex dynamical system   211
12.2   Phase space for two players in a tennis rally; Serena Williams (left)
       Justine Henin (right); $\triangle$, $\square$ = strokes of Williams; $\blacksquare$, $\blacklozenge$ = strokes of
       Henin; going for the ball to strike and returning to a neutral position
       results in cyclical structures in a speed/position phase space   212
12.3   Longitudinal team centres, differences and relative phase for Italy and
       France during the first half of the 2006 World Cup final game   215
12.4   Separating a constellation of players on the playground into its
       formation and position   217
12.5   A trajectory of formations on the net and its reduction to a formation
       type trajectory   218
12.6   Frequencies of formations and their correlations   219
12.7   Distribution of a typical pair of formations between minutes 21
       and 30   220
12.8   Example of a typical tactical pattern produced between the two teams 221
12.9   Prototype of the tactical pattern from Figure 12.5, together with
       success values   222
13.1   The constraint of goal location on coordination processes in dyadic
       systems presented in decomposed format: (left column) distances of

each player to the centre of the goal; (right column) angles of each player to the centre of the goal; (a) and (b) exemplar data from attacker five [A5] and nearest defender [Def]; (A) and (B) exemplar data from attacker five [A5] and nearest defender [D]; (C) and (D) dynamics of the relative phase of the exemplar data from A5 and nearest D; (e) and (f) frequency histograms of the relative phases of all A–D dyadic systems ($n = 52$)   234

13.2   Mean values and standard error of the required velocity for intercepting the ball of (A) defender and (B) goalkeeper in shots that ended in a defender's interception, in a goalkeeper's save and in a goal. The represented levels of statistical significance are $P < 0.05$ (*), $P < 0.01$ (**) and $P < 0.001$ (***). Note that the required velocity of the goalkeeper was not measured when the defender intercepted the ball, since it is impossible to compute the goalkeeper's interception point   235

15.1   Schematic (i.e. one-dimensional) presentation of the corrugated hierarchically soft-assembled potential landscape with two confining barriers on both sides   263

15.2   (Top) snapshots of the four metastable states of dancers for the first 35 seconds of improvisation; (middle): overlaps q of the four metastable body configurations with principal components (axis Y) and pathway of their dynamics. Overlap values are given in the legend on right; (bottom): reconfigurations are given as nonzero Hamming distances of the dancer's action system; after some reconfigurations take place, the action system relaxes and dwells in a state where no further reconfigurations occur for some time; i.e. zero reconfiguration; this process represents the metastable attractor configurations (movement/posture pattern)   268

15.3   The profile of the average dynamic overlap $q_d(t)$ for different time lags; its dynamics proceed on three timescales (from seconds to several minutes) and does not converge to zero during the observation time scale   269

16.1   Continuous relative phase (CRP) between elbow and knee through a complete cycle for 24 beginners (left panel) and for 24 expert swimmers (right panel), showing lower inter-individual variability for experts   281

16.2   Angle between horizontal, left limb and right limb (left panel); modes of limb coordination as regards the angle value between horizontal, left limb and right limb (right panel). The angle between the horizontal line and the left and right limbs was positive when the right limb was above the left limb and negative when the right limb was below the left limb   283

16.3   Trajectory plots from O'Donovan *et al.* (2011)   285

17.1   Waddington's (1957) schematic of the epigenetic landscape   296

17.2   The landscape dynamics of the basic equation of the HKB (Haken-Kelso-Bunz) model, with the same parameters as in Kelso

(1995, Figure 2.7)   297

17.3   (a) Landscape of learning the 90-degree phase task of the HKB model; at the beginning of practice (C = 0.4) only temporary stabilization of the target phase x0 = 0.25 can be achieved when starting from special initial conditions close to C; (b) right at the transition (C = 0.425) the target phase x0 = 0.25 shows one-sided stability: initial conditions close to C will be attracted to the new attractor. Note that, in this situation, the system is very sensitive to noise perturbations; (c) after sufficient practice (C = 0.525), all initial conditions close to the target attractor x0 = 0.25 will converge to the fixed point   298

17.4   A two-timescale landscape model associated with Snoddy's (1926) score data (black dots) as elevation levels. The four clusters correspond to the four practice sessions. The *x* behavioural variable corresponds to the slow timescale (shallow dimension), whereas the *y* variable corresponds to the fast timescale (steep dimension)   300

17.5   Initial and final performance of the mirror tracing task; (A) breakdown of one-dimensional performance score measure into movement time and spatial error (movement time) components. Filled and open symbols indicate outcome score on trial 1 and trial 50, respectively. Triangle, circle and square symbols reflect movement time (MT), mixed (MIXED) and spatial error (SE) group assignment (see text for detailed explanation); (B) performance score on trial 1 and trial 50 as a function of group; error bars indicate standard error   302

18.1   (left) Angles identified for the horizontal planes of the left and right limbs in the upper and lower body of ice climbers; (right) modes of limb coordination as regards the angle value between horizontal, left limb and right limb   310

19.1   The role of Brunswik's lens model in understanding informational variables for complex systems in sport – analysis of a tennis serve   320

19.2   Principles for the assessment of representative learning design   324

Tables

3.1   Categories of coordination and their associated coupling angle (γ) ranges   51

4.1   Summary of the four experiments performed until the fatigue-induced spontaneous termination point   66

11.1 Summary of the results of all trajectories of all three groups (hockey, soccer, control)   204

Contributors

Alexandar Aceski is currently Assistant Professor at the Faculty of Physical Education, University of Ss. Cyril and Methodius, Skopje, Republic of Macedonia. He has research interests in methods of qualitative analysis and modelling used in biomechanics, particularly as applied to transfer in motor learning.

Daniel Aragonés is a PhD student at the National Institute of Physical Education of Catalonia, University of Barcelona, Spain. His research is currently focused on the psychobiological integration of exercise-induced fatigue.

Duarte Araújo is Associate Professor at the Faculty of Human Kinetics of the University of Lisbon, Portugal. He is the Director of the Laboratory of Expertise in Sport. He is the President of the Portuguese Society of Sport Psychology and a member of the National Council of Sports. His research on ecological dynamical approaches to expertise and decision making in sports has been funded by the Fundação para a Ciência e Tecnologia.

Natàlia Balagué Serre is Professor of Exercise Physiology at INEFC University of Barcelona, Spain. Her field of research is complex systems in sport, with special focus on dynamic integrative approaches to exercise-induced fatigue and the nonlinear psychobiological integration during exercise. In 2003, she organized the first Complex Systems in Sport Congress, which was held in Barcelona. Co-author of *Complejidad y Deporte* and papers relating to the effects of exercise-induced fatigue on attention focus, perceived exertion and exercise termination.

Scott Bonnette received a BA in psychology from Wheeling Jesuit University, USA, in 2009 and a MA in experimental psychology from the University of Cincinnati, USA, in 2013. He is currently a graduate student at the University of Cincinnati. He has been involved with research and publications concerning the nonlinear analysis of postural control and with research on how exploratory movements facilitate perception.

Eric Brymer is a psychologist and Senior Lecturer in the Faculty of Health at Queensland University of Technology, Australia. His research focuses on investigating nature-based activities, adventure and extreme sports. Eric is interested in the broad psychological understanding of the experience, the development of skill and how such activities enhance positive health and well-being. He is particularly interested in the role of the physical environment and how to design and facilitate nature-based experiences so that positive outcomes for the environment and people are optimised.

Chris Button is Associate Professor of Motor Learning at the University of Otago, New Zealand. His research interests include the ecological dynamics approach to motor learning and human behaviours in relation to water safety.

Jia Yi Chow is Assistant Professor at the Physical Education and Sports Science Department, National Institute of Education, Nanyang Technological University, Singapore. His area of specialization is in motor control and learning. Jia Yi's key research work includes nonlinear pedagogy, investigation of multiarticular coordination changes, analysis of team dynamics from an ecological psychology perspective and examining visual–perceptual skills in sports expertise.

Vanda Correia is Assistant Professor at the University of Algarve in Faro, Portugal. She did her PhD in Sport Sciences at the Faculty of Human Kinetics of the University of Lisbon, Portugal. Specializing in decision making in team sports, Vanda is particularly concerned with understanding how the dynamics of players' interactions express adaptive behaviours to performance constraints and are coupled with key information sources. She has been conducting research both in the field and in virtual reality settings.

Cathy Craig is Head of the School of Psychology of Queens University Belfast, Northern Ireland, and Director of the Movement Innovation Laboratory of that institution. She completed her PhD at the University of Edinburgh under the supervision of Professor Dave Lee in the Perception in Action Laboratories.

Keith Davids is Professor of Motor Learning at the Centre for Sports Engineering Research at Sheffield Hallam University in the UK. He currently holds additional appointments at the University of Jyväskylä in Finland (FiDiPro) and at the Queensland University of Technology in Australia. He is a graduate of the University of London and gained a PhD at the University of Leeds in 1986. Between 1993 and 2001, he led the Motor Control group at the Department of Exercise and Sport Science at Manchester Metropolitan University, UK. In 2002 he moved to the University of Otago in New Zealand before taking up an appointment at the Queensland University of Technology in Australia. Currently he supervises doctoral students from Portugal, UK, Australia and New Zealand. His major research interest involves the study of movement coordination and skill acquisition in sport. He is particularly focused on understanding how to design representative learning and perform-ance evaluation environments in sport.

Ana Diniz is a teacher and researcher at the Department of Mathematics of the Faculty of Human Kinetics, University of Lisbon, Portugal. Her investigation includes mathematical methods and models related to motor control and inter-personal coordination processes.

Ricardo Duarte is Lecturer in Training Methods of Soccer at Faculdade de Motricidade Humana, Portugal. His academic career involves mentoring young football coaches, developing research on tactical behaviours in soccer with applications to training and performance analysis and presenting his perspective in applied soccer training courses, congresses and seminars around the world.

Orlando Fernandes is Assistant Professor at the Department of Sport and Health of the University of Évora, Portugal. He is an expert in biomechanics of human movement, with particular interest in signal processing and nonlinear analysis of time-series data. His expertise has been also transferred to the preparation of some elite athletes in track and field sports.

Hugo Folgado is Lecturer at the Department of Sport and Health, University of Évora, Portugal, and collaborator at the Research Center for Sport Sciences, Health and Human Development, Portugal. He is currently working on his PhD studies about football players' movement synchronization. His research interests are performance analysis and expertise in team sports.

Sofia Fonseca has a degree in statistics from the Faculty of Sciences of Lisbon (1999), a PhD in statistics from the University of Aberdeen (2004) and a PhD in sports science from the University of Lisbon (2012). Sofia has been Assistant Professor at the Faculty of Physical Education and Sports, Lusofona University, Lisbon, Portugal, since 2006. Her research interests are team sports behavior, particularly modelling players' and teams' spatial organization.

Paul Glazier is a Research Fellow at the Institute of Sport, Exercise and Active Living, Victoria University, Melbourne, Australia. He has expertise in sports biomechanics, motor control, skill acquisition and performance analysis of sport. He has authored or co-authored over 40 peer-reviewed journal articles, invited book chapters and published conference papers in these areas. Paul also has a wealth of practical experience, having provided sports biomechanics and performance analysis services to a wide range of athletes and teams, from regional juniors to Olympic and World Champions, in a variety of sports.

Jonathon Headrick is a PhD scholar at the School of Exercise and Nutrition Sciences, Queensland University of Technology, Australia. His research interests include the application of an ecological dynamics approach for studying the role of emotion in learning and skill acquisition in sport.

Robert Hristovski is currently Professor at the Faculty of Physical Education, University of Ss. Cyril and Methodius, Skopje, Republic of Macedonia. He obtained his MSc degree in 1994 and a PhD degree in 1997 at the Faculty of Physical Education. In 2001 he had a five-month research visit at the Institute of Nonlinear Science at the University of California, San Diego. He has research interests in methods of analysis and modelling in nonlinear dynamics, particularly as applied to human action selection and adaptation during training. He is also an invited lecturer on masters and soctoral courses at several European universities.

J. A. Scott Kelso is a neuroscientist and Glenwood and Martha Creech Chair in Science, Professor of Complex Systems and Brain Sciences, Florida Atlantic University, Boca Raton, Florida, USA, and Professor of Psychology, Biological Sciences and Biomedical Science at the University of Ulster (Magee Campus), Derry, Northern Ireland. He has worked on coordination dynamics, the science of coordination and on fundamental mechanisms underlying voluntary movements and their relation to the large-scale coordination dynamics of the human brain. His experimental research in the late 1970s and early 1980s led to the HKB model (Haken–Kelso–Bunz), a mathematical formulation that quantitatively describes and predicts how elementary forms of coordinated behaviour arise and change adaptively as a result of nonlinear interactions among components.

Nikita Kuznetsov received a BA in psychology from California State University, Northridge, in 2008, and a PhD in experimental psychology from the University of Cincinnati in 2013. He is currently a post-doctoral associate at Northeastern University, USA. His research focuses on perception–action from the complex/dynamical systems perspective and the application of nonlinear methods in motor control.

Peter Lamb was born in Canada and obtained a PhD in biomechanics from the University of Otago, New Zealand, in 2010. Currently, Peter is Associate Researcher at the Technische Universität München (TUM), Germany. As head of research and diagnostics at the TUM Golf Laboratory, Peter works with national-level golf teams and their coaches, as well as private golfers. Part of his work includes applying the constraints-led perspective to coordination of the golf swing in search of critical boundaries of stability. The implications are both for theoretical aspects of human movement, as well as golf-specific applications to training and on-course strategies. Peter is an avid golfer, skier, cyclist and ice-hockey player.

Martin Lames is full Professor at the Faculty of Sports and Health Science at the Technical University of Munich, Germany. His main research interests are modelling of sports performances, talent research and top-level sports, with special focus on information technology support. He has served as President of the International Association of Computer Science in Sport (IACSS) since 2013.

Yeou-Teh Liu was born and raised in Taipei. She received her PhD in kinesiology from the University of Illinois at Urbana-Champaign, USA, and is currently Professor in the Department of Athletic Performance, National Taiwan Normal University. Her research focuses on the dynamics of motor skill acquisition, movement adaptation and motor control. Her other research interest is in the performance analyses in competitive sports including both team and individual sport events.

Tim McGarry is Associate Professor in the Faculty of Kinesiology, University of New Brunswick, Canada. He has published many journal articles and book chapters on various aspects of movement control and sports performance. He serves as an advisory editorial board member on the *Journal of Sports Sciences* and the *International Journal of Performance Analysis in Sport* and is co-editor of the *2013 Routledge Handbook of Sports Performance Analysis*.

Daniel Memmert is Professor and Head of the Institute of Cognitive and Team/Racket Sport Research, German Sport University of Cologne. His research interests are cognitive science, human movement science, computer science and sport psychology. He has 15 years of teaching and coaching experience, has published more than 100 publications, 20 books or book chapters and is a recognised figure through his multi-keynotes in football. He is a reviewer for several international journals and has transferred his expertise to business and to several professional soccer clubs within the Bundesliga.

Karl M. Newell PhD is the Marie Underhill Noll Chair of Human Performance and Professor, Department of Kinesiology, Pennsylvania State University, State College, USA. His research focuses on the coordination, control and skill of normal and abnormal human movement across the life span; developmental disabilities and motor skills; and the influence of drug and exercise on movement control. One of the specific themes of his research is the study of variability in human movement and posture, with specific reference to the onset of aging and Parkinson's disease. His other major research theme is processes of change in motor learning and development that is the focus of his chapter contribution to this book.

David O'Donovan is a postgraduate student who currently works for High Performance New Zealand as a knowledge editor. He completed his Masters in 2011 in which he examined the throwing kinematics of elite athletes with cerebral palsy. He has worked as a coach and sport science provider for Boccia New Zealand and he has supported athletes participating in World Championships, Commonwealth and Paralympic Games.

Dominic Orth is a PhD student at the University of Rouen, France, and Queensland University of Technology (QUT), Australia. He completed his undergraduate and Masters degree by research at the School of Exercise and Nutrition Science at QUT. His research programme examines the role of adaptive movement variability in skilled climbers.

Pedro Passos is Assistant Professor at the Faculty of Human Kinetics, University of Lisbon, Portugal. He gained his PhD in sport sciences in 2008. His research involves the study of the dynamics of interpersonal coordination in team sports, which led him to produce several papers accepted for publication in scientific journals, book chapters, as well as communications in scientific meetings. He currently maintains his research work regarding interpersonal coordination in social systems as team sports and extending the paradigm of analysis to video games cooperative tasks, searching for new methods of analysis and extending his collaboration with researchers in Portugal, across Europe, Singapore, Australia and New Zealand. He supervises masters' and doctoral students from Portugal. Parallel with his research activity, he is also technical coordinator of a rugby union club. In his leisure time, he practices mountain biking, surfing and alpine skiing.

Jürgen Perl is Professor Emeritus of Computer Science, University of Mainz, Germany. His main research interests using modelling and simulation methods include pattern recognition of game behaviours and player movements, as well as physiological load performance dynamics. He is a founding member of the International Association of Computer Science in Sport, serving as President from 2003–2007 and as Honorary President thereafter.

Elissa Phillips is Senior Biomechanist at the Australian Institute of Sport. Elissa's responsibility includes implementing a programme of biomechanical services and research for athletes and coaches to enhance performance. Recent research has focussed on feedback technology and coordination profiling in expert performance.

Ross Pinder is Lecturer in Sport and Exercise Sciences at the University of the Sunshine Coast, Australia. He is primarily interested in maximising skill learning in sport through the design of representative experimental and practice environments. He currently works as a skill acquisition and high-performance consultant for the Australian Paralympic Committee.

Ian Renshaw is Senior Lecturer, Queensland University of Technology, Brisbane, Australia. Ian's teaching and research interests are centred on applications of ecological dynamics to sport settings. Given Ian's background in physical education and coaching, he is particularly interested in enhancing pedagogical practice. Recent research has focussed on developing the links between sport psychology and skill acquisition; implementing constraints-led approaches in physical education; emotions and learning in sport; talent development; developing expertise in cricket and visual regulation of run-ups. Ian has worked with numerous sports providing coach education and skill acquisition advice.

Michael A. Riley received a BA in psychology from the University of Louisiana-Monroe, USA, in 1994 and a PhD in experimental psychology from the University of Connecticut, USA, in 1999. He is currently Professor of Psychology and Director of the Center for Cognition, Action and Perception, University of Cincinnati, USA, where he has been on the faculty since 2000. His research on ecological and complex dynamical systems approaches to perception–action has been funded by the National Science Foundation and the US Army Medical Research and Materiel Command.

Wolfgang I Schöllhorn is Professor for Movement and Training Science and Director of the Institute of Sport Science at the University of Mainz, Germany. With a background in physics, sports, pedagogy and neurophysiology his research areas include dynamic systems, adaptive behaviour, learning and brain states, biomechanics, signal analysis and pattern recognition.

Ludovic Seifert is Associate Professor at the Faculty of Sport Sciences, University of Rouen, France. He conducts his research in the field of motor learning and motor control regarding expertise in sport, movement variability and temporal dynamics of learning. He gained a PhD in expertise and coordination dynamics in swimming at the University of Rouen in 2003, then a certification to direct research in 2010 entitled 'Motor coordination and expertise: A complex and dynamical system approach of sport and physical education', for which he exhibited numerous publications in this field. He is also a mountain guide certified by the International Federation of Mountain Guides Associations and now investigates expertise and motor learning in climbing.

Carlota Torrents is a teacher of expressive movement and dance and a researcher at the Human Motor Behavior and Sport Laboratory, National Institute of Physical Education of Catalonia, University of Lleida, Spain. She completed her PhD in complex systems applied to training methods and has published international books and papers related to complex systems, dance and sport.

Bruno Travassos is Assistant Professor at the Department of Sport Sciences, University of Beira Interior, Portugal, and member of the group of performance analysis at CIDESD – Research Centre in Sports, Health Sciences and Human Development, Portugal. His research interests are in the area of game analysis and also in the learning processes and decision-making behaviour of players in team sports with special emphasis in futsal and soccer.

Alexandar Tufekcievski is Professor at the Faculty of Physical Education, University of Ss. Cyril and Methodius, Skopje, Republic of Macedonia. He has research interests in methods of qualitative analysis and modelling used in biomechanics, particularly as applied to transfer in motor learning.

Alfonsas Vainoras is Professor at the Lithuanian University of Health Sciences. He investigates novel methods of analysis of the electrocardiograph using complex systems approach and analysis tools. Has participated in the development of the E-Health program in Lithuania and Europe.

Pablo Vázquez is a PhD student at the National Institute of Physical Education of Catalonia, University of Barcelona, Spain. The focus of his research is the application of complex systems principles on processes related to motor and performance changes under fatigue.

Luis Vilar completed his PhD in sports sciences, investigating the informational constraints on attacker and defender performance in futsal. Currently, he is

Assistant Professor at the Faculty of Human Kinetics, University of Lisbon, Portugal, and at the Faculty of Physical Education and Sports, Lusófona University of Humanities and Technologies, Portugal. He teaches UEFA-pro courses for coaches. He is also head of youth football department and coach at Colégio Pedro Arrupe. He was a football and a futsal player.

Gareth Watson gained a BSc in psychology from Queens University Belfast, Northern Ireland, and concluded his PhD in mechanical and aeronautical engineering and psychology at the same university.

Jon Wheat is a Principal Research Fellow in Biomechanics, Centre for Sports Engineering Research (CSER), Sheffield Hallam University, UK. He gained his undergraduate degree in sport and exercise science from Manchester Metropolitan University before completing his PhD at Sheffield Hallam University. Jon works on biomechanics research and consultancy projects in CSER and teaches on the MSc sports engineering and MSc sport and exercise science degrees. His work is influenced by the ecological approach to motor control and dynamical systems theory and he has a keen interest in the development and application of biomechanics measurement systems for use outside the laboratory, in more representative settings. He leads the Biomechanics Research Group in CSER which has several research and consultancy projects in this area.

Acknowledgements

We give our profound thanks to all the chapter authors for their willingness to share their comprehensive knowledge of the complexity sciences. We also thank all the individuals who helped with reviewing the text and compiling the index, especially Dominic Orth, José Pedro Silva, Rens Meerhoff, Pablo Vázquez Justes, Sergi Garcia Retortillo.

Keith Davids: I acknowledge the efforts of my fellow co-editors for their wonderful professionalism in seeing this project through from conceptualisation to completion. They showed exemplary patience in dealing with my endless requests. Finally, as always, I dedicate this book to my family (Anna, Mike, Jake, Charlie and India) for their love and support.

Robert Hristovski: I dedicate this book to my family who supported me each step of the way.

Duarte Araújo: This book is dedicated to those students who taught me the meaning of inter-independence: Bruno Travassos, Vanda Correia, Ricardo Duarte, Luis Vilar, Pedro Esteves and João Carvalho. I also acknowledge the students of SportLab for stretching their autonomy to offer me more time for the book.

Natàlia Balagué Serre: I dedicate to this book to Dani, Gerard and Pau.

Chris Button: This book has been an amazing act of teamwork. As such I give my thanks to my offsiders, the chapter reviewers, and the authors. You've made my editorial role a pleasure. And to the most important dyad in my life: Ange and Melanie, thanks for your support.

Preface

Complex systems in nature are those with many interacting parts, all capable of influencing global system outcomes. There is a growing body of research that has modelled sport performance from a complexity sciences perspective, studying the behaviour of individual athletes and sports teams as emergent phenomena which self-organize under interacting constraints. This literature has been published in journals covering physical education, sport science and sports medicine, coaching science, psychology and human movement science.

This book was conceived over many years of discussion and research, when it became apparent that there was a need to bring together the conceptual creativity and innovative ideas of many experts studying complex systems in the context of sport performance from across the world. The intention is to provide a coherent summary of where we currently stand with regards to theory, current methodologies and empirical data concerning the understanding of sport performance from a complexity sciences perspective. Our rationale is to complete a comprehensive overview of complex systems in sport for advanced undergraduate students, postgraduate students and academics in a range of disciplinary areas. The authors contributing chapters to this edited textbook have undertaken comprehensive overviews to summarize the key ideas that have appeared in many excellent empirical reports, reviews and theoretical position papers in the extant literature. The aims of the various chapters in this book include the presentation of key ideas from the complexity sciences and a summary of how these ideas might be adopted in the organization of sport practice. In this way, this textbook builds on existing material to provide a comprehensive foundation for students of complex systems in sport.

This is a timely endeavour, since the study of complex systems in sport has gained increasing prominence in recent years, leading to a deep interest from students from a range of different disciplinary backgrounds. For example, there is an increasing number of physicists and mathematicians involved in this field of work and this book showcases research in sport science and performance analysis that will enhance their understanding of the applications of methodologies from the complexity sciences. Conversely, within the sport sciences, there is a need to document the range of new methods of analysis used for investigating representative complex sport movements and actions at an individual and team level. These requirements cannot be adequately captured by experimental designs and methods of analysis that already exist in the basic movement sciences.

The proposed structure of the book has been carefully designed to equip readers with the basic theoretical knowledge of complex, nonlinear dynamical systems (Part 1: Theoretical bases for understanding complex systems in sport) prior to delivering an understanding of current methods for studying such systems in sport performance environments (Part 2: Methodologies and techniques for data analyses in investigating complex systems in sport). In the final parts of the book (Part 3: Complexity sciences and sport performance and 4: Complexity sciences and training for sport), the emphasis is on expanding knowledge of practical applications of ideas and methods in the study of training and performance in individual and team sports.

Many of the chapters deliberately explore common themes, although each chapter attempts to provide a unique and detailed contribution to the topic of complexity in sports. The interaction of many authors across multiple chapters allows the overall book to develop collective themes, which emerge throughout the whole text. This collective approach has been a deliberate strategy of the editors, meaning that comprehension of the whole book provides much more than the sum of each chapter in isolation. Typical complexity science thinking!

This book supports a burgeoning area of academic interest. There is now a biennial international scientific congress dedicated to this area of study, which attracts around 250 delegates to each meeting. The proposed book neatly complements the research presented at this meeting. There are also academic journals newly emerging to support this field of work. The editors acknowledge the powerful and influential role that every one of the chapter authors of this book have played in bringing together theoretical material and practical applications which will further develop our understanding of complex systems in sport.

Keith Davids
Robert Hristovski
Duarte Araújo
Natàlia Balagué Serre
Chris Button
Pedro Passos

Part 1

Theoretical bases for understanding complex systems in sport

1 Basic notions in the science of complex systems and nonlinear dynamics

Robert Hristovski, Natàlia Balagué Serre and Wolfgang Schöllhorn

The historical roots of the complexity sciences can be traced back to ancient philosophers such as Aristotle (384–322 BC), whose famous saying, 'The whole is more than the sum of its parts', indicated the duality of holism versus reductionism in science. The beginning of modern Western science is mostly associated with the development of a mechanistic world view, originating in contributions from Galileo, Kepler and Newton in the seventeenth century. The mathematico-experimental method became trend setting and in the same period Newton created the mathematical basis of dynamical systems theory. By showing explicitly that, celestial mechanics, Earthly tides and falling bodies were governed by the same law of universal gravity, he actually paved the way to what later became a foundation of general systems theory and particularly synergetics: the search for the same principles acting at different levels in the organization of matter. This world view may be conceived as a special kind of holism where general principles manifest themselves through different contexts, i.e. levels of organization. The whole manifests itself through different partial phenomena, owing to different contexts in which these phenomena are embedded.

These ideas have been influential in the movement sciences and, during the 1970s and 1980s, concepts of dissipative structures and self-organization were incorporated in explanations of movement coordination (e.g. Kugler *et al.* 1980). General predictions of this theoretical approach, such as non-equilibrium phase transitions and critical fluctuations enhancement in cyclic movements, were corroborated (Kelso 1984), and modelled (Haken *et al.* 1985; Schöner *et al.* 1986) with great success. These papers became milestones in the search for principles of motor behaviour from a complexity sciences and dynamical systems perspective, which made direct contact with theory in sport science. Principles of self-organization were successfully applied to multi-limb cyclic movements before they were experimentally corroborated (Fuchs *et al.* 1992) and mathematically modelled (Jirsa *et al.* 1994) at the level of the central nervous system, as well as in learning processes (Zanone and Kelso 1992). Self-organizing phenomena were also discovered in studies of social coordination (Schmidt *et al.* 1990). In 2005, a unified model of rhythmic and discrete movements was published (Jirsa and Kelso 2005), predicting as a generic consequence the possibility of the emergence of false starts. In the past two decades, the complex dynamic systems paradigm became a fruitful experimental and theoretical approach in capturing and explaining many phenomena of motor behaviour that are closely related, although not equal, to problems in sports science. This relatedness and prospects of the dynamical systems approach to sports science problems were advocated in the works of Davids and colleagues (see e.g. Davids *et al.* 1994, 2003).

In the following sections, we define complex systems and point to some main differences between non-living and living systems. We then discuss in more detail the differences between linear and nonlinear dynamical systems and point to some necessary concepts important for understanding why nonlinear dynamics is important in explaining sports phenomena. The material is presented in a way suitable for unfamiliar readers to be acquainted with basic terms and meanings from the complex dynamical systems approach to sports.

What are complex systems?

Complex systems consist of many components which interact among themselves and, as a whole, interact with their environments. Complex systems may be homogenous or heterogeneous. For example, a piece of ice contains innumerable interacting components, i.e. water molecules. These are complex but homogenous systems. Living complex systems, besides having many interacting elements, consist of structurally and functionally heterogeneous (neural, muscle, tendinous, etc.) components, so they belong to the class of heterogeneous complex systems. Biological systems also contain parts existing in different physical phases: fluid (e.g. blood), semi-rigid (muscles have properties of liquid crystals) and rigid (e.g. bones). Social systems, as well, consist of interactions between heterogeneous agents. Thus, whereas between water molecules there is one kind of interaction, i.e. hydrogen bonds, between heterogeneous components there may be different kinds of interactions (generally informational or/and mechanical). These may have varying intensities, and span different spatiotemporal scales, which immensely increases the level of complexity of description of such systems. In such systems, each single component can 'perceive' a different environment. There is another important difference between non-living and living complex systems. In non-living systems one can isolate a large portion of the larger system and study it because the behaviour of the system will be the same. This is one of the main advantages that make statistical physics feasible, and in living systems this is not possible. One cannot isolate an organ that will function independently of the organism. Living complex systems are also adaptive and goal directed, while one cannot find an argument to claim the same for the non-living systems. Adaptive systems are those which evolve, develop and learn to negotiate with their environments by changing and fitting their behaviour to emerging constraints.

Besides these qualitative differences, there are universal features that are valid for either living or non-living complex systems. Both kinds of systems possess mutual interactions and interdependence between constituent components. It seems that interactions are largely responsible for the possibility of capturing both kinds of systems within similar formal frameworks because mutual interactions, and recursive self-interactions that result from these, form the nonlinear character of such systems. As a consequence, complex systems, living or non-living, exhibit nonlinear dynamical properties and form the class of complex nonlinear dynamical systems. How these interactions change depends largely on the constraints embedded within the complex systems. Under some constraints, new forms of behaviour emerge spontaneously, without being previously designed and imposed on the system's behaviour, and this is a property of all complex systems, regardless whether they are living or non-living. Complex systems may exhibit complex or simple behaviour. An athlete may perform simple arm-curl rhythmic movements but also may be able to perform complex sequences of dribbling actions. On the other hand, simple systems like a single-component nonlinear pendulum may produce simple oscillatory behaviours but also a very complex pattern of chaotic behaviour. Hence, the complexity of behaviour should not be confused with the complexity of the system. Complex systems may behave in a simple fashion because their interacting components, under certain constraints, may form large coalitions of cooperative elements, which reduces the dimensionality of the behaviour. In this way, a complex system attains simple behaviour and may be treated as a simple system on a macroscopic level. We get simplicity from complexity. There are unifying principles that make possible to treat complex systems in a relatively simple fashion.

Linear and nonlinear complex dynamical systems

Dynamical systems are systems that change over time. Because all systems change over time, although on different timescales, it follows that all systems are dynamical. They are usually represented by differential or difference equations but also by cellular automata and networks, or even by a mixture of some of these. Dynamical or *behavioural variables* converge in their evolution to a *stable state* in which they can dwell infinitely under given sets of constraints. This stable state is called an *attractor*, because it attracts all nearby initial states of the system (Figure 1.1).

If the system is placed into different initial positions, it will converge to one state that is stable, i.e. the attractor. The set of initial states that converge toward the attractor form its *basin of attraction*. The attractor can be conceived as a source of forces that pull all initial states toward it. Its antipode is the *unstable state* called a *repeller*. The repeller repels all the nearby initial states further away from it. If the system is placed into different initial positions close to the repeller, they will diverge far from it (see Figure 1.1).

Dynamical systems consist of two broad classes: linear and nonlinear. Linear dynamical systems are those whose rate of change of the relevant behavioural variable is a linear function of that same variable. These systems are *proportional*, in the sense that a small change of the constraints influencing them brings about a small change in the behavioural variable. A large change in constraints is needed to produce a large change in the behavioural variable. In a sense, linear systems

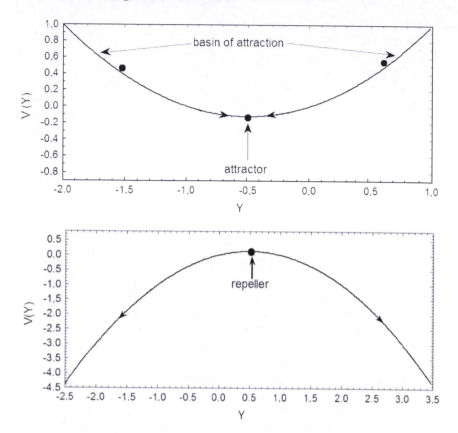

Figure 1.1 Top: a stable linear system with one attractor and one basin of attraction (see converging arrows). Bottom: unstable linear system with one repeller and diverging flows toward infinity. There are no alternative stable states (attractors) for the behavioural variable Y

are overly flexible because of their proportional response to changing constraints. However, they are monostable (see Figure 1.1); i.e. under any set of constraints they either converge to a well-defined attractor or diverge to infinity if they become unstable. In this sense, linear systems are too rigid.

Nonlinear systems, although containing unstable states, i.e. repellers, do not send nearby states to infinity but enable other alternative, behavioural stable finite states (Figure 1.2). Moreover, nonlinear dynamical systems enable more than one stationary behavioural solution for one and the same set of constraints supporting *multi-stability* of behaviour. Nonlinear systems are safe from exploding to infinity and their behaviour is confined to a set of finite behavioural modes.

Because of this stabilizing property, nonlinear systems enable multiple stable behavioural solutions. In such a way, they are multifunctional and such multi-functionality may be reached and changed by changing system's influential

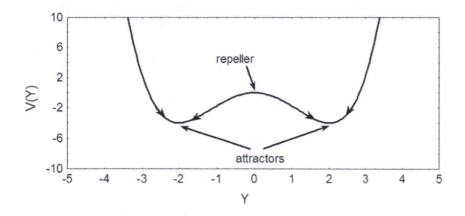

Figure 1.2 Nonlinear systems can possess repeller(s), but also two or more stable states
of the behavioural variable Y and associated basins of attraction shown by
converging arrows toward the attractors

parameters. Hence, multi-functionality of nonlinear system may be harnessed by
parametric control.

Collective variables, instability and bifurcations (phase transitions)

Consider a complex system comprising many, say thousands, of components and
their connections, enabling a vast set of interactions among them. If we seek to
capture the dynamics of that system we have to formulate thousands of equations
describing the dynamical laws governing their behaviour and then solve them to
deduce the behaviour of each of those components. This kind of microscopic
approach to capturing complex systems behaviour seems quite unreasonable.
Think of the complexity of description if we are to deduce the macroscopic
behaviour of a biological system, say running, starting from microscopic
biochemical processes in each cell of the organism. Fortunately, large masses of
cells in living systems perform in coherent and cooperative ways so that they
create much smaller numbers of mesoscopic and macroscopic behavioural variables, which render their comprehension easier. These macroscopic variables are
those which are essential for describing the coordinated behaviour of the system
as a *whole* and, because they emerge from the cooperative behaviour of collectives of components, they are called *collective variables*. Since they arise from
the collective task dependent cooperation among components, they capture the
order, i.e. coordination, present within the system and hence they are called *order
parameters*.

Now, how are these collective variables or order parameters connected to
stability and instability properties of the system? It happens that these variables
are best detected in the vicinity of the instability points of the system. In this

region, the system, after a *perturbation*, incrementally returns (relaxes) back to the attractor, as some parameter is varied, a property known as a *critical slowing down*. The increase of the local relaxation time shows that components of the system behave less cooperatively, i.e. they are losing their coherent synergic action and attain a larger degree of independence. As the control parameter nears a critical value, any initial perturbation grows and leaves the previous stable state. This point is called a *critical point*. At this point, the system suffers a *loss of stability* and the local *relaxation time* becomes infinite, since the system never relaxes back to the previous attractor. This growth is due to the self-enhancing, positive feedback process. Positive feedback exists when the subsequent influences enhance the initial change. At critical points, a qualitative discontinuous change in a system's behaviour occurs – a *bifurcation* or a *phase transition* – and the values of influential parameters at those points are called *bifurcation* or *critical values*.

An example of this critical phenomenon in the sports domain concerns the interstrike time intervals of phase-free boxing actions used to strike a target (Chow *et al.* 2009). Consider when performers initiate strikes in a parallel stance from different scaled distances to the target. Scaled distance D may be measured as a ratio between the physical distance of a performer's tip of the toes from the target and their arm's length. The forward performer's strikes toward the target act as unidirectional perturbations on their centre of mass, tentatively considered as a collective variable. For increasing scaled distances D from the target, the forward lean is increasingly less quickly restored, so the inter-strike time intervals increase too. The restoration time of the forward-leaned trunk position back to an upright two-foot parallel stance slows down and tends to infinity for critical scaled performer–target distances region D > 1.35, i.e. $D_0 - D < 0.05$, with $D_0 = 1.4$, i.e. exhibits a critical slowing down effect (Figure 1.3, left panel). In fact, the curve has a typical critical behaviour form: $\langle\tau\rangle = A(D_0 - D)^{-\alpha} + B$, where $\langle\tau\rangle$ is the average inter-strike time interval; $A = 0.63$; $B = 0.19$ and the critical exponent $\alpha = 0.456$.

In other words, below $D_0 = 1.35$, a qualitative coordination change from the parallel to the more stable diagonal stance, by stepping forward, takes place (Figure 1.3, right panel), settling the centre of mass to a more stable state. This posture-to-posture transition, which places the centre of mass in a more stable state, is obviously preceded by increasing of the relaxation, (i.e. restoration) time of the forward lean toward backwards as the scaled distance D was increased. In the newly formed coordination, not only does the centre of mass become more stable but the new stance is also more functional and affords a more stable position adjacent to the target-striking position.

In general, it has been shown (Haken 1987) that, at a transition point, only one or few collective modes of the system become unstable and grow (like the centre of mass). The other system degrees of freedom, such as the leg components, become dependent on these collective modes and start to be governed by them. In other words, collective modes enslave the rest of the components and force them to organize in a certain way (e.g. a step forward). This is the well-known

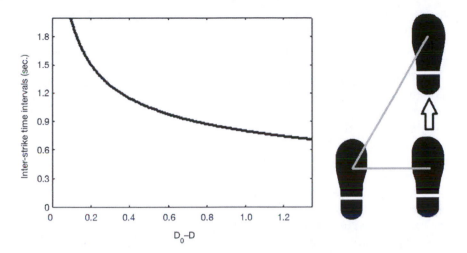

Figure 1.3 Left panel: the increase of the inter-strike time interval for increasing of D control parameter (right-to-left direction). The whole cycle of leaning forward to strike – upright posture restoration – leaning forward to strike, increases, showing increase in the relaxation time toward the upright parallel-foot stance. For $D_0 - D < 0.05$, the relaxation time towards parallel stance tends to become infinite; that is, no relaxation toward the parallel stance exists anymore. The parallel stance loses its stability and transits to a more stable diagonal stance; see right panel (modified from Chow *et al*. 2009, with kind permission from *Nonlinear Dynamics, Psychology and Life Sciences*)

slaving principle introduced by Herman Haken (e.g. Haken 1987). These enslaved components stabilize the value of the collective variables by nonlinear interactions to a finite stable value (the newly formed body position). That is why, instead of growing infinitely, the behavioural variable converges to a finite value, which is the new stable state of organization, i.e. the attractor, of the system. A temporal hierarchy is settled in a spontaneous way. The collective variable (e.g. the centre of mass) takes the role of a slowly varying top-down influence and the enslaved elements, i.e. the leg components, adopt the role of fast variables that follow the behaviour of the collective variable. Enslaved components, by their cooperative behaviour, maintain the collective variable and the collective variable governs the components. The system spontaneously splits into a two-level hierarchy; i.e. on variable(s) that govern and those that are being governed. This is the meaning of the *circular causality* present in complex systems. In this way, a pattern emerges from the interaction of components that is greater than and different from the individual components themselves. *Emergence* means that the macroscopic pattern has properties that cannot be found in the components that form it. A parallel or diagonal stance cannot be reduced to properties of individual motor units, metabolic processes or single neural firings. Motor units, metabolic processes and neurons do not possess a stance themselves. This is how synergetics solves the problem of the part and the whole, which we have already discussed briefly.

Because the components of a complex system are mutually interacting, any influence of one component affects a large set of other components. However, this influence is recurrently fed back to the same component because it is itself under the influence of the rest of the components in the system. This *self-interaction* is the root of nonlinearity and circular causality. Hence, each component self-interacts through its influence on other components. An illustrative example of a self-interaction is the co-adaptive behaviour of two players. Player A reacts to the actions of the player B and player B adapts his actions with respect to player A's actions (see, e.g. Passos *et al.* 2008). In this sense, each of them changes their behaviour by changing the behaviour of the other.

Now, let us assume that, at some critical value of the influential parameter, a small initial seed of behaviour has been formed by a few components. These affect other components in such a way that makes them behave in the same way or some kind of cooperative fashion. The bottom-up cooperation of the components forms a macroscopic collective order. As more and more components are recruited in this recurrent way, the top-down influence of the macroscopic collective order becomes increasingly stronger. New components are recruited in a bottom-up fashion in an ever increasing rate. These newly recruited components add to the strength of the collective macroscopic order that has emerged and, in turn, recruit more components. It is important to note how top-down and bottom-up processes cooperate. However, depending on the value of the constraints impinging on the system, this recruitment process will be stabilized around some value. Then, the same entangled recurrent interactions of components will act as a *negative feedback*, stabilizing the newly formed collective order. If some small subset of components for some reason tries to change its behaviour, the collective interaction field will force it to behave in a collective fashion. The collective field governs the components that form macroscopic patterns of behaviour. This is why self-organization is proclaimed to be a spontaneous *pattern-forming process*.

In this way, an enormous amount of information contained in the large number of degrees of freedom becomes reduced and the system deals with one or only few of them. This is the reason for calling these events *self-organization*. The complex system self-organizes by reducing its large dimensionality to only one or a few variables without the information bearer, a designer, imposing order from outside. Such variables are of great importance for researchers and coaches because they contain the compressed information about a system's component behaviours. In this sense, collective variables are essential because they are relevant for guiding the innumerable microscopic components which depend on them. That is why the search for such macroscopic variables is important in sports science research. Their behaviour informs us about the behaviour of the microscopic components; i.e. about their macroscopic task-dependent functional role. Examples of self-organizing systems within biological systems and their levels and processes are many: human movement (Kelso 1984), the human brain (Fuchs *et al.* 1992), central pattern generators (Wojcik *et al.* 2011), intracellular organization (Daga *et al.* 2006), cell aggregates and tissue formation (Garfinkel *et al.* 2004) to name a few.

We have seen that the stability properties of the system depend on the values of influential constraints of the system. They are the generators of stability and instability in complex systems, being able to control a system's stability properties. That is why these influential parameters are known as *control parameters* (e.g. scaled distance D in the previous example). Such parameters are non-specific, meaning that they do not refer to the specific properties of the system's collective variables. In complex dynamical systems, a large set of control parameters may be present, each one acting on different spatial or time scales. In sport settings, such control parameters are usually formed by confluences of informational task, personal and environmental constraints. For example, hormonal, neuromodulator and neurotransmitter concentrations, synaptic strengths, network topologies, morpho-anatomical properties, psychological states and motor abilities may play a role as personal constraints.

A vast set of variables may play the role of collective variables, i.e. order parameters, owing to their context dependence, task specificity or level of analysis. Collective variables may take the form of, for example, the *amplitude* of oscillations (Haken 1987), *concentrations* in reaction–diffusion processes (Meinhardt and Gierer 2000) and *phase relations* between neurobiological system components (Kelso 1984; Haken *et al.* 1985). In complex networks and actions, these may include local (e.g. Arenas *et al.* 2006; Hristovski *et al.* 2011,) or non-local *correlation* quantities (e.g. Endres *et al.* 2011), orientations and directions (Hristovski *et al.* 2006), *density differences* (e.g. in gas–liquid transitions). Generally, angle variables (of real or formal spaces) are good candidates for order parameters. In particular, useful collective variables may be eigenvectors extracted by principal component analysis (Jirsa *et al.* 1994; Maisuradze *et al.* 2009; Balasubramaniam and Turvey 2004), which may be subsequently dynamically modelled.

Bifurcations are discontinuities in functional dependence

One of the properties of bifurcation or phase-transition points is the onset of *discontinuity* of a behavioural state variable with respect to some control parameter (or set of control parameters). This discontinuity, i.e. singularity, may be manifested as a change of the *functional dependence* of the behavioural variable for a certain value of the control parameter. This is why bifurcations are known as points of qualitative system change. In linear systems, knowing the law of change of the representative curve at one point, we can extrapolate its value at any other point. This provides the feasibility of extrapolating our knowledge about one region of a system's behaviour to any other. This is not always the case for the behaviour of nonlinear systems. For certain values of control parameter(s), a point of discontinuity arises. By knowing the curve of change in one parameter region, we are *not* able to infer anything about its behaviour in the other region and vice versa, unless we know the basic dynamic characteristics of the system.

This is called a non-analyticity of the function, i.e. behaviour. In the sport context, it points to the *non-proportionality* of stimulus–response (or dose–effect) relationship present in nonlinear biological systems such as athletes. The property of non-analyticity may often lead coaches wrongly to extrapolate the behaviour of athletes, knowing their behaviours only in a certain control parameter range. This kind of extrapolation may be a frequent cause of the emergence of overtraining states in athletes, where the role of a control parameter is usually some workload quantity (e.g. Hristovski *et al.* 2010). Moreover, we may wonder how these discontinuities arise in the first place when, e.g. physiological functions within athletes or the workload change more or less continuously during exercise. Such questions bring us to the second important characteristic of bifurcation points. In such points, old stable behaviours die and new ones occur and the number of possible behaviours may change.

Notice here the difference between linear and nonlinear systems. We have already noted that linear systems respond to any minute change of the control parameter with a minute change in their behaviour. In nonlinear systems, such minute changes may accumulate and no detectable or only a small effect may be noticed. Then, with a further small change, a qualitative dynamic change may emerge. It is as if the system slowly accumulates a residual potential for change and then releases it in the form of discontinuous reorganization of behaviour. This behaviour cannot be captured by linear or nonlinear regression procedures.

Rearrangement and breaking of symmetry

At bifurcation points, the symmetry of the state of the system may change. Before the bifurcation, the system may be in a monostable state of symmetry. For example, consider a team sport situation in which all your teammates are well marked by opponents and you have ball possession. Each teammate's action is fully compensated by an opponent's actions. You see the same environment wherever you look. This is a symmetrical state of the system. No passing opportunity emerges. Hence, no game starts. The situation is stable. Then, one of your teammates succeeds in avoiding a marker. You pass the ball to her/him. The system symmetry is broken and the game starts, all over again. The game dwells on broken symmetries.

But the previous symmetry may simply *rearrange* itself into two (or more) equally attractive symmetrical states. Two players simultaneously lose their markers and your decision may be again stuck, at least for a moment – an instance of the 'Buridan's donkey' problem in sport. In symmetrical cases, the system usually switches to one of the newly emerging states because of any random event. So, although there are two equally attractive states, the system selects the behavioural solution spontaneously, as if by chance, relaxing into one of the equally attractive states. This process is an instance of *spontaneous symmetry breaking* because there is no clearly discernible constraint that forces the system to prefer one of the solutions more than the other. This kind of bifurcation is connected to what is referred to as a *second-order phase transition* or a *pitchfork bifurcation*.

However, usually in any performance context there exists a bias in informational constraints. Such events are connected to what is referred to as a *first-order phase transition* or a *saddle-node bifurcation*. In this case, asymmetry is induced into the system by some asymmetric control parameter. This kind of symmetry breaking is called *forced symmetry breaking*, because some kind of bias forces the system to contain asymmetric behavioural solutions. In sports settings, an example of this kind of symmetry breaking emerges when one of the teammates has a better position to score a goal or point than the other. The difference in the positions of the two teammates induces a bias which constrains the decision of the player in possession of the ball, so s/he passes the ball to the one who is better positioned. The diagonal stance in martial arts also may play a role of a symmetry breaking parameter, i.e. a bias-inducing constraint, forcing either left- or right-handed punches to be more used, respectively.

In forced symmetry breaking systems, an interesting effect can arise – *hysteresis*. Hysteresis could arise in the previous example if the player who is in possession of the ball continues to pass the ball to one of the teammates, although the other teammate attains a better position to score. At one moment, the player who has ball possession decides to pass it to the player who is better positioned for a score. But, now he becomes stuck by passing to this teammate, even though the other teammate becomes better positioned for scoring. This type of inertia or system 'memory' is typical for systems with forced symmetry breaking. As we stated earlier, this phenomenon cannot be found in pitchfork bifurcations, i.e. the second-order phase transitions.

When initial symmetry is broken and the system becomes unstable owing to combinations of control parameters, dynamic systems become *weakly unstable* or *metastable* and dwell for a long time close to the remnants of the attractor points. This happens when, under the influence of control parameter(s), the stability of the system is lost but the dynamics are trapped in the vicinity of the previously stable point, i.e. attractor. The system eventually escapes to be temporarily trapped in the vicinity of another attractor remnant. This semi-transient behaviour is a result of purely deterministic dynamics and is a case of *relative coordination* (Kelso 1995), where components are not tightly integrated but only weakly so, allowing them to flexibly decouple and form new transient relations. More information on this extraordinary mechanism of system flexibility may be found in previous published works (e.g. Bressler and Kelso 2001 and the references therein and, particularly in sport contexts, Chow *et al.* 2011).

The overall message is that bifurcations, i.e. thresholds in nonlinear systems, may be of different kinds and they cannot be thought of as fixed set points given once for all time but as points that depend on the combinations of control parameter values and symmetries of the system. Because these parameters are formed by combinations of natural constraints impinging on the system, this would mean that the dynamics of such complex systems and threshold values are guided by those constraints.

Fluctuations, exploration and rugged potential landscapes

In the deterministic approach to dynamical systems when a system reaches a stable state, it keeps that value for an infinitely long time if control parameters are not changed. However, all complex systems in nature possess intrinsic noise, that is, random-like processes that live on timescales faster than the one observed or researched. Such processes do not allow the system, described by some behavioural variable, to stay in an attractor state but push it on the both sides of this state. They counteract the stabilizing, negative feedback loops, 'forces' which try to pull the system into the attractor state. Close to instability points such fluctuations are enhanced, owing to the larger decoupling tendencies among the system components. This phenomenon is called *critical fluctuation enhancement* and together with critical slowing down are hallmarks of phase-transition phenomena.

When noise is present, the system exhibits *fluctuations* around the attractor, i.e. around the steady value or trajectory. In this case, the attractor can be defined as the *most probable* point (or trajectory) of the dynamics. Since the different values of the behavioural variable actually refer to different configurations, i.e. patterns, of the components that form them, it follows that the attractor is the most probable configuration of the system. Depending on the shape of the attractor basin, other configurations take less probable values. The larger the deviation from the attractor, the larger is the amount of component reconfiguration that occurred. It seems that fluctuations make the system *explore* its own capacity for pattern production.

At the beginning of exploration, the system has not well explored all its available configurations and is in a non-equilibrium state. After some longer time period, it has produced all of the available patterns many times and it has reached some stationary probability distribution. The system has equilibrated. However, in nonlinear systems, there may be two or more attractor basins separated by hills or barriers, on top of which the repeller is located (see Figure 1.2). So, while the system has explored the basin of attraction where it was first located and equilibrated there, it may still not reach other available attractor basins. The system has locally equilibrated but not globally. The rate of this global equilibration depends on the height of the barriers and on the strength of fluctuations. It is proportional to the strength of fluctuations and inversely proportional to the height of the barriers. This kind of dynamics of exploration is also called metastability (e.g. Baker 1998). If the system is *weakly stable*, i.e. there exist large fluctuations and low barriers between stable attractors, the rate of exploration may be very large and vice versa, high barriers and low fluctuations would lead to small exploratory rates. These ideas highlight the functionality of system fluctuations for adaptive behaviours, for example, motor learning (Schöllhorn *et al.* 2009). In complex systems, control parameters may be themselves subject to noise. Interesting phenomena may arise around critical points, which may smear the critical point (i.e. the threshold) of the system and produce two- instead of one-phase transitions, i.e. noise-induced transitions. For example, lactate thresholds are sometimes difficult to locate with respect to the load intensity taken as control parameter.

Complex systems often have a complex structure of attractor basins. There may be basins within basins within basins of attraction. In this case, we speak of *rugged potential landscapes* (e.g. Hristovski *et al.* 2011). These systems have a large spectrum of relaxation times and the equilibration process may be very slow. They may never explore the whole space of possible state configurations, i.e. patterns. For example, a non-gymnast would never reconfigure his/her action into a Tsukahara vault or a gymnast may never engage the fat system of energy production during workouts. These systems are *non-ergodic*. *Ergodicity* signifies that, if the system starts with any initial configuration, during the equilibration, i.e. exploration, process, it will visit *all* other configurations many times in some large time limit. For non-ergodic systems, some or even many possible configurations are unavailable. Task and other constraints acting on the system do not allow this to happen and break the ergodicity, allowing the system to equilibrate only locally within relatively small regions. Specific constraints combine to arrest the system within limited configuration space and, if noise strength is small compared with barrier heights, make the system explore for a longer time only a limited set of patterns before it transits to another basin of attraction, where it will face even larger barriers. Over larger time scales, the relaxation becomes increasingly slower. Thus, the trapping role of the constraints may produce *correlated fluctuations*. Depending on the distribution of the barrier height hierarchy, the global relaxation (equilibration) times of patterns or time correlations may take a form of a stretched exponential, power law, show plateau or even logarithmic relaxation. In this sense, athletes may be viewed as non-ergodic, out of equilibrium systems, exploring larger and larger regions of the state space but eventually getting trapped within some relatively small set of the whole state space by the constraints of their sport discipline. Within such regions, some local equilibration may be attained in the long run.

From a practical point of view, these noise phenomena may explain why precise values of thresholds or threshold points in complex biological systems, such as athletes, are hard or sometimes impossible to define. They may be changed by different combinations of control parameters values, as we have noted earlier, but also they may be smeared around some mean value by the influence of intrinsic biological fluctuations. They may have narrower or wider threshold regions instead of threshold points, pointing to the intertwined nature of stochastic and deterministic processes in nonlinear complex dynamical systems. Finding an abrupt change of the probability distribution function as a consequence of a small control parameter change is one possible way to test the critical behaviour of nonlinear systems.

One can also see how the unpredictable behaviours of complex systems arise. The multistability of the system, which is a product of nonlinearity, enables the system to be in more than one state for the same value of parameter. A random event, i.e. a fluctuation, may push the system into a less expected state of organization, perhaps indicative of a lower performance level. Hence, nonlinearity and noise in weakly stable systems might synthesize a behaviour that does not always have to have 'a good reason' to emerge. The only way to reduce the probability of such erratic behaviours is to make attractors more stable by changing the control parameter(s) in an adequate direction. But sometimes such weakly stable behaviours are desirable because they may produce novel functional performance behaviours which no one knew existed. In this way, complex systems are also creative, a valuable resource in sport performance.

References

Arenas, A., Guilera, A. D., and Perez-Vicente, C. (2006) Synchronization reveals topological scales in complex networks. *Physical Review Letters*, 96 (11): 114102.

Baker, D. (1998) Metastable states and folding free energy barriers. *Nature Structural Biology*, 5: 1021–4.

Balasubramaniam, R. and Turvey, M. T. (2004) Coordination modes in the multisegmental dynamics of hula hooping. *Biological Cybernetics*, 90: 176–90.

Bressler, S. L. and and Kelso, J. A. S. (2001) Cortical coordination dynamics and cognition. *Trends in Cognitive Sciences*, 5 (1): 26–36.

Chow, J.-Y., Davids, K., Button, C., Rein, R., Hristovski, R. and Koh, M. (2009) Dynamics of multi-articular coordination in neurobiological systems. *Nonlinear Dynamics, Psychology and Life Sciences*, 13 (1): 27–55.

Chow, J.-Y., Davids, K., Hristovski, R., Araújo, D. and Passos, P. (2011) Nonlinear pedagogy: learning design for self-organizing neurobiological systems, *New Ideas in Psychology*, 29 (2): 189–200.

Daga, R., Lee, K.-G., Bratman, S., Salas-Pino, S. and Chang, F. (2006) Self-organization of microtubule bundles in anucleate fission yeast cells. *Nature Cell Biology*, 1108–13.

Davids, K., Handford, C. and Williams, M. (1994) The natural physical alternative to cognitive theories of motor behaviour: an invitation for interdisciplinary research in sports science? *Journal of Sport Sciences*, 12 (6): 495–528.

Davids, K., Glazier, P., Araújo, D. and Bartlett, R. M. (2003) Movement systems as dynamical systems: the role of functional variability and its implications for sports medicine. *Sports Medicine*, 33: 245–60.

Endres, M., Chenau, M., Fukuhara,T., Weitenberg, C., Schauß, P., Gross, C., Mazza, L., Bañuls, M. C., Pollet, L., Bloch, I. and Kuhr, S. (2011) Observation of correlated particle-hole pairs and string order in low-dimensional mott insulators. *Science*, 334 (6053): 200–3.

Fuchs, A., Kelso, J. A. S. and Haken, H. (1992) Phase transitions in the human brain: spatial mode dynamics. *International Journal of Bifurcation and Chaos*, 2: 917–39.

Garfinkel, A., Tintut, Y., Petrasek, D., Bostrom, K. and Demer, L. L. (2004) Pattern formation by vascular mesenchymal cells. *PNAS*, 101 (25): 9247–50.

Haken, H. (1987) Synergetics: an approach to self-organization in self-organizing systems, in *Self-organizing Systems: The Emergence of Order*, F. Eugene Yates (ed.) Life Science Monographs 21. New York: Plenum, pp. 417–34.

Haken, H., Kelso, J. A. S. and Bunz, H. (1985) A theoretical model of phase transitions in human hand movements. *Biological Cybernetics*, 51: 347–56.

Hristovski, R., Davids, K. and Araújo, D. (2006) Affordance – controlled bifurcations of action patterns in martial arts. *Nonlinear Dynamics, Psychology and Life Sciences*, 4: 409–44.

Hristovski, R., Venskaityte, E., Vainoras, A., Balagué, N. and Vázquez, P. (2010) Constraints-controlled metastable dynamics of exercise-induced psychobiological adaptation. *Medicina*, 46: 447–53.

Hristovski, R., Davids, K., Araújo, D. and Passos, P. (2011) Constraints-induced emergence of functional novelty in complex neurobiological systems: a basis for creativity in sport. *Nonlinear Dynamics, Psychology and Life Sciences*, 15 (2): 175–206.

Jirsa, V. K. and Kelso, J. A. S. (2005) The Excitator as a Minimal Model for Coordination Dynamics of Discrete and Rhythmic Movement Generation. *Journal of Motor Behaviour*, 37 (1): 35–51.

Jirsa, V. K., Friedrich, R., Haken, H. and Kelso, J. A. S. (1994) A theoretical model of phase transitions in the human brain. *Biological Cybernetics*, 71: 27–35.

Kelso, J. A. S. (1984) Phase transitions and critical behavior in human bimanual coordination. *American Journal of Physiology: Regulatory, Integrative and Comparative*, 15: R1000–4.

Kelso, J. A. S. (1995) *Dynamic Patterns*. Cambridge, MA: MIT Press.

Kugler, P. N., Kelso, J. A. S. and Turvey, M. T. (1980) On the concept of coordinative structures as dissipative structures: I. Theoretical lines of convergence. In G. E. Stelmach and J. Requin (eds) *Tutorials in Motor Behaviour*. Amsterdam: North Holland, pp. 49–70.

Maisuradze, G. G., Liwo, A. and Scheraga, H. S. (2009) Principal component analysis for protein folding dynamics. *Journal of Molecular Biology*, 385 (1): 312–29.

Meinhardt, H. and Gierer, A. (2000) Pattern formation by local self-activation and lateral inhibition. *BioEssays*, 22: 753–60.

Passos, P., Araújo, D., Davids, K., Gouveia, L., Milho, J. and Serpa, S. (2008) Information-governing dynamics of attacker–defender interactions in youth rugby union. *Journal of Sports Sciences*, 26 (13): 1421–9.

Schmidt, R. C., Carello, C. and Turvey, M. T. (1990) Phase transitions and critical fluctuations in the visual coordination of rhythmic movements between people. *Journal of Experimental Psychology: Human Perception and Performance*, 16 (2): 227–47.

Schöllhorn, W. I., Mayer-Kress, G., Newell, K. M. and Michelbrink M. (2009) Time scales of adaptive behavior and motor learning in the presence of stochastic perturbations. *Human Movement Science*, 28 (3): 319–33.

Schöner, G., Haken, H. and Kelso, J. A. S. (1986) A stochastic theory of phase transitions in human hand movement. *Biological Cybernetics*, 53: 247–57.

Wojcik, J., Clewley, R. and Shilnikov, A. (2011) Order parameter for bursting polyrhythms in multifunctional central pattern generators. *Physical Review E, Statistical, Nonlinear, and Soft Matter Physics*, 83 (5 Pt 2): 056209.

Zanone, P. G. and Scott Kelso, J.A. (1992) Evolution of behavioral attractors with learning: nonequilibrium phase transitions. *Journal of Experimental Psychology: Human Perception and Performance*, 18 (2): 403–21.

2 Coordination dynamics and cognition[1]

J. A. Scott Kelso

Could he whose rules the rapid comet bind, describe or fix one movement of his mind?

Alexander Pope

In his preface to the *Principia*, Isaac Newton speculated that not just the motions of the planets, the Moon and the tides could be explained by the forces of attraction and repulsion but all other natural phenomena as well (Pope's eulogy to Newton, quoted above, was rather more sceptical). Although Newton himself was cautious about these as yet unknown forces, others in many fields set out to become the Newtons of their time. After all, if Newton could explain celestial events through a simple gravitational force, more mysterious areas of inquiry should be open to the same approach.

For the eighteenth century Scottish philosopher David Hume, all the sciences bore a relation to the human mind. In his *Treatise of Human Nature* (1738), Hume first divided the mind into its contents: ideas and impressions. Then he added dynamics, noting the impossibility that simple ideas could not form more complex ones without some bond of union between them. Hume's three dynamical laws for the association of ideas – resemblance, contiguity and cause and effect – were thought to be responsible for controlling all mental operations. A kind of attraction, Hume thought, existed in the mental world: the motion of the mind was conceived as analogous to the motion of a body. Mental 'stuff' was governed (somehow) by dynamics.

It is practically a cliché that human cognition and behaviour, not to speak of human social interactions, unfold in time. Human behaviour is emergent: patterns of behaviour arise from the way that individual parts or processes are coordinated. Context is crucial. Nonlinearity rules: small changes sometimes produce large effects and large changes no effect at all. Interactions, nonlinearity, emergence and meaningful contextual information, although ubiquitous in the cognitive,

---

1 The present chapter is a slightly revised and updated version of Kelso, J. A. S. (2003). Cognitive coordination dynamics, in W. Tschacher and J. P. Dauwalder (eds) *The Dynamical Systems Approach to Cognition: Concepts and Empirical Paradigms Based on Self-Organization, Embodiment and Coordination Dynamics*. Singapore: World Scientific, pp. 45–71.

brain and behavioural sciences have proven remarkably resistant to understanding. Yet such understanding is obviously central to the development of a truly dynamic cognition (Kelso 2000, 2008, 2012a).

In this chapter, the path towards a dynamic cognition is deemed to lie in *coordination dynamics*, a line of scientific enquiry that aims to understand, through theory, analysis and experiment, how patterns of coordinated behaviour emerge, persist, adapt and change in living things in general and human beings (and brains) in particular (Kelso 1995). Cognition arises from the coevolution of brains, bodies and the environment in which they are immersed; tempered, of course, by developmental and learning processes. Specific cognitive functions require coordination *within* and *between* specialized regions of the brain. The dual nature of this coordination, how the numerous parts of the brain retain their local individualized functions while interacting to form global context-dependent spatiotemporal patterns of neural activity may be understood through coordination dynamics, especially, as we shall see, in its multi- and metastable regimens. This theme of *duality* or *coexistence* permeates the entire chapter. Complementary pairing is fundamental to coordination dynamics (Kelso and Engstrom 2006). Conceptual distinctions such as 'programmes' versus 'self-organization', 'representations' versus 'dynamics' evaporate in very much the same way as the wave/particle duality in quantum mechanics. Within coordination dynamics itself, basic dynamical concepts like attractor and repeller, stability and instability, etc., go together like bread and cheese: one does not make any sense without the other. The coordination dynamics of complex systems in biology, psychology and the social sciences thus embraces a fundamental complementarity (Kelso 1995). In complex systems and the science of coordination, dichotomy is seldom if ever the path to understanding.

In the next section, this dual, complementary nature of coordination dynamics is described, since it is crucial to the development of a truly (spatiotemporal) dynamic cognition. Self-organizing dynamics creates information and information modifies and directs dynamics. The following section stresses the need to identify relevant variables, parameters and their dynamics on a given level of description and articulates a research strategy ('constructive reduction') for doing just that, and for relating levels. A brief and non-inclusive summary of evidence is then presented for the first conceptual foundation of coordination dynamics, *spontaneous self-organizing processes*. Following this, the second, coexistent foundation of coordination dynamics is addressed: meaningful, often directed, information. Emphasis is placed on *metastable coordination dynamics*. This is the regimen in which the tendency of individual component parts and processes to function independently (sometimes called segregation) coexists with the tendency to coordinate together (sometimes called integration). The metastable regimen is also where new information is created without any need for amplification. In coordination dynamics, information may take the form of specific perceptual, cognitive, linguistic and emotional constraints on behaviour. The concepts and tools of coordination dynamics are elaborated further in a section on the context of human skill learning, especially the particularly thorny problem of identifying pre-existing biases that influence and are influenced by the learning process. A possible neural coordination dynamics for handling the joint influences of learning and attention is proposed. In the brain, changes in synaptic weights during learning are accompanied by attention-related neuromodulatory changes that take place in cell bodies, the soma. It may be that cell bodies, including astrocytes and synapses function as a bi-directionally coupled unit (Wade, *et al.* 2011). In the final section of the chapter, some of the main messages of the coordination dynamics of learning are briefly presented, in the hope that these may be useful to practitioners and education policy makers, together with a short summary and some concluding remarks.

The two coexistent foundations of coordination dynamics: spontaneous tendencies and meaningful information

Coordination is not just matter in motion. It refers to different kinds and degrees of *functional* (dis)ordering among interacting parts and processes in space and time. Such functional ordering comes in many guises, from genes to cells to neural ensembles to behaviour (both individual and group) and cognition. Coordination dynamics seeks to identify the laws, principles and mechanisms underlying the coordinated behaviour of a variety of different systems at multiple levels of description (for a comprehensive set of encyclopaedia articles, see Fuchs and Kelso 2009; Oullier and Kelso 2009; Kelso 2009a). Coordination dynamics contains two *coexistent* aspects, a self-organizing, 'undirected' aspect and a 'directed' aspect. Coexistence is inherent to the coordination dynamics of cognition because cognitive function is inherently informational: information, as we shall see later in this chapter, is created by self-organizing dynamical processes and, in turn, modifies or directs the dynamics (Kelso 2002).

The first conceptual foundation of coordination dynamics, synergetic self-organization, refers originally to collective or cooperative effects that arise spontaneously when ordinary matter takes on novel properties, as in lasers and superconductors, or when new forms of organization among water molecules arise, as in the weather (e.g. Haken 1977; Nicolis and Prigogine 1977). In such pattern forming systems, cooperation among the many microscopic components emerges, not because of some special coordinating agent or instruction set residing inside the system but rather as a result of the system's ability to organize itself under specific boundary constraints. The second, coexistent root of coordination dynamics, complementing spontaneous self-organizing processes, concerns the special nature of the boundary constraints (parameters, initial conditions) in human cognition and behaviour. This 'directed' aspect of coordination dynamics deals with how information is created *de novo* and how information guides, directs, modulates and is modulated by self-organizing processes (Kelso 1995). 'Directed' informational terms, such as 'plans', 'programmes', 'intentions', and so forth, common in cognitive science, are embraced rather than reified in coordination dynamics. Unlike the behaviour of inanimate things, the self-organizing dynamics of human brains and the behaviour they produce is fundamentally informational, although not in the standard sense of data communicated across a channel (Shannon and Weaver 1949). Rather, in coordination dynamics, the *coordination variables are themselves context dependent and intrinsically meaningful*. Context dependence does not imply lack of reproducibility, nor does it mean that every new context requires new coordination variables and dynamics. What it does mean is that specific information (situational context, perception of a task to be learned, intention to change behaviour, attention devoted to particular task components, a template or memory of the pattern to be produced, etc.) can be expressed in terms of parameters acting on system-relevant coordination variables. Thus, the full coordination dynamics contains a term defining 'informational forcing' and a term expressing spontaneous, self-organizing processes (see Kelso 1995, p. 163). In recent theoretical developments, such as so-called parametric *stabilization* (Jirsa *et al.* 2000), parameters and variables may act multiplicatively, meaning that a parameter can directly affect a relevant variable and vice versa. It is also possible that the coordination variable or 'order parameter' can act back on to parameters and modify them; a kind of nonlinear feedback process. In terms of scientific understanding, the benefit of identifying relevant variables is that one knows what to parametrically modify. Likewise, the structure of the self-organizing dynamics – prior to the introduction of new information – influences how that information is used. Thus, information is not lying out there as mere data: information is meaningful and specific to the extent that it modifies and is modified by the underlying dynamics.

Identifying coordination dynamics in complex systems

In the brain, cognitive, behavioural and social sciences, neither the key coordination quantities nor their coordination dynamics are known a priori and have to be identified. Brain structure and function, for example, appears to be hierarchically organized; the component elements on multiple levels of description are heterogeneous and the relevant coordination variables characterizing ongoing neural and cognitive processes are invariably context, task or function dependent.

How do we discover relevant coordination variables in such complex systems? And which, if any, can we reasonably discard as not relevant? In the following, the six-step research strategy of coordination dynamics is presented, which can be (and has been) applied to different fields of study. A possible limitation of this strategy is that it appears to be restricted to laboratory settings. However, many of the same steps – or at least the questions raised by these steps – may be adopted in other contexts, such as observational or field studies, including sports (see, e.g. Duarte, *et al.* 2012; Passos *et al.* 2008).

Step 0: Choose a level of description

In coordination dynamics, the key is to choose a level of description and understand the (coupling) relation between adjacent levels, not (or not only) reducing to some 'fundamental' lower level. The choice of a level of description is the scientist's and can only be made with informed insight. Choice of a level of description is not an issue of a 'top-down' versus 'bottom-up' approach. In coordination dynamics, the first step at any level of description, whether one is studying biomolecular processes or social behaviour, requires the identification of relevant coordination variables and their dynamics.

Step 1: Prune away complications

Science always needs special entry points; places where irrelevant details may be pruned away while retaining the essential aspects of the phenomena that one is trying to understand. One may call this the Galilean strategy. By studying balls rolling down an inclined plane and abstracting away friction, Galileo was able to provide deep insights into the nature of falling bodies and planetary motion. There is no formula or recipe that may be applied to this step. One has to find or even invent experimental model systems or situations that distil away irrelevant aspects, leaving the ones that really matter.

Step 2: Use qualitative change

Unique to the perspective of self-organizing coordination dynamics is its focus on *qualitative change*, places where behaviour bifurcates or a phase transition occurs (Haken *et al.* 1985; Kelso 1984). Qualitative change is important for both theoretical and empirical reasons. Theoretically, dynamic instability is the generic mechanism underlying spontaneous self-organized pattern formation and change in all systems coupled to their internal or external environment (Haken 1983; Nicolis and Prigogine 1977). Experimentally, qualitative change affords a clear distinction between one pattern and another, thereby enabling one to identify the key coordination variables that characterize patterned states. In a typical situation, many variables may be changing some smoothly and linearly. However, the one(s) that change(s) abruptly are likely to be the most informationally meaningful, both for the system itself and for the scientist trying to understand them (Kelso 1994b). Qualitative change may also be used to infer relevant quantities in more naturalistic settings (for a lovely example, see Beekman *et al.* 2001). Instead of driving the system toward instabilities, for example, one can examine time series of complex interacting systems for places where abrupt changes occur and use these to identify the underlying dynamics – a kind of reverse engineering approach.

Step 3: The coordinative level

Finding collective or coordination variables on a chosen level of description (neural, behavioural, cognitive) is the 'yin' of the coordination dynamics research strategy. The 'yang' is identifying the control parameter(s) that cause coordinative change. Naturally occurring environmental conditions or intrinsic, endogenous factors may qualify as *control parameters*.

Technically speaking, a parameter is a control parameter if, when it changes smoothly and continuously, the coordinative behaviour of the system changes qualitatively and abruptly. Thus, when a control parameter crosses a critical value, *instability* occurs, leading to the formation of new (or different) patterns. The payoff from knowing coordination variables and control parameters is high: they enable one to obtain the dynamical rules, i.e., the equations of motion that describe the stability and change of patterned coordinative states on a given level of description. Coordination variables and control parameters (whether specific or nonspecific) are complementary: you do not have one without the other and vice versa. Moreover, they may be interchangeable, depending on level of description (Kelso 1995). For example, in studies of phase transitions in bimanual coordination movement, frequency is a control parameter at the coordinative level and a coordination variable at the component level.

Step 4: The component level

By adopting the same strategy at the next level down, the individual component dynamics may be studied and identified. In general, in complex systems, it is difficult to isolate the components and study their dynamics. The reason is that the individual components seldom exist outside the context of the functioning whole and have to be studied as such. Just as an example, recent work on interpersonal coordination (Oullier *et al.* 2008) shows that individuals retain a memory of the interaction with a partner, even when they are no longer coupled.

Step 5: Establish relations among levels

A 'final' but nontrivial step is to derive the coordinative level dynamics from the, in general, nonlinear coupling between the individual components. This is what some people call 'emergence' and it allows for a bridge to be built across different levels of description in a systematic fashion. It should be clear that no level is any more or less 'fundamental' than any other. Likewise, there are no absolute 'macro' or 'micro' levels. The complete coordination dynamics on a given level of description always requires three adjacent tiers: the specific boundary conditions and control parameters that establish the context for a particular phenomenon to arise; the coordinative level and its dynamics; and the component level and its dynamics. Notice that the descriptors at each level are always different from each other. However, the language of coordination dynamics serves to bridge different domains. I call this *constructive reductionism*: by starting with a coherent description of behaviour on one level and by focusing on adjacent levels 'above' (boundary constraints) and 'below' (individual component parts and processes), the behaviour of the whole may be seen as 'emerging' from the nonlinear interactions among component subsystems. The strategy of constructive reductionism can be implemented at least 'one level down'. In recent times, a complementary picture has been forming – namely that *laws of coordination in neurobehavioural systems deal with collective properties that emerge from microscopic dynamics but are not deducible from them.* Such 'mesoscopic protectorates' (after Laughlin and Pines 2000) are generic, emergent behaviours that are reliably the same from one system to another, regardless of details, and are repeatable within a system on multiple levels and scales (Kelso 2012b; see also Turvey and Carello 2012). The notion that laws of coordination are truly emergent and sui generis suggests that it may not be possible – even in principle – to deduce psychological-level descriptions from (more microscopic) neural- or molecular-level descriptions. As stressed here in step 5, this does not mean that we should not try to understand the relationships between different levels. Rather, the task is to come up with lawful descriptions that allow us to understand emergent behaviour at all levels and to respect the autonomy of each.

The self-organizing nature of coordination dynamics

Are the foundational concepts of self-organization in physical, chemical and biochemical systems relevant to cognitive and behavioural function? Over the last three decades, starting with experiments on people (Kelso 1981, 1984) and theoretical modelling of such (Haken et al. 1985), it has been shown that the same coordination dynamics (equations of motion whose parameters alter the stability and change of coordination patterns over time, together with the nonlinear coupling among components that gives rise to them) apply to the functional coordination among anatomically different parts and processes, including but not limited to: intentional movements of two or more fingers and limbs (Carson et al. 1995; Fuchs and Kelso 1994; Haken et al. 1985; Kelso 1984; Kelso and Jeka 1992; Peper et al. 1995; Schöner et al. 1990; Swinnen et al. 1997; Treffner and Turvey 1996); coupling among the joints of a single, multi-jointed limb (Buchanan and Kelso 1993; Carson et al. 1999; Kelso et al. 1991); perception-action coupling between visual auditory and tactile stimuli and motor responses (Kelso et al. 1990, 1998; Lagarde and Kelso 2006; Stins and Michaels 1999; Wimmers et al. 1992); postural sway (Bardy et al. 1999; Dijkstra et al. 1994; Jeka et al. 1997); visually mediated coordination between two people (Amazeen et al. 1995; Dumas et al. 2010; Naeem et al. 2012; Riley et al. 2011; Schmidt et al. 1990; Tognoli et al. 2007); between humans and computers (Kelso et al. 2009); and even between humans and other species (Lagarde et al. 2005). In numerous situations, the coordination dynamics – at both the coordinative level and at the level of the nonlinear interactions among the components – explicitly incorporates the role of specific neuromuscular–skeletal constraints. For instance, eigenfrequency differences between coupled limb movements (Fuchs and Kelso 1994; Kelso and Jeka 1992; Sternad et al. 1995) as well as neurally based informational couplings between auditory, tactile or visual stimuli and movement are known to shape or sculpt the form of coordination observed (Kelso et al. 1990; Kelso 2010; Riley et al. 2011).

Neural correlates of the stability and change of behavioural coordination have been revealed using a high-density superconducting quantum interference device and electroencephalograph arrays (Banerjee et al. 2012; Daffertshofer et al. 2000;

Fuchs *et al.* 1992, 2000a,b; Kelso *et al.* 1991, 1992; Mayville *et al.* 1999, 2001; Frank *et al.* 2000; Wallenstein *et al.* 1995), as well as functional magnetic resonance imaging and positron emission tomography (DeLuca *et al.* 2010; Jantzen *et al.* 2008, 2009; Meyer-Lindenberg *et al.* 2002; Swinnen 2002; Swinnen and Wenderoth 2004; Ullen *et al.* 2000; Fuchs *et al.* 2000c). Theoretical work at the neural level has progressed from phenomenological modelling at behavioural (Beek *et al.* 1995; Fuchs and Jirsa 2001; Haken *et al.* 1985; Jirsa *et al.* 2000; Kelso *et al.* 1990, 1993; Schöner *et al.* 1986, 1990; Treffner and Turvey 1996) and brain levels (Jirsa *et al.* 1994; Uhl *et al.* 1995) to neurobiologically grounded accounts of both unimanual (Jirsa and Haken 1997; Fuchs *et al.* 2000; Frank *et al.* 2000) and bimanual coordination (Jirsa *et al.* 1998) that are based on known cellular and neural ensemble properties of the cerebral cortex. Recent work has extended this neural theory to include the heterogeneous connectivity between neural ensembles in the cortex (See 'Neural coordination dynamics of learning and attention' below; Jirsa and Kelso 2000). In all these circumstances, once general laws at behavioural and brain levels have been identified, it has proved possible to derive them from a deeper theory grounded in neuroanatomical and neurophysiological data, thereby causally connecting different levels of description (Kelso *et al.* 1999 for review). In showing that stability and change of coordination at both behavioural and neural levels is due to nonlinear interactions among interacting components some of the mysticism behind the contemporary terms 'emergence' and 'self-organization' has been removed.

The informational nature of coordination dynamics

It may be said that the self-organizing nature of coordination dynamics possesses 'universal' properties (Haken 1996; Kelso 1995), seemingly unrelated systems behaving in essentially the same way. Individual components or features of complex coordinative systems may be coupled by material forces, by light, by sound, by touch and by intention (Kelso 2009b; Kelso *et al.* 2001 for review and experimental evidence). How then does information arise? And what does it do? How are the central concepts of cognitive science terms such as 'plans', 'programmes', 'intentions' and so forth, handled in coordination dynamics? Let us first consider the creation of information question.

Elsewhere (Kelso 1995, 2002), I have proposed that the origins of information lies in the *metastable regimen of the coordination dynamics*. This is the regimen in between the idealized states of complete interdependence between interacting components (such as patterns of phase and frequency synchronization between neural regions of the brain) and total independence of the component parts from each other (i.e., each local region of the brain expresses its own dynamic properties without any interaction with other local regions).

In the metastable regimen, there are no attractors or repellers in the coordination dynamics but there is still *attraction* to where the attractors used to be. The reason is that intrinsic differences between the individual components are sufficiently large that they do their own thing, while still retaining a *tendency* to cooperate. Thus, the relative phase between the components may drift in time, but is occasionally trapped near 'remnants' or 'ghosts' of patterned coordination states. This, I propose, is how global integration, in which component parts are locked together, is reconciled with the tendency of the parts to function as locally specialized autonomous units. Because of metastable coordination dynamics, the brain is able to exhibit a far more variable, plastic and fluid form of coordination in which *tendencies* for integration and segregation *coexist*. Metastable coordination dynamics is characteristic of successful organizations (let the parts remain semi-autonomous while still cooperating loosely) and is especially evident in the functional organization of the human brain (e.g. Bressler and Kelso 2001; Friston 2000; Kelso 1992, 1995, 2002, 2012a; Kelso and Tognoli 2007; Tognoli and Kelso 2009) and cognition (e.g. Chen *et al.* 1997, 2001; Ding *et al.* 2002; Kello *et al.* 2010; Tuller *et al.* 1997; van Orden *et al.* 2005).

How does metastable coordination dynamics relate to the issue of the origins of information? If the brain is metastable (and the evidence is compelling at both behavioural and neural levels) *it may be conceived as a measuring device that is poised to create information*. Analogous to effective devices for measuring quantal events (Green 2000), in order to be sensitive to the world, the brain must exist in the metastable regimen, where the slightest fluctuation or change in parameters will nudge it into and out of coordinative states. Such coordinative states are *intrinsically meaningful*. What could be more relevant to the brain than information that communicates the relationship between its component parts? Information can never be known fully in advance. It must be discovered. The remarkable aspect of metastable coordination dynamics is that no amplification of microscopic events (as in quantal emission) is warranted or required. The essentially nonlinear nature of the coupling between the individual parts and the intrinsic nature of the parts themselves gives rise to metastability in a natural way. Indeed, in the Kelso *et al.* (1990) elaboration of the HKB (Haken–Kelso–Bunz) model, metastable coordination dynamics is caused by the interplay of two factors, the intrinsic properties of the component features themselves and the nonlinear coupling between them. Akin to quantum theory, after the measurement of information the metastable brain is in a coordinated (read pure, idealized) state that (importantly) is quantified by the values of collective states). Selection among meaningful coordination states may occur in several ways. First, an extremum principle may govern the selection or choice between equally available collective or coordinated states (Blekhman 1988). Second, selection may occur via parametrically induced instability, the selection via instability principle enunciated earlier (Kelso 2000). (Still another selection mechanism – selection via matching – has been revealed in studies of sensori-motor learning, see Kostrubiec *et al.* 2012.)

Once created due to the metastability of self-organizing coordination dynamics and expressed in terms of system-relevant coordination states, what does information do? Again, cognitive information can play the dual role of stabilizing and destabilizing behaviour depending on context (initial conditions). Early and more recent research shows that information is capable of *stabilizing* the coordination dynamics even under conditions in which patterns of coordinated activity typically become unstable and switch. For example, internally generated intentions (Kelso *et al.* 1988; Lee *et al.* 1996) and cognitive strategies (Kelso *et al.* 1990; see also Chen *et al.* 2001) enable the cognitive system to stay longer in a pattern of behaviour than it normally would or could. Intention to stay in a pattern can simultaneously recruit new biomechanical degrees of freedom and annihilate ones that were formerly engaged (Buchanan and Kelso 1999; Buchanan *et al.* 1997; Fink *et al.* 2000a; Kelso *et al.* 1993). Perceptual information also serves to stabilize coordinated behaviour, as in the well-known 'anchoring' effect (Byblow *et al.* 1994; Fink *et al.* 2000b) in which specific, attended to perceptual inputs are selectively coupled to specific aspects of activity. Such so-called 'parametric stabilization' effects have been modelled mathematically within the current framework of coordination dynamics (Fink *et al.* 2000b; Jirsa *et al.* 2000). *Multimodal* information from auditory, haptic and intentional sources is bound together in time in a coherent way that serves to stabilize coordinative actions (Kelso *et al.* 2001; Lagarde and Kelso 2006). In more recent work by Kovacs *et al.* (2010), a so-called Lissajous template may serve to stabilize apparently arbitrary phasing patterns between the limbs.

Likewise, perceptual, cognitive, emotive and linguistic information can also *destabilize* behaviour. Depending on task context and parameters, such as stimulation rate, perceptual information can destabilize the cognitive system, causing it to switch from one pattern of behaviour to another (Kelso *et al.* 2001). For example, haptic input that is counterphase to a rhythmic auditory stimulus can cause a switch in behaviour such that haptic and auditory inputs coincide with intended movement, forming a spatiotemporally coherent bond. In a similar vein, intentions can destabilize behaviour and cause it to switch (DeLuca *et al.* 2010; Kelso *et al.* 1988; Lee *et al.* 1996; Scholz and Kelso 1990). Perceptually available spatial information can readily overcome apparent neuromuscular biases such as preferences for coactivation of homologous muscles (e.g. Kelso and Jeka 1992; Kelso *et al.* 1991; Meschner *et al.* 2001; but see Salter *et al.* 2004) or one muscle group over another (Kelso *et al.* 2001), at least up to a point.

In short, the parameters of cognitive coordination dynamics emerge from a variety of sources that mutually constrain behaviour and behavioural choice. These informational sources contribute to what we typically refer to under the umbrella term, *context*. They include the perceptual requirements of the task, information that arises during performance of the task, intention to perform a particular behavioural pattern, allocation of attentional resources (Temprado *et al.* 1999), memory of previous experiences and even 'low-level' neuromuscular–skeletal factors. All of these constraints have been connected to the concept of stability of the coordination dynamics in one form or another (including metastability, multistability and instability; see Kelso 2012a) and measurements thereof. Many of these constraints are prevalent in the context of learning, a topic to which we now turn.

The coordination dynamics of skill learning

The organism, so goes the truism, is not a blank slate. Every individual enters the learning situation with a history of pre-existing capacities. A key idea of the coordination dynamics of the learning process is that learning involves a modification of the learner's pre-existing capacities in the direction of the skill to be learned. However, although other theorists also stress that learning and development proceed in the context of pre-existing biases (e.g. Sporns and Edelman 1993), ways to evaluate this pre-existing movement repertoire prior to learning are lacking or, more usually, totally ignored in theories of skill acquisition. Because discovering the nature of pre-existing capabilities is so difficult, investigators have tried to use tasks that are as novel as possible and hence they are completely unrelated to any existing coordination tendencies that the learner might possess. Ironically, this strategy may prevent us from understanding the features of the learned representation that are *shared* across tasks and the level at which they are specified. In addition, rather than studying a group of people performing a novel task and averaging across them, coordination dynamics studies the individual learner, searching instead for learning mechanisms that are common *across* individuals.

Starting in 1987, Pier-Giorgio Zanone and I developed methods to overcome the difficult problem of evaluating the pre-existing capabilities of the learner by scanning – before learning begins; throughout the learning process; and after practice is over – the space of the coordination variable proven to be valid for visuomotor coordination tasks, namely, the relative phase between the interacting components (Haken *et al.* 1985; Kelso 1984; Schmidt and Turvey 1995; Swinnen *et al.* 1997). This technique allows us to set the learning task on an individual basis such that it does or does not correspond to pre-existing coordination tendencies, which, whether innate or acquired, may already exist in the individual learner's repertoire. According to coordination dynamics, new task requirements may cooperate or compete with pre-existing tendencies, thereby influencing the nature and rate of the learning process. As the task is learned, the stability of the performed pattern increases (indexed by shifts in the mean relative phase toward the learned pattern, a sharpening of the distribution of phasing fluctuations and faster relaxation times to the pattern). At the same time, the memorized relative phase evolves on a slower timescale, biasing the performed pattern toward the to-be-learned relative phase (for formal details, see Schöner and Kelso 1988; Schöner *et al.* 1992).

In our initial work (Zanone and Kelso 1992; see also Fontaine *et al.* 1997; Kelso 1990, 1995 chapter 6; Magne and Kelso 2008; Zanone and Kostrubiec 2004), we showed not only that a new attractive state is established as memorized information gains strength but also that the learning process may take the form of a non-equilibrium phase transition or bifurcation: stabilization of the learned pattern increased the number of coordination patterns available to the learner and destabilized others (at least temporarily). *Learning, in other words, not only altered behaviour in the direction of the to-be-learned pattern but also changed the entire layout of the coordination dynamics* (see Schöner *et al.* 1992, for the formal details). More recently, we have provided evidence that learning may delay or even eliminate instabilities along with neurophysiological correlates of such (Jantzen *et al.* 2001, 2002).

An important issue in theories of skill acquisition and learning concerns the nature of what is learned. Coordination dynamics constitutes a lawful representation that governs how the central nervous system assembles coordinated patterns of activity on different levels of description. How abstract this representation is may be ascertained by determining the effectiveness of transfer or generalization from one (trained) effector system to another (untrained) effector system. In previous work, we established that transfer of timing relations occurs spontaneously between two components within the same effector system (Zanone and Kelso 1994, 1997). We then tested whether transfer of learning also occurs across different effector systems, causing similar alterations in their respective coordination dynamics (Kelso and Zanone 2002). The task was to learn a specific phase relationship through practice with the arms or the legs. In order to assess modifications induced by learning and transfer, the coordination dynamics of both effector systems were evaluated before and after practice through scanning probes aimed at revealing underlying attractive states of the coordination dynamics.

We predicted that transfer and generalization of learning should occur across different effector systems to the extent that they share comparable coordination dynamics. Thus, if this hypothesis is correct, both the trained and the untrained effector combination should simultaneously exhibit stabilization of the to-be-learned phasing pattern. Moreover, other phasing relations are predicted to be biased toward the to-be-learned pattern, if as our theory predicts, the entire coordination dynamics is altered by the learning process. Such a result is not typically examined in work from other traditions because the full range of task-related coordination tendencies and how these may change with learning is not explored. That is, traditional approaches seldom measure how other timing relations, beyond the task to be learned, are influenced by the learning process (for discussion, see Schmidt and Lee 1998 pp. 382–3).

Whether complete transfer occurs, of course, may depend on whether the learning task is accomplished by components that are biomechanically similar (e.g. the two arms or the two legs and their neural activation) or different (e.g. an arm and a leg). The extended form of the HKB dynamics (Kelso *et al.* 1990) contains a term ($\delta\omega$) that respects asymmetries, such as those caused by biophysical differences between limbs (Jeka and Kelso 1995; Kelso and Jeka 1992; Sternad *et al.* 1996) or differences between stimulus and response components (Kelso *et al.* 1990; Wimmers *et al.* 1992), whereas the original form (Haken *et al.* 1985) does not. Given the many differences of neural and biomechanical origin between arms and legs, no one, of course, expects perfect transfer. Nevertheless, evidence that the unpractised pattern is learned and stabilized would bolster the view that coordination dynamics constitutes a single abstract representation for an entire equivalence class of coordinated actions, specifically those dealing with the relative timing between coordinating components.

Results of the Kelso and Zanone (2002) study indicated that learning a novel relative phase with one effector system spontaneously transferred to the other *untrained* effector system. Not only was transfer seen as performance improvements in both systems when the to-be-learned phasing was required but it was also revealed by qualitative modifications of their underlying coordination dynamics. That is, the dynamics of both the trained and untrained limb pairs exhibited either comparable phase transitions, themselves a signature of learning (Kelso 1990; Zanone and Kelso 1992) or similar shifts in pre-existing attractive states, a further, parametric sign of learning (Zanone and Kelso 1997). Irrespective of which form the learning process actually took, the perceptually required phasing pattern was learned and remembered, creating a new attractive state in both the practised and unpractised coordination dynamics.

An important provision taken in the present approach is that the pattern selected as a learning task does not coincide with already existing attractive states (or preferences) of the underlying coordination dynamics. Theoretically, before learning, any contribution to the coordination dynamics owing to the novel task requirement should compete with any pre-existing, so-called 'intrinsic' coordination tendencies. Such competitive interaction between behavioural task demands and individual coordination tendencies leads to observed biases and increases in variability of the performed pattern. Our results strongly suggest that a common mechanism underlies learning and transfer, namely reduction of the competition that initially arises between task requirements and intrinsic coordination tendencies. How such competition is instantiated in the central nervous system is an interesting question. It is now well-established that different behavioural phasing patterns have their expression in spatiotemporal patterns of brain activity, quantified (using time-averaging techniques) in terms of spatial modes and their time-dependent amplitudes (e.g. Fuchs *et al.* 1992; Fuchs *et al.* 2000; Jirsa *et al.* 1998; Kelso *et al.* 1992, 1998) or (in the frequency domain) as patterns of power and coherence, particularly in the beta (15–30 Hz) range (Chen *et al.* 1999, 2003; Jantzen *et al.* 2001; Mayville *et al.* 2001). Still other evidence using positron emission tomography has found that neural areas such as the sensorimotor cortex are quite effector-specific, whereas activity in parietal cortex remains high after transfer has occurred from fingers to arms in a sequencing task (Grafton *et al.* 1998). Our findings that similar alterations occur in the coordination dynamics of both the trained and untrained effector systems confirm the hypothesis that learning and transfer occur at a rather abstract level of system function. It may well be that parietal areas are involved in generating action sequences at this abstract level, quite independent of the effectors used. The latter statement is not meant to minimize specific neuromuscular–skeletal factors that have been shown to sculpt the coordination dynamics (Carson and Riek 1998; Kelso *et al.* 2001; Kelso and Jeka 1992; Jeka and Kelso 1995).

How does the present work relate to more classical views of skill acquisition and learning? In most, if not all previous views, the outcome of learning is addressed in terms of abstract, task-specific entities such as schemas, images of achievement and generalized programs (e.g. Bartlett 1932; Bernstein 1967;

Schmidt 1975). For example, the aim of schema theory was to explain how variable experiences with a skill allow the learner to parameterize it in the form of a generalized motor programme. This generative, rule-like feature of schema theory is intrinsic to even the most elementary form of the coordination dynamics. The HKB (1985) equation, for example, incorporates not only the so-called 'invariance' properties of the generalized motor programme but also the crucially important dynamic features of multistability, phase transitions and hysteresis. For neurobehavioral dynamical systems (Kelso 1991, 2012a), the latter correspond respectively to multi-functionality (different behavioural patterns for the same parameter values), switching or 'decision making' (one behavioural pattern is selected over another at critical parameter values) and a primitive kind of memory (the history of system behaviour affects the current state), respectively. Whereas data suggesting that the temporal structure of movement is preserved across various kinds of parameterizations are used as *prima facie* evidence for a generalized motor programme (as it was for the earlier notion of coordinative structure, e.g. Kelso *et al.* 1979; Turvey *et al.* 1978), coordination dynamics rationalizes why this is so in terms of the concept of stability. For example, in coordination dynamics loss of stability provides a selection mechanism in the form of bifurcations or phase transitions for the emergence of novel behavioural patterns. Fluctuations or variability are not 'errors' or 'noise' in the output of the motor programme but rather a fundamental way for the system to test its own stability under the current circumstances. Thus, in coordination dynamics, fluctuations are an essential part of the 'decision-making' mechanism determining whether the system switches behaviour or not (e.g. Kelso *et al.* 1986). These theoretical differences notwithstanding, a persistent issue in cognitive science has been to define equivalence classes of processes in order to understand how two different processes may be accomplished by the same higher-level mechanism or 'algorithm' (Marr 1982). Viewed in the context of coordination dynamics, this problem reduces to identifying the ensemble of behaviours that share the same task- or function-specific coordination dynamics (Kelso 2009a,b). By showing task-level transfer, the Kelso and Zanone (2002) study provided an indication of just how abstract and generalizable the coordination dynamics is and what form it takes. A more recent summary of this entire research programme, including a specific theoretical model that accommodates old as well as newer experimental observations on learning, memory and attention may be found in Kostrubiec *et al.* (2012).

Neural coordination dynamics of learning and attention

Coordination dynamics and its theoretical extensions, e.g. which model observations of human brain and behavioural activity in terms of dynamic neural fields (Fuchs *et al.* 2000; Jirsa *et al.* 1994, 1998; Jirsa and Haken 1996; Jirsa and Kelso 2000; Kelso *et al.* 1999) may mark the genuine arrival of a new kinematics and dynamics for psychological states and cognitive processes (Churchland 1988). Once the laws are known at the behavioural level, it has proved possible to derive them from the excitatory and inhibitory dynamics of neural populations and their long- and short-range connections. The neural theory, in turn, poses a number of challenges to experiment, such as how synaptic and cellular properties are influenced by learning, arousal and attention (Kelso 2000). Let us pursue that challenge a bit further and delve into what it entails.

It is well-known that spontaneous macroscopic reorganization of activity occurs in both behavioural and brain dynamics (e.g. Chialvo 2010; Daffertshofer *et al.* 2000; Frank *et al.* 2000; Fuchs *et al.* 1992; Jantzen *et al.* 2001; Jirsa *et al.* 1998; Kelso 2010; Kelso *et al.* 1991, 1992; Mayville *et al.* 1999, 2001; Meyer-Lindenberg *et al.* 2002; Plenz and Thiagarian 2007; Wallenstein, Kelso and Bressler 1995). Such phase transitions are described by the destabilization of a macroscopic activity pattern when neural populations are forced to reorganize their spatiotemporal behaviour. Destabilization is typically controlled via unspecific control parameters. In contrast, traditional neuroscience describes reorganization of neural activity as changes of spatial and timing relations among neural populations. Both views are tied together by neural field theory; here, the spatiotemporal evolution of neural activity is described by a nonlinear retarded integral equation, which has a heterogeneous integral kernel. The latter describes the connectivity of the neocortical sheet and incorporates both continuous properties of the neural network as well as discrete long-distance projections between neural populations. Mathematical analysis (Jirsa and Kelso 2000) of such heterogeneously connected systems shows that local changes in connectivity alter the timing relationships between neuron populations. These changes enter the equations as a topological control parameter and can destabilize neural activity patterns globally giving rise to macroscopic phase transitions. Heterogeneous connectivity also addresses the stability–plasticity dilemma: a stable transmission of directed activity flow may be achieved by projecting directly from area A to area B and from there to area C (stability). However, if necessary, area A may *recruit* neighbouring populations of neurons (plasticity). See also Banerjee *et al.* (2012) for a postulated recruitment mechanism for the case of bimanual interactions between the limbs.

On the basis of our integral formulation of neural coordination dynamics, we are currently addressing the following two aspects of brain functioning, namely learning and attention/intention. Learning is approached via local changes of synaptic weights resulting in a temporal dependence of the connectivity function; i.e., the integral kernel. Two dynamics may be distinguished: 1) the learning dynamics in which we employ established methods usually based on unsupervised modified Hebbian learning; and 2) the neural dynamics itself.

Reorganization of spatiotemporal neural activity can be controlled via learning (Jirsa and Kelso 2000). Attention and intention are approached via local changes in the sigmoidal response curves of neural ensembles, the so-called conversion operations. These conversion operations have been investigated in quantitative detail as a function of attention (e.g. Freeman 1975). The main result is that the slope and the height of the sigmoid vary by a factor of 2.5 between minimal and maximal attention. The sigmoidal variation of the ensemble response is realized biochemically by different concentrations of neuromodulators such as dopamine and norepinephrine. Mathematically, the neural dynamics described by the spatiotemporal integral equations can be coupled to a one-dimensional concentration field in which elevated values designate increased values of slope and height of the sigmoidal response curve of neural ensembles. An increased slope and height of the sigmoid typically causes increased amplitude and excitability of the neural sheet.

The following line of thought allows an operationalization of the above concepts, both experimentally and theoretically: a novel (or more difficult) task requires more attention/arousal than an automated behavioral pattern (Jantzen *et al.* 2001; Temprado *et al.* 1999). Increased attention demand is realized in the cortical sheet via a larger concentration of neurotransmitter substance resulting in a steeper slope and larger height of the sigmoid response function. As a consequence, excitability and amplitude of neural activity are increased in task conditions requiring more attention. During learning, changes in connectivity occur. After learning, the task condition is no longer novel but rather more 'automated', reflected in decreased concentrations of neurotransmitters and thus decreased excitability and amplitude of ongoing neural activity (see also Jantzen *et al.* 2001).

Implications and applications of coordination dynamics

Since this volume deals with applications of complex, self-organizing dynamical systems to sport and since sport involves highly skilled activity, it may be useful to summarize the 'bottom line' or message of coordination dynamics in the context of skill learning. Although much remains to be understood about the learning process and the brain mechanisms that underlie it, the following summary statements are based on results obtained thus far within the context of coordination dynamics. Several propositions are still under detailed experimental scrutiny.

- The individual, not the group is the significant unit of analysis (this statement contradicts practically all of the twentieth century experimental psychology of learning).
- The individual is not a blank slate. Every individual enters a new learning situation with an existing set of capabilities ('repertoire' or 'signature') unique to her/him.
- In order to understand the nature of learning, these pre-existing capabilities need to be identified before the introduction of a novel task/new material. The reason is that they influence the way new skills are learned and remembered. As all good teachers know, 'you have to have hooks'.
- Learning, fundamentally, means the modification (expansion/elaboration) of pre-existing capabilities. It is not (or not only) a reinforcement/repetition/ associative process.
- New information (e.g. from task demands, the environment) either cooperates or competes with the existing capabilities (the current coordination

dynamics) of the learner. Cooperative and competitive mechanisms determine the rate of learning: fast for the former, slow for the latter.

- Learning is not necessarily a smooth gradual process. Rather, depending on the strength of cooperative and competitive mechanisms it may involve smooth shifts in parameter space (the shift route) or highly nonlinear, abrupt transitions ('Eureka!') – the bifurcation route.
- Remembering refers to the *stability* of learned states, a process that can be and has been precisely quantified. Notice, remembering is a process, memory is a thing.
- When the human brain is learning a skill, activity in local neural populations and the coordination among distant neural areas is dramatically reorganized. Moreover, the individual brain, after it has learned, is functioning far more economically than one that has not.
- The degree of brain plasticity (changes in the size and distribution of active regions in the cerebral cortex following learning) is remarkable, unexpected and warrants serious investigation in children *and* adults.

The above brief and incomplete list amounts to (at least a partial) re-evaluation of the psychological and neuronal basis of learning. The focus on individual pre-existing capabilities as constraints on the learning process and the need to structure the learning environment in light of them has significant consequences for education and educational policy, as well as implications for sports training, therapy and rehabilitation (e.g. in learning disabilities and recovery of function following stroke or brain disease).

Summary and conclusions

Most theories in cognitive psychology and cognitive neuroscience tend to view the mind in terms of fairly static representations. Symbolic representation, by definition, is discrete and time independent. Yet many perceptual and cognitive processes unfold in time. Indeed, in many processes – such as perceiving, learning, remembering, forgetting, decision-making and moving – time and timing are essential. Over the last few decades, a new foundation for understanding spatiotemporally organized behaviour on multiple levels has emerged, called coordination dynamics. Coordination dynamics is both a theory and a research programme. In its mature form, it contains two complementary conceptual themes. One concerns the cooperative and competitive mechanisms that give rise to the spontaneous formation of patterns and pattern change in complex cognitive and social systems. The other deals with how information is created *de novo* in such complex systems and how it modulates and is modulated by spontaneous, pattern forming processes.

Dynamics is the language of understanding and transcends levels bridging individual and collective processes. Dynamics, however, is not a panacea. In every case, dynamical tools must be filled with conceptual content. It is not enough to talk about the 'dynamical systems approach' to motor control, development, cognition, and so forth, without the crucial concepts and methods of self-organization, identifying meaningful pattern variables, and informational specificity in the form of parameters of the coordination dynamics. Although every system is different, what we learn about one may aid in understanding another. Indeed, such an approach led to the recognition of universality and mesoscopic protectorates in coordination dynamics.

Although the theoretical concepts of self-organizing dynamical systems now enjoy some popularity in the social, behavioural, cognitive and brain sciences, their usage is still quite restricted and still largely metaphorical – though times, it must be said, are changing. One reason for the inertia was that the tools are difficult to learn and require a degree of mathematical sophistication. Their implementation in real systems is nontrivial, requiring a different approach to experimentation and observation. Another reason is that coordination dynamics (and the dynamical perspective in general) are often cast (or cast themselves) in opposition to more conventional theoretical approaches, instead of as an aid to understanding. On a personal note, the author has been invited on many occasions over the years to write papers on 'programmes' versus 'dynamics'. Selforganizing dynamics tends to emphasize decentralization, collective decision making, spontaneous and cooperative behaviour among many interacting elements. Conventional cognitive psychology tends to focus on individual psychological processes such as intention, perception, attention, memory, action, and so on, as if they were clearly separable aspects of the goal-directed coordination of living things. Yet, as evidence and theory now show, processes that we associate with meaningful information such as intending, perceiving, attending, deciding and remembering – as well as spontaneous self-organizing processes – prove to be essential, coexisting aspects of the coordination dynamics of cognition. Representation and dynamics are complementary: two sides of the same coin.

Acknowledgements

Much of the research described herein was originally supported by NIMH (Neurosciences Research Branch) grants MH42900, MH01386 and the Human Frontier Sciences Program and, more recently, by grants from the National Institute of Mental Health (MH080838), the National Science Foundation (BCS0826897), the US Office of Naval Research (N000140510117) and the Chaire d'Excellence Pierre de Fermat. I am extremely grateful to all of these agencies for their support over many years and to my colleagues and students for their tireless work and freely given talents which are an inspiration.

References

Amazeen, P. G., Schmidt, R. C. and Turvey, M. T. (1995) Frequency detuning of the phase entrainment dynamics of visually coupled rhythmic movements. *Biological Cybernetics*, 72: 511–18.

Amazeen, E. L., Amazeen, P. G., Treffner, P. J. and Turvey, M. T. (1995) Attention and handedness in bimanual coordination dynamics. *Journal of Experimental Psychology: Human Perception and Performance*, 23: 1552–60.

Banerjee, A., Tognoli, E., Kelso, J. A. S. and Jirsa, V. K. (2012) Spatiotemporal reorganization of large-scale neural assemblies mediates bimanual coordination. *NeuroImage*, 62 (3): 1582–92.

Bardy, B. G., Marin, L., Stoffregen, T. A. and Boutsma, R. J. (1999) Postural coordination modes considered as emergent phenomena. *Journal of Experimental Psychology: Human Perception and Performance*, 25: 1284–96.

Bartlett, F. C. (1932) *Remembering: A Study in Experimental and Social Psychology*. New York: Cambridge University Press.

Beek, P. J., Peper, C. E. and Stegeman, D. F. (1995) Dynamical models of movement coordination. *Human Movement Science*, 14: 573–628.

Beekman, M., Sumpter, D. J. and Ratnieks, F. L. W. (2001) Phase transition between disordered and ordered foraging in pharaohs' ants. *Proceedings of the National Academy of Sciences of the United States of America*, 98 (17): 9703–6.

Bernstein, N. (1967) *The Coordination and Regulation of Movements*. Oxford: Pergamon.

Blekhman, I. I. (1988) *Synchronization in Science and Technology*. New York: ASME Press.

Bressler, S. L. and Kelso, J. A. S. (2001) Cortical coordination dynamics and cognition. *Trends in Cognitive Sciences*, 5: 26–36.

Buchanan, J. J. and Kelso, J. A. S. (1993) Posturally induced transitions in rhythmic multijoint limb movements. *Experimental Brain Research*, 94 (1): 131–42.

Buchanan, J. J. and Kelso, J. A. S. (1997) To switch or not to switch: recruitment of degrees of freedom stabilizes biological coordination, *Journal of Motor Behavior*, 31 (2): 126–44.

Buchanan, J. J., Kelso, J. A. S., DeGuzman, G. C. and Ding, M. (1997) The spontaneous recruitment and suppression of degrees of freedom in rhythmic hand movements. *Human Movement Science*, 16: 1–32.

Byblow, W. D., Chua, R. and Goodman, D. (1995) Asymmetries in coupling dynamics of perception and action, *Journal of Motor Behavior*, 27 (2): 123–37.

Carson, R. G. and Riek, S. (1998) The influence of joint position on the dynamics of perception-action coupling. *Experimental Brain Research*, 121: 103–14.

Carson, R. G., Goodman, D., Kelso, J. A. S. and Elliot, D. (1995) Phase transitions and critical fluctuations in rhythmic coordination of ipsilateral hand and foot. *Journal of Motor Behavior*, 27 (3): 211–24.

Carson, R. G., Chua, R., Byblow, W. D., Poon, P. and Smethurst, C. S. (1999) Changes in posture alter the attentional demands of voluntary movement. *Proceedings of the Royal Society of London B Biological Sciences*, 266: 853–7.

Chen, Y., Ding, M. and Kelso, J. A. S. (1997) Long term memory processes (1/f type) in human coordination. *Physics Review Letters*, 79: 4501–4.

Chen, Y., Ding, M. and Kelso, J. A. S. (1999) Alpha (10 Hz), Beta (20 Hz) and Gamma (40 Hz) networks in the human brain and their functions in a visuomotor coordination task revealed by MEG. *Society for Neuroscience*, 25: 1893.

Chen, Y., Ding, M. Z. and Kelso, J. A. S. (2001) Origins of human timing errors. *Journal of Motor Behavior*, 33: 3–8.

Chen, Y., Ding, M. and Kelso, J. A. S. (2003) Task-related power and coherence changes in neuromagnetic activity during visuomotor coordination. *Experimental Brain Research*, 148: 105–16.

Chialvo, D. (2010) Emergent complex neural dynamics. *Nature Physics*, 6: 744–50.

Churchland, P. M. (1988) *Matter and Consciousness*. Cambridge, MA: MIT Press.

Daffertshofer, A., Peper, C. E. and Beek, P. J. (2000) Power analysis of event-related encephalographic signals. *Physics Letters A*, 266: 290–302.

DeLuca, C., Jantzen, K. J., Comani, S., Bertollo, M. and Kelso, J. A. S. (2010) Striatal activity during intentional switching depends on pattern stability. *Journal of Neuroscience*, 30 (9): 3167–74.

Ding, M., Chen, Y. and Kelso, J. A. S. (2002) Statistical analysis of timing errors. *Brain and Cognition*, 48: 98–106.

Dijkstra, T. M. H., Schöner, G., Geise, M. A. and Gielen, C. C. A. M. (1994) Frequency-dependence of action-perception cycle for postural control in a moving visual room: relative phase dynamics. *Biological Cybernetics*. 71: 489–501.

Duarte, R., Araújo, D., Freire, L., Folgado, H., Fernandes, O. and Davids, K. (2012) Intra- and inter-group coordination patterns reveal collective behaviours of football players near the scoring zone. *Human Movement Science*, 31 (6): 1639–51.

Dumas, G., Nadel, J., Soussignan, R., Martinerie, J. and Garnero, L. (2010) Inter-brain synchronization during social interaction. *PloS One* 5 (8): e12166; doi:10.1371/journal.pone.0012166.

Edelman, G. M. (1987) *Neural Darwinism*. New York: Basic Books.

Fink, P., Kelso, J. A. S., Jirsa, V. K. and DeGuzman, G. C. (2000a) Recruitment of degrees of freedom stabilizes coordination. *Journal of Experimental Psychology: Human Perception and Performance*, 26: 671–92.

Fink, P. W., Kelso, J. A. S., Foo, P. and Jirsa, V. K. (2000b) Local and global stabilization of coordination by sensory information. *Experimental Brain Research*, 134: 9–20.

Fontaine, R. B., Lee, T. D. and Swinnen, S. P. (1997) Learning a new bimanual coordination pattern: Reciprocal influences of intrinsic and to-be-learned patterns. *Canadian Journal of Experimental Psychology*, 51 (1): 1–9.

Frank, T. D., Daffertshofer, A., Peper, C. E., Beek, P. J. and Haken, H. (2000) Towards a comprehensive theory of brain activity: Coupled oscillator systems under external forces. *Physica D*, 144: 62–86.

Freeman, W. J. (1975) *Mass Action in the Nervous System*. New York: Academic Press.

Friston, K. (2000) The labile brain. III. Transients and spatio-temporal receptive fields. *Philosophical Transactions of the Royal Society of London Series B, Biological Sciences*, 355 (1394): 253–65.

Fuchs, A. and Jirsa, V. K. (2001) The HKB model revisited: how varying the degree of symmetry controls dynamics. *Human Movement Science*, 19: 425–49.

Fuchs, A. and Kelso, J. A. S. (1994) A theoretical note on models of interlimb coordination. *Journal of Experimental Psychology: Human Perception and Performance*, 20 (5): 1088–97.

Fuchs, A. and Kelso, J. A. S. (2009) Movement coordination, in R. A. Meyers (ed.) *Encyclopedia of Complexity and System Science*, Heidelberg: Springer.

Fuchs, A., Kelso, J. A. S. and Haken, H. (1992) Phase transitions in the human brain: spatial mode dynamics. *International Journal of Bifurcation and Chaos*, 2: 917–39.

Fuchs, A. Mayville, J., Cheyne, D., Weinberg, H., Deecke, L. and Kelso, J. A. S. (2000a) Spatiotemporal analysis of neuromagnetic events underlying the emergence of coordinative instabilities. *NeuroImage*, 12: 71–84.

Fuchs, A., Deecke, L. and Kelso, J. A. S. (2000b) Phase transitions in the human brain revealed by large SQuID arrays. *Physics Letters A*, 266, 303–8.

Fuchs, A., Jirsa, V. K. and Kelso, J. A. S. (2000) Theory of the relation between human brain activity (MEG) and hand movements. *NeuroImage*, 11: 359–69.

Grafton, S. T., Hazeltine, E. and Ivry, R. B. (1998) Abstract and effector-specific representations of motor sequences identified with PET. *Journal of Neuroscience*, 18: 9420–8.

Green, H. S. (2000) *Information theory and Quantum Physics*. Berlin: Springer.

Haken, H. (1983) *Synergetics, an Introduction: Non-equilibrium Phase Transitions and Self-organization in Physics, Chemistry and Biology*. Berlin: Springer.

Haken, H. (1996) *Principles of Brain Functioning*. Berlin: Springer.

Haken, H., Kelso, J. A. S. and Bunz, H. (1985) A theoretical model of phase transitions in human hand movements. *Biological Cybernetics*, 51: 347–56.

Jantzen, K. J., Fuchs, A. Mayville, J. M. and Kelso, J. A. S. (2001) Neuromagnetic activity in alpha and beta bands reflects learning-induced increases in coordinative stability. *Clinical Neurophysiology*, 112: 1685–97.

Jantzen, K. J., Steinberg, F. L. and Kelso, J. A. S. (2002) Practice-dependent modulation of neural activity during human sensorimotor coordination: A Functional Magnetic Resonance Imaging study. *Neuroscience Letters*, 332: 205–9.

Jantzen, K. J., Oullier, O. and Kelso, J. A. S. (2008) Neuroimaging coordination dynamics in the sports sciences. *Methods*, 45: 325–35.

Jantzen, K. J., Steinberg, F. L. and Kelso, J. A. S. (2009) Coordination dynamics of large-scale neural circuitry underlying sensorimotor behavior. *Journal of Cognitive Neuroscience*, 21: 2420–33.

Jeka, J. J. and Kelso, J. A. S. (1995) Manipulating symmetry in the coordination dynamics of human movement. *Journal of Experimental Psychology Human Perception and Performance*. 21 (2): 360–74.

Jeka, J. J. and Lackner, J. R. (1994) Fingertip contact influences human postural control, *Experimental Brain Research*, 100 (3): 495–502.

Jirsa, V. K. and Haken, H. (1996) Field theory of electromagnetic brain activity. *Physical Review Letters*, 77: 960–3.

Jirsa, V. K. and Haken H. (1997) A derivation of a macroscopic field theory of the brain from the quasi-microscopic neural dynamics, *Physica D (Nonlinear Phenomena)*, 99: 503–26.

Jirsa, V. K. and Kelso, J. A. S. (2000) Spatiotemporal pattern formation in neural systems with heterogeneous connection topologies. *Physical Review E*, 62: 8462–5.

Jirsa, V. K., Fuchs, A. and Kelso, J. A. S. (1998) Neural field theory connecting cortical and behavioral dynamics: bimanual coordination. *Neural Computation*, 10: 2019–45.

Jirsa, V. K., Friedrich, R., Haken, H. and Kelso, J. A. S. (1994) A theoretical model of phase transitions in the human brain. *Biological Cybernetics*, 71: 27–35.

Jirsa, V. K., Fink, P. W., Foo, P. and Kelso, J. A. S. (2000) Parametric stabilization of biological coordination: A theoretical model. *Journal of Biological Physics*, 26: 85–112.

Kello, C. T., Brown, G. D. A., Ferrer-i-Cancho, R., Holden, J., Linkenkaer-Hansen, K., Rhodes, T. and Van Orden, G. C. (2010) Scaling laws in cognitive sciences. *Trends in Cognitive Sciences*, 14: 223–32.

Kelso, J. A. S. (1981) On the oscillatory basis of movement. *Bulletin of the Psychonomic Society*, 18: 63.

Kelso, J. A. S. (1984) Phase transitions and critical behavior in human bimanual coordination. *American Journal of Physiology: Regulatory, Integrative and Comparative*, 15: R1000–4.

Kelso, J. A. S. (1990) Phase transitions: Foundations of behaviour, in H. Haken (ed.) *Synergetics of Cognition*. Berlin: Springer, pp. 249–68.

Kelso, J. A. S. (1991) Behavioral and neural pattern generation: the concept of neurobehavioral dynamical system (NBDS), in H. P. Koepchen (ed.) *Cardiorespiratory and Motor Coordination*. Berlin: Springer, pp. 224–38.

Kelso, J. A. S. (1992) Theoretical concepts and strategies for understanding perceptual-motor skill: from information capacity in closed systems to self-organization in open, nonequilibrium systems. *Journal of Experimental Psychology General*, 121 (3): 260–1.

Kelso, J. A. S. (1994a) Elementary coordination dynamics, in S. Swinnen, H. Heuer, J. Massion and P. Casaer (eds) *Interlimb Coordination: Neural, Dynamical and Cognitive Constraints*. Academic Press: San Diego, pp. 301–18.

Kelso, J. A. S. (1994b) The informational character of self-organized coordination dynamics. *Human Movement Science*, 13: 393–413.

Kelso, J. A. S. (1995) *Dynamic Patterns: The Self Organization of Brain and Behavior*. Cambridge: MIT Press.

Kelso, J. A. S. (1997) Relative timing in brain and behavior: Some observations about the generalized motor program and self-organized coordination dynamics. *Human Movement Science*, 16: 453–60.

Kelso, J. A. S. (2000) Principles of dynamic pattern formation and change for a science of human behaviour, in L. R. Bergman, R. B. Cairns, L.-G. Nilsson, L. and Nystedt, *Developmental Science and the Holistic Approach*. Mahwah, NJ: Erlbaum, pp. 63–83.

Kelso. J.A.S. (2001) Metastable coordination dynamics of brain and behavior. *Brain and Neural Networks (Japan)* 8: 125–30.

Kelso, J. A. S. (2002) The complementary nature of coordination dynamics: self-organization and the origins of agency. *Journal of Nonlinear Phenomena in Complex Systems*, 5: 364–71.

Kelso, J. A. S. (2008) An essay on understanding the mind. *Ecological Psychology*, 20: 180–208.

Kelso, J. A. S. (2009a) Coordination dynamics, in R.A. Meyers (ed.) *Encyclopedia of Complexity and System Science*. Heidelberg: Springer, pp. 1537–64.

Kelso, J. A. S. (2009b) Synergies: Atoms of brain and behavior. *Advances in Experimental Medicine and Biology*, 629: 83–91.

Kelso, J. A. S. (2010). Instabilities and phase transitions in human brain and behavior. *Frontiers in Human Neuroscience,* 4: 23. doi:10.3389/fnhum.2010.00023

Kelso, J. A. S. (2012a) Multistability and metastability: Understanding dynamic coordination in the brain. *Philosophical Transactions of the Royal Society B Biological Sciences*, 367: 906–18.

Kelso, J. A. S. (2012b) Criticality reveals emergence ('mesoscopic protectorates') in neural and behavioral systems, in *Criticality in the Nervous System*, D. Plenz and E. Niebur (eds). Bethesda, MD: National Institutes of Health.

Kelso, J.A.S. and Engstrom, D. A. (2006) *The Complementary Nature*. Cambridge, MA: MIT Press.

Kelso J. A. S. and Jeka, J. J. (1992) Symmetry breaking dynamics of human multilimb coordination. *Journal of Experimental Psychology: Human Perception and Performance*, 18 (3): 645–68.

Kelso, J. A. S. and Tognoli, E. (2007) Toward a complementary neuroscience: metastable coordination dynamics of the brain, in R. Kozma and L. Perlovsky (eds) *Neurodynamics of Cognition and Consciousness*. Heidelberg: Springer, pp. 39–60.

Kelso, J. A. S. and Zanone, P. G. (2002) Coordination dynamics of learning and generalization across different effector systems. *Journal of Experimental Psychology: Human Perception and Performance*, 28: 776–97.

Kelso, J. A. S., Southard, D. and Goodman, D. (1979) On the nature of human interlimb coordination. *Science*, 203: 1029–31.

Kelso, J. A. S., Scholz, J.P. and Schöner, G. (1986) Non-equilibrium phase transitions in coordinated biological motion: Critical fluctuations. *Physics Letters A*, 118: 279–84.

Kelso, J. A. S., Scholz, J. P. and Schöner, G. (1988) Dynamics governs switching among patterns of coordination in biological movement. *Physics Letters A*, 134: 8–12.

Kelso, J. A. S., DelColle, J. and Schöner, G. (1990) Action perception as a pattern formation process, in M. Jeanerod (ed.) *Attention and Performance XIII*. Hillsdale, NJ: Erlbaum, pp. 139–69.

Kelso, J. A. S., Buchanan, J. J. and Wallace, S. A. (1991) Order parameters for the neural organization of single, multijoint limb movement patterns. *Experimental Brain Research*, 85: 432–44.

Kelso, J. A. S., Bressler, S. L., Buchanan, S., DeGuzman, G. C., Ding, M., Fuchs, A. and Holroyd, T. (1992) A phase transition in human brain and behavior. *Physics Letters A*, 169: 134–44.

Kelso, J. A. S., Buchanan, J. J., DeGuzman, G. C. and Ding, M. (1993) Spontaneous recruitment and annihilation of degrees of freedom in biological coordination. *Physics Letters A*, 179: 364–8.

Kelso, J. A. S., Fuchs, A., Holroyd, T., Lancaster, R., Cheyne, D. and Weinberg, H. (1998) Dynamic cortical activity in the human brain reveals motor equivalence. *Nature*, 392: 814–18.

Kelso, J. A. S., Fuchs, A. and Jirsa, V. K. (1999) Traversing scales of brain and behavioral organization. I–III, in C. Uhl (ed.) *Analysis of Neurophysiological Brain Functioning*. Berlin: Springer, pp. 73–125.

Kelso, J. A. S., Fink, P., DeLaplain, C. R. and Carson, R. G. (2001) Haptic information stabilizes and destabilizes coordination dynamics. *Proceedings of the Royal Society of London B: biological Sciences*, 268: 1207–13.

Kelso, J. A. S., DeGuzman, G. C., Reveley, C. and Tognoli, E. (2009) Virtual partner interaction (VPI): exploring novel behaviors via coordination dynamics. *PLoS ONE*, 4 (6): e5749; doi: 10.1371/journal.pone.0005749

Kostrubiec, V., Zanone, P.-G., Fuchs, A. and Kelso, J. A. S. (2012) Beyond the blank slate: routes to learning new coordination patterns depend on the intrinsic dynamics of the learner: experimental evidence and theoretical model. *Frontiers in Human Neuroscience*, 6: 222.

Kovacs, A. J., Buchanan, J. J. and Shea, C. H. (2010) Impossible is nothing: 5:3 and 4:3 multi-frequency bimanual coordination. *Experimental Brain Research*, 201: 249–59.

Lagarde, J. and Kelso, J. A. S. (2006) Binding of movement, sound and touch: multimodal coordination dynamics. *Experimental Brain Research*, 173: 673–88.

Lagarde, J., Peham, C., Licke, T. and Kelso, J. A. S. (2005) Coordination dynamics of the horse–rider system. *Journal of Motor Behavior*, 37: 419–24.

Laughlin, R. B. and Pines, D. (2000) The theory of everything. *Proceedings of the National Academy of Sciences of the USA*, 97: 28–31.

Lee, T. D., Blandin, Y. and Proteau, L. (1996) Effects of task instruction and oscillation frequency on bimanual coordination. *Psychological Research*, 59: 100–6.

Magne, C. and Kelso, J. A. S. (2008) A dynamical framework for human skill learning. *Advances in Psychology*, 139: 189–203.

Marr, D. (1982) *Vision*. San Francisco: Freeman.

Mayville, J. M., Bressler, S. L., Fuchs, A. and Kelso, J. A. S. (1999) Spatiotemporal reorganization of electrical activity in the human brain associated with a phase transition in rhythmic auditory-motor coordination. *Experimental Brain Research*, 127: 371–81.

Mayville, J. M., Fuchs, A., Ding, M., Cheyne, D., Deecke, L. and Kelso, J. A. S. (2001) Event-related changes in neuromagnetic activity associated with syncopation and synchronization tasks. *Human Brain Mapping*, 14: 65–80.

Mechsner, F., Kerzel, D., Knoblich, G. and Prinz, W. (2001) Perceptual basis of bimanual coordination, *Nature*, 414: 69–73.

Meyer-Lindenberg, A., Zieman, U., Hajak, G., Cohen, L. and Faith Berman, K. (2002) Transition between dynamical states of differing stability in the human brain. *Proceedings of the National Academy of Sciences of the USA*, 99: 10948–53.

Naeem, M., Prasad, G., Watson, D. R. and Kelso, J. A. S. (2012) Electrophysiological signatures of intentional social coordination in the 10–12Hz range. *NeuroImage* 59: 1795–803.

Nicolis, G. and Prigogine, I. (1977) *Self-organization in Nonequilibrium Systems*. New York: Wiley.

Oullier, O. and Kelso, J. A. S. (2009) Social coordination from the perspective of coordination dynamics, in R. A. Meyers (ed.) *Encyclopedia of Complexity and Systems Science*, Heidelberg: Springer, pp. 8198–212.

Oullier, O., DeGuzman, G. C., Jantzen, K. J., Lagarde, J. and Kelso, J. A. S. (2008) Social coordination dynamics: measuring human bonding. *Social Neuroscience*, 3: 178–92.

Passos, P., Araújo, D., Davids, K., Gouveia, L., Milho, J. and Serpa, S. (2008) Information-governing dynamics of attacker–defender interactions in youth rugby union. *Journal of Sports Sciences*, 26 (13): 1421–9.

Peper, C. E., Beek, P. and van Wieringen P. C. (1995) Frequency-induced phase transitions in bimanual tapping. *Biological Cybernetics*, 73 (4): 301–9.

Plenz, D. and Thiagarian, T. (2007) The organizing principles of neuronal avalanche activity: cell assemblies and cortex. *Trends in Neurosciences*, 30: 101–10.

Riley, M. A., Richardson, M. C., Shockley, K. and Ramenzoni, V. C. (2011) Interpersonal synergies. *Frontiers in Psychology (Movement Science and Sports Psychology)*, 2: 38; doi: 10.3389/fpsyg.2011.00038

Salter, J, Wishart, L. R., Lee, T. D. and Simon, D. (2004) The perceptual and motor basis for bimanual coordination. *Neuroscience Letters*, 363: 102–7.

Schmidt, R. A. (1975) A schema theory of discrete motor skill learning. *Psychological Review*, 82: 225–60.

Schmidt, R.A. and Lee, T. D. (1998) *Motor Control and Learning: A Behavioral Emphasis* (3rd ed.). Champaign IL: Human Kinetics.

Schmidt, R. C., Carello, C. and Turvey, M. T. (1990) Phase transitions and critical fluctuations in the visual coordination of rhythmic movements between people. *Journal of Experimental Psychology Human Perception and Performance*, 16 (2): 227–47.

Scholz, J. P. and Kelso, J. A. S. (1990) Intentional switching between patterns of bimanual coordination depends on the intrinsic dynamics of the patterns. *Journal of Motor Behaviour,* 22 (1): 98–124.

Schöner, G. and Kelso, J. A. S. (1988) Dynamic pattern generation in behavioral and neural systems. *Science*, 239: 1513–20.

Schöner, G., Haken, H., Kelso, J. A. S. (1986) A stochastic theory of phase transitions in human hand movement. *Biological Cybernetics*, 53: 442–52.

Schöner, G., Jiang, W. Y. and Kelso, J. A. S. (1990) A synergetic theory of quadrupedal gaits and gait transitions. *Journal of Theoretical Biology*, 142: 359–91.

Schöner, G., Zanone, P. G. and Kelso, J. A. S. (1992) Learning as change of coordination dynamics: theory and experiment. *Journal of Motor Behavior*, 24: 29–48.

Shannon, C. E. and Weaver, W. (1949) *A Mathematical Model of Communication*. Urbana, IL: University of Illinois Press.

Sporns, O. and Edelman, G. M. (1993) Solving Bernstein's problem: a proposal for the development of coordinated movement by selection. *Child Development*, 64: 960–81.

Sternad, D., Collins, D. and Turvey, M. T. (1995) The detuning factor in the dynamics of interlimb rhythmic coordination. *Biological Cybernetics*, 73: 27–35.

Sternad, D., Amazeen, E. L. and Turvey, M. T. (1996) Diffusive, synaptic and synergetic coupling: an evaluation through in-phase and antiphase rhythmic movements, *Journal of Motor Behavior*, 28 (3): 255–69.

Stins, J. F. and Michaels, C. F. (1999) Strategy differences in oscillatory tracking: stimulus–hand versus stimulus–manipulandum coupling. *Journal of Experimental Psychology: Human Perception and Performance*, 25: 1793–812.

Swinnen, S. P. (2002) Intermanual crosstalk: From behavioural models to neural-network interactions. *Nature Neuroscience*, 3: 350–61.

Swinnen, S. P. and Wenderoth, N. (2004) Two hands, one brain: cognitive neuroscience of bimanual skill. *Trends in Cognitive Sciences*, 8: 18–25.

Swinnen, S. P., Lee,T. D., Verschueren, S., Serrien, D. J. and Bogaerds, H. (1997) Interlimb coordination: learning and transfer under different feedback conditions. *Human Movement Science*, 16 (6): 749–85.

Temprado, J. J., Zanone, P. G., Monno, A. and Laurent, M. (1999) Attentional load associated with performing and stabilizing preferred bimanual patterns. *Journal of Experimental Psychology: Human Perception and Performance*, 25: 1595–608.

Tognoli, E. and Kelso, J. A. S. (2009) Brain coordination dynamics: true and false faces of phase synchrony and metastability. *Progress in Neurobiology*, 87: 31–40.

Tognoli, E., Lagarde, J., DeGuzman, G. C. and Kelso, J. A. S. (2007) The phi complex as a neuromarker of human social coordination. *Proceedings of the National Academy of Sciences*, 104: 8190–5 [from the cover; see also *Scientific American Mind*, August, 2007].

Treffner, P. J. and Turvey, M. T. (1996) Symmetry, broken symmetry and handedness in bimanual coordination dynamics. *Experimental Brain Research*, 107 (3): 463–78.

Tuller, B., Ding, M. and Kelso, J. A. S. (1997) Fractal timing of phonemic transforms. *Perception*, 26: 913–28.

Turvey, M. T. and Carello, C. (2012) On intelligence from first principles: guidelines for inquiry into the hypothesis of physical intelligence (PI). *Ecological Psychology*, 24: 3–32.

Turvey, M. T., Shaw, R. E. and Mace, W. M. (1978) Issues in the theory of action: degrees of freedom, coordinative structures and coalitions, in J. Requin (ed.) *Attention and Performance VII*. Hillsdale, NJ: Erlbaum, pp. 557–95.

Uhl, C., Friedrich, R. and Haken, H. (1995) Analysis of spatiotemporal signals of complex systems. *Physical review E, Statistical Physics, Plasmas, Fluids and Related Interdisciplinary Topics*, 51 (5): 3890–900.

Ullen, F., Ehrsson, H. H. and Forssberg, H. (2000) Brain areas activated during bimanual tapping of different rhythmical patterns in humans. *Society for Neuroscience Abstracts*, 26: 458.

van Orden, G. C., Holden, J. G. and Turvey, M. T. (2005) Human cognition and 1/f scaling. *Journal of Experimental Psychology General*, 134 (1): 117–23.

Wade, J. J., McDaid, L. J., Harkin, J. G., Crunelli, V. and Kelso, J. A. S. (2011) Bidirectional coupling between astrocytes and neurons mediates learning and dynamic coordination in the brain: a multiple modeling approach. *PLoS ONE*, 6: e29445; doi:10.1371/journal.pone.0029445

Wallenstein, G. V., Kelso, J. A. S. and Bressler, S. L. (1995) Phase transitions in spatiotemporal patterns of brain activity and behavior. *Physica D*, 84, 626–34.

Wimmers, R. H., Beek, P. J. and van Wieringen, P. C. W. (1992) Phase transitions in rhythmic tracking movements: a case of unilateral coupling. *Human Movement Science*, 11: 217–26.

Zanone, P. G. and Kelso, J. A. S. (1992) The evolution of behavioral attractors with learning: Nonequilibrium phase transitions. *Journal of Experimental Psychology: Human Perception and Performance*, 18/2: 403–21.

Zanone, P.G. and Kelso, J. A. S. (1994) The coordination dynamics of learning: theoretical structure and experimental agenda, in S. P. Swinnen, H. Heuer, J. Massion and P. Casaer (eds) *Interlimb Coordination: Neural, Dynamical and Cognitive Constraints*. San Diego. CA: Academic Press, pp. 461–90.

Zanone, P. G. and Kelso, J. A. S. (1997) The coordination dynamics of learning and transfer: collective and component levels. *Journal of Experimental Psychology: Human Perception and Performance*, 23: 1454–80.

Zanone, P. G. and Kostrubiec, V. (2004) Searching for (dynamic) principles of learning, in V. Jirsa and J. A. S. Kelso (eds) *Coordination Dynamics: Issues and Trends*. Berlin: Springer, pp. 57–89.

3 Why coordination dynamics is relevant for studying sport performance

Chris Button, Jon Wheat and Peter Lamb

The role of coordination dynamics in understanding movement behaviour in sport is focused on identifying key parameters that describe system organization (order parameters), as well as variables that act as information to constrain the way that systems adapt to key environmental objects and events (control parameters). Coordination dynamics has been used to study human movement behaviour over the past three decades and more recently it has been applied to the study of performance in team games. This chapter reviews and summarizes current research in this area.

Sports performers coordinate their actions in many different ways to achieve their goals. Coordination is a universal feature of sport common to the graceful, precise actions of an ice dancer through to the explosive, physical power of a shot putter. When watching elite sport performers, their coordination patterns simultaneously entertain us and also remind us of the incredible dexterity of the human body. Coordination dynamics offers a new and potentially valuable lens through which our understanding of sports performance can be developed. Indeed, movement scientists are only just beginning to appreciate the complex, coalition of constraints that engulfs and enables a sports performer. In this chapter, we explain what coordination dynamics represents, with recourse to research that has applied a dynamical systems approach to human movement behaviour. We then discuss why coordination dynamics are relevant for sports performance in relation to optimization, adaptation to constraints and rehabilitation from injury and learning.

In writing this chapter, we conducted a critical review of relevant literature before developing some practical implications based on this information. Combining general search terms including 'coordination dynamics', 'sport performance' and 'movement' in several online search engines (ProQuest Central [3,438], SportsDiscus [2,617] and Science Direct [2,582]) it was possible to identify a relatively large body of literature. In fact, using the same search terms, the open access search engine, Google Scholar, returned a staggering over 25,000 research citations (admittedly not all quality-assured outputs). A high percentage of this body of research appears to have been published since 2000; for instance, in the case of ProQuest Central, this proportion was 93%. Clearly, a significant amount of research using the term 'coordination dynamics' has been published in the new millennium, reflecting the growing interest in this topic. Incidentally, ScienceDirect lists the most-cited article statistics of this body of literature, identifying an impressive 78 citations for the coordination dynamics review article of Davids *et al.* (2003), with most other articles being cited less than 30 times.

To explain why coordination dynamics is relevant for studying movement underlying sport performance, one must first describe the challenges that this field of study has historically faced. In the field of skill acquisition, scientists spent most of the twentieth century preoccupied with addressing theoretically driven issues in laboratory controlled environments with applied sport research very much on the fringes (Williams and Ford 2009). Simple, closed tasks have proven to be popular vehicles through which to test specific theoretical predictions. Admittedly, limitations in technology and restrictions in relation to athlete tracking in competition have curtailed the extent to which movement analysis could be conducted in naturalistic sports environments.

Human movement scientists have been typically inclined to adopt a reductionist (or positivist) philosophy in terms of analyzing sport performance from the relative comfort of their laboratories. Notational analysis of video footage is an excellent example of how the scientific method has permeated sport performance research (Glazier 2010). It is likely that the underlying assumption that sport performance can be optimized for a given set of constraints perpetuates this traditional philosophy (Brisson and Alain 1996; Glazier and Davids 2009). However, in setting out to identify the best way to move, scientists have conveniently put to one side the more fundamental issue of understanding how people move. Glazier and Davids (2010) suggest that sports biomechanists working to optimize human movement need to reconceptualize the athlete as a nonlinear, stochastic, biological system.

Important issues such as these have meant that the subdisciplines of biomechanics and motor control have historically rested in the shadows of their more prominent, peer disciplines (i.e. physiology and psychology) when it comes to supporting sports performance (Williams and Hodges 2005). However, Button and Farrow (2012) point out that skill acquisition has made considerable strides in recent times with notable developments in research techniques, theory, practical implications and technology. Indeed, increasing recognition of the importance of experimental design that is representative of the context to which the results are to be generalized has demonstrated that sport can provide an excellent vehicle for the progression of theory (Davids *et al.* 2006; Pinder *et al.* 2011). As we aim to demonstrate in this chapter, the advent of coordination dynamics may herald a new era in sports performance research.

What is coordination dynamics?

Defined broadly as the science of coordination (Kelso 2009), coordination dynamics can describe, explain and predict the patterns of coordination that form, adapt, persist and dissolve in complex systems. Using nonlinear structural equations to model behaviour, scientists have demonstrated how seemingly complex, disordered systems adhere to simple, elegant principles. Mutual information exchange between system components is required for the system to organize itself. The field of coordination dynamics is founded upon several important concepts which merit further discussion here, namely synergies, self-organization, collective variables and control parameters, and metastability.

Synergies

Synergies are functional groupings of components which are temporarily assembled as a single unit. Synergies reflect nature's propensity for animate objects to reduce their organizational complexity. For example, brain synergies can be identified in the presence of a perturbation to one part of the synergy (or network) and the subsequent reorganization of putatively linked brain areas (Jantzen *et al.* 2008). Bernstein (1967) recognized the existence of synergies in all forms of human movement, preferring the term 'coordinative structure' in explaining how humans solve the degrees of freedom problem. That being said, given the complexity of the movement system, how can the human movement system arrive at a single solution for a task, given the infinite possible solutions?

Self-organization

Complex systems have many independent parts which communicate in different ways but primarily in terms of information exchange. Such systems have a tendency to form patterned behaviour (synergies) which is not prescribed externally nor indeed controlled by a central manager. Instead, behaviours are said to spontaneously organize at a macroscopic level as a result of the microscopic fluctuations of individual components. Whilst sports teams are influenced to varying extents by the instructions of key figures such as a coach or captain, the spatiotemporal trajectories of each player can be thought of as a product of self-organization (Duarte *et al.* 2012a).

Collective variables and control parameters

Coordination dynamics is expressed through the interrelated behaviour of collective variables and control parameters. Collective variables are high-order, relational properties that capture or characterize the system at different levels of analysis. As we shall discover in the next section, the relative phase between two oscillating components (e.g. legs in gait) has been a popular choice for a collective variable. Control parameters are naturally occurring environmental conditions or intrinsic factors that can move the system through its repertoire of patterns. For example, the gradient of a hill or an intention to run can qualitatively change the value of the collective variable (i.e. interlimb phasing), resulting in a phase transition to a new stable state. Hence, control parameters act to influence the macroscopic (self-)organization of a system which result from the collective variables that characterize the microscopic levels. The reciprocity of this nested relationship allows the system to settle in stable states, while still adapting functionally to external factors when required.

Metastability

Complex systems are typically composed of multiple stable states. Consequently, they exhibit periods of stability and instability, as they transit between them in response to changing control parameter dynamics. A particularly important property arises when pre-existing stable states dissolve (i.e. bifurcations) to create remnants or 'ghosts' of these stable states. In a metastable performance region, one or several movement patterns are weakly stable (when there are multiple attractors) or weakly unstable (when there are only attractor remnants) and switching between two or more movement patterns occurs according to interacting constraints. A metastable system can simultaneously realize a number of different competing patterns and thus has the potential to exhibit novel and independent solutions (i.e. creativity) as well as stable, coordinated behaviour. The neural dynamics of the brain capitalize upon the metastability of the system, to flexibly reorganize thoughts, memories and intentions on a moment-to-moment basis. This allows appropriate online guidance of our actions.

Particular impetus to the field of coordination dynamics has been provided by studies of bimanual coordination in identifying the role of key constructs of self-organization, collective variables and control parameters, as well as transitions between stable states of neurobiological organization (see Kelso 1984; Schöner and Kelso 1988). The construction and adaptation of movement patterns has been successfully modelled and investigated by means of synergetic theoretical concepts since Haken, Kelso and Bunz (HKB; 1985) applied them in investigations of brain and behaviour. In their pioneering HKB model and its subsequent development (e.g. Schöner *et al.* 1986), abrupt changes in bimanual and multi-limb oscillatory movement patterns (Jeka and Kelso 1995) were explained by a 'loss of stability' mechanism, which produced spontaneous phase transitions from less stable to more stable states of motor organization with changes in critical control parameters.

Together, these theoretical and empirical advances have provided a sound rationale for a coordination dynamics-based explanation of how processes of perception, cognition, decision making and action underpin intentional movement behaviours in dynamic environments (e.g. van Orden *et al.* 2003). This framework proposes that the most relevant information for decision making and regulating action in dynamic environments is emergent during performer–environment interactions.

Traditional investigations of limited-degree-freedom actions have provided some useful models for understanding how control systems may operate during neurobiological action. But they have shed fewer insights on understanding how many biomechanical degrees of freedom are managed in complex actions prevalent in dynamic performance environments common to sport (Davids *et al.* 2006). Although many initial studies of coordination dynamics tended to favour analysis of actions involving a limited number of degrees of freedom, over multi-articular movement patterns (for a review of that body of work see Davids *et al.* 1999), investigation of complex multi-articular movements has proceeded rapidly in the last two decades (see for example: Chen *et al.* 2005 on learning a pedalo task; Forner-Cordero *et al.* 2007 on postural control). Interesting issues in neurobiological coordination and control concern the specific order parameter/collective variable dynamics that have been studied in this body of work and how coordination training shapes its manifestation over time.

How has coordination dynamics been analyzed in movement science?

Coordination dynamics have been studied in the movement sciences at several scales of analysis. These scales range from the study of intralimb coordination to examine interactions between players in sports. Various methods and techniques have been used to analyze coordination dynamics at these different scales. In addition to providing a brief account of the details of the methods and techniques in this section, pertinent issues related to their application in different contexts are highlighted.

Cross-correlations

Similar to commonly used correlation techniques such as Pearson's product-moment, cross-correlations assume that a linear relationship exists between the two time series under analysis – for example hip and knee flexion–extension angles during gait. However, unlike other correlation techniques, cross-correlations do not assume that the variables change in synchrony during motion (Mullineaux *et al.* 2001). Rather, by time shifting one relative to the other, the 'time lag' at which the correlation between two time series is greatest can be identified. As such, in addition to identifying the strength of the relationship or degree of linkage between the time series, cross-correlation analyses reveal the type of relationship (the degree to which the time series are in-phase or anti-phase). Indeed, if expressed relative to the period of the motion, the time lag associated with the greatest correlation coefficient indicates the phase relationship between the two segments (Temprado *et al.* 1997) and is analogous to the measure of discrete relative phase – discussed later in this section.

As Mullineaux *et al.* (2001) highlighted, cross-correlations have been suggested as being particularly suited to the study of human movement, as the coordinated actions of body segments and joints are often time shifted relative to each other. However, several issues need to be considered before conducting cross-correlation analyses in the study of coordination dynamics. Firstly, cross-correlations are not suited to the analysis of two-time series that have a non-linear relationship (Sidaway *et al.* 1995). It is prudent that cross-correlations are interpreted alongside more qualitative indications of the relationship between the time series, such as variable–variable plots (known as angle–angle plots if the time series concerns body segment/joint angles). Secondly, as Pohl and Buckley (2008) highlighted in their study of foot and shank motion during running, cross-correlation techniques provide information about only the temporal similarity of, but not the ratio of the coupling between, two time series. In other words, cross-correlation techniques do not take account of excursion magnitudes (Pohl and Buckley 2008). Thirdly, there is disagreement regarding the recommended maximum number of time lags that should be applied when estimating cross-correlations. Mullineaux *et al.* (2001) highlighted that the probability of type-I statistical errors inflates with an increasing number of lags. To reduce the risk of a type-I error, they cited a recommendation that a maximum of plus or minus seven lags be used. Alternatively, as a general rule, Derrick and Thomas (2004) recommended a maximum time lag of $n/2$ (where n is the number data points in the time series) but acknowledge that factors specific to the time series under investigation should be considered when defining a maximum number of time lags. A final point to consider before using cross-correlations in the study of coordination dynamics is that they provide only one, discrete, measure of coordination per movement cycle.

Vector coding

Angle–angle diagrams provide a convenient means for qualitatively analyzing coordination dynamics. The shape of the angle–angle trace reveals important information about the interaction and coupling between the body joint/segment angles of interest. Several techniques have been developed to provide a quantitative measure of the shape of the angle–angle trace; the techniques are collectively referred to here as vector coding methods.

An early vector coding technique was presented by Freeman (1961). By superimposing a grid on to the angle–angle curve and defining an eight-element direction convention, a chain of integers (0–7) is established to represent the shape of the curve. Although the integer chains capture the shape of the trace and this technique has been used to study human movement (e.g. Hershler and Milner 1980; Whiting and Zernicke 1982), a limitation of the approach is that ratio data (joint/segment angles) are reduced to the nominal scale (Tepevac and Field-Fote 2001). More recent vector coding methods have addressed this issue. Hamill *et al.* (2000) reported a modification of a technique presented by Sparrow *et al.* (1987), in which the shape of the angle–angle trace is quantified by calculating a 'coupling angle'; the angle formed by the vector connecting two adjacent data points on an angle–angle trace and the right horizontal.

The coupling angle provides information about the shape of the angle–angle trace and the interaction/coupling between body segments. Figure 3.1 illustrates how coupling angles can be interpreted. Coupling angles of 0° and 180° indicate movement solely in the body segment/joint angle represented on the x axis of the angle–angle diagram – where 0° indicates positive and 180° indicates negative, angular motion. Similarly, coupling angles of 90° and 270° indicates movement solely in the body/segment angle represented on the y axis of the angle–angle

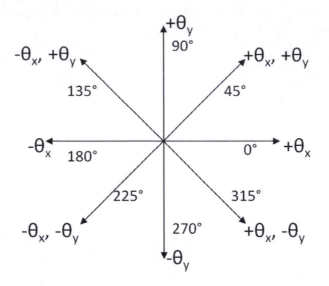

Figure 3.1 The interpretation of coupling angles; arrows represent the direction of a vector connecting data points on an angle-angle diagram

diagram (90° indicates positive and 270° indicates negative, angular motion). Coupling angles of 45° and 225° indicate that both body segment/joints are moving at the same rate in the same direction (in-phase). Finally, coupling angles of 135° and 315° indicate that the body segments/joints are moving at the same rate but in opposite directions (anti-phase).

Coupling angles have been used to analyze coordination in a variety of contexts. For example, Wilson *et al.* (2009) used vector coding methods to determine the degree to which specific training drills represented lower-extremity coordination patterns seen during triple jumping. Also, many studies have used coupling angles to investigate coordination in gait (e.g. Pohl and Buckley 2008; Ferber *et al.* 2005; Ong *et al.* 2011; Chang *et al.* 2008). For example, Ferber *et al.* (2005) investigated the effect of foot orthotics on the coupling between the rearfoot and tibia during running. In many studies, interpretations of coupling angles regarding coordination are made directly using the approach outlined in Figure 3.1. However, it is rare for coupling angles to be exactly equal to those highlighted in Figure 3.1, making interpretation more complex. Recently, Chang *et al.* (2008) introduced an approach to aid the interpretation of coordination, whereby the range of possible coupling angles (0–360°) represented in Figure 3.1 is split into four quadrants. The quadrant within which a particular coupling angle lies is used to categorize coordination patterns and indicate the type of coordination present (Table 3.1).

Table 3.1 Categories of coordination and their associated coupling angle (γ) ranges; *x*-axis phase and *y*-axis phase denote the phases in which movement is predominantly associated with the joint/segment rotations represented on the on the *x* and *y* axis of the angle–angle diagram, respectively

Type of coordination	Coupling angle ranges
Anti-phase	$112.5° \leq \gamma < 157.5°$, $292.5° \leq \gamma < 337.5°$
In-phase	$22.5° \leq \gamma < 67.5°$, $202.5° \leq \gamma < 247.5°$
x-axis phase	$0° \leq \gamma < 22.5°$, $157.5° \leq \gamma < 202.5°$, $337.5° \leq \gamma < 360°$
y-axis phase	$67.5° \leq \gamma < 112.5°$, $247.5° \leq \gamma < 292.5°$

Source: adapted from Chang *et al.* (2008)

Vector coding techniques have the advantage that they are more intuitive and easier to relate to than more complex techniques such as relative phase (Field-Fote and Tepavac 2002). However, it is important to note that the most commonly used vector coding methods involve calculating a coupling angle, which is a circular variable, requiring directional statistics to be used when further analysing the data (Batschelet 1981).

Relative phase

Coordination dynamics have also been investigated by calculating the relative phase between oscillating system components. Both discrete relative phase (DRP) and continuous relative phase (CRP) methods have been used. DRP estimates the latency of the motion of one system component relative to another (Kelso 1995). It is calculated by estimating the time difference between an event common to both system components, relative to the period of oscillation. For example, where the system components of interest are joint angles, the common event might be the time at which the maximum joint angles occur and the period would be the time to complete a joint rotation cycle. DRP has been used to investigate the coordination between, for example, respiration and stride rate during gait (O'Halloran *et al.* 2012), pelvis and thorax rotations during treadmill walking (Lamoth *et al.* 2002) and upper-arm segments during field hockey drives (Brétigny *et al.* 2011). DRP is simple to calculate and, generally, does not require data normalization (Hamill *et al.* 2000; Wheat and Glazier 2006; Krasovsky and Levin 2010). However, similar to the coupling angle, DRP is a circular variable and should be analyzed using directional statistics (Batschelet 1981). Finally, a disadvantage of DRP is that it provides only one measurement of coordination per movement cycle.

A continuous measure of relative phase has also been used in the study of coordination dynamics: CRP. CRP indicates the phase relation between two oscillating system components at each time point of a cycle of movement. Based on phase plane plots – a plot of velocity against position – phase angles are calculated by obtaining the arctangent of the ratio between velocity and position. In other words, the angles between vectors connecting the origin and each data point on the phase plane and the right horizontal identify phase angles time series for each system component. The CRP between two system components is then calculated as the difference between their phase angles ($0°$ represents in-phase and $180°$ represents anti-phase coupling).

In addition to providing a continuous measure of coordination, as velocity is included in the calculation of phase angles, CRP offers the potential for a rich and more detailed analysis of coordination (Hamill *et al.* 1999). Many studies have used CRP to study coordination dynamics. For example, Silfies *et al.* (2009) used CRP to investigate differences in movement strategies during reaching in participants with and without lower-back pain. Irwin and Kerwin (2007) used CRP to identify effective skill progressions for developing the long swing on the high bar in men's gymnastics. Also, numerous studies have used CRP in the study of bimanual coordination and nonlinear phase transitions originating from the seminal studies of Kelso *et al.* (1981, 1984). In addition to studying intra- and intersegmental coordination, CRP has also been used on a macro scale to investigate interactions between players in sports such as squash (McGarry *et al.* 1999) and tennis (Palut and Zanone 2005).

There are important factors to consider before CRP is used. First, position and velocity data used in the calculation of phase angles can require normalization and the resulting CRP values vary dependent on the normalization used – see Peters *et al.* (2003) for more information. Related to this, an assumption of CRP is that the time series used in the calculation are sinusoidal. Data that violate the sinusoidal assumption can make interpretation of CRP difficult (Peters *et al.* 2003). Alternative methods have been developed to address this limitation, including those based on the Hilbert transform (Rosenblum and Kurths 1998) and relative Fourier phase (Lamoth *et al.* 2002).

Principal components analysis

Much of the coordination dynamics literature has focused on studying the coordination between pairs of joints. When movements involving several degrees of freedom are analyzed, multiple pairwise analyses of coordination are performed. However, this approach can fail to grasp the global perspective on the coordination task as a whole (Forner-Cordero *et al.* 2005). The analysis of more complex coordination patterns, involving many degrees of freedom, is becoming increasingly possible given advances in data acquisition technology. Daffertshofer *et al.* (2004) suggested that multivariate analysis techniques can be useful for analyzing these complex coordination patterns. Principal components analysis (PCA) is one such technique that can be used to reduce the dimensionality of high-dimensional multivariate datasets. Based on the covariance between variables, PCA identifies mutual information. In an n-dimensional space (where n is the number of variables in a dataset), PCA first identifies the orientation of an axis that explains the most variability in the data – the first principal axis. Subsequently, by removing the variability in the dataset associated with the first principal axis, the axis that explains the next greatest variability in the data is identified –

variability associated with the first principal axis is removed by ensuring that the second principal axis is orthogonal to the first. This process continues, with each succeeding principal axis accounting for as much of the remaining variability in the dataset as possible. In other words, PCA converts the input data variables into new, uncorrelated, principal components; where principal components are the linear combinations of the input variables with maximal variance (Forner-Cordero *et al.* 2005).

For many human movements, much of the variability in the dataset can be explained by only a few principal components. For example, in a study of lower body kinematics during walking, 90% of the variance in the data was represented by the first two principal components (Lee *et al.* 2009). By analyzing the relatively small number of principal components that explain maximal variance, the dimensionality of the original input data set is reduced.

Daffertshofer *et al.* (2004) presented a tutorial which provided a detailed account of PCA calculations and examples of how PCA can be applied to study coordination. They highlighted how PCA can be used to study coordination during gait; examples with kinematic and electromyographic data are presented. Daffertshofer *et al.* (2004) also demonstrated how PCA can be used as a 'data-driven filter' to help isolate deterministic and random components of a dataset. There are many further examples of the use of PCA to study coordination dynamics. For example, Forner-Cordero and colleagues have used PCA to study the global coordination of the arms during complex multi-joint coordinative movements (Forner-Cordero *et al.* 2005) and examine the interaction between multi-joint coordinative movements and postural control (Forner-Cordero *et al.* 2007). PCA has also been used to study coordination during gait in, for example, people with stroke (Olney *et al.* 1998) and lower back pain (Lamoth *et al.* 2006) and participants carrying external loads (Lee *et al.* 2009).

PCA enables the analysis of global coordination in high-dimensional systems. However, several issues related to PCA must be considered. Firstly, PCA assumes that linear relationships between variables and the relationships between biological signals can be nonlinear (Krasovsky and Levin 2010). Secondly, as variations in the amplitude between variables in the input dataset can have a large effect on the calculated principal components, the issue of normalizing the input variables should be considered before conducting PCA (Lamoth *et al.* 2006). The interpretation of PCA can also be difficult. When the predominant mode of coordination is either in- or anti-phase, interpretation can be relatively straightforward (Forner-Cordero *et al.* 2005). For example, Forner-Cordero *et al.* (2005) prescribed experimental motions that required either in- or anti-phase movements of the arm joints. In this situation, the first principal component can be used to study overall global coordination. However, when coordination is not predominantly in- or anti-phase, interpretation/classification of principal components becomes more difficult. In their study of gait in participants with stroke, Olney *et al.* (1998) related the first principal component to locomotion speed (this accounted for 41% of the variance in the data), the second to interlimb symmetry (accounting for 13% of the variance) and the third to postural flexion bias. The remaining principal components accounted for minimal variability and were not interpretable. Although interpretation/classification of principal components is possible, the process is often based on prior knowledge and expertise (Krasovsky and Levin 2010). Furthermore, sometimes interpretation/classification of principal components is not possible.

Self-organizing maps

Self-organizing maps (SOMs) are a specific type of artificial neural network most commonly used for dimensionality reduction and pattern classification (Kohonen 2001). A SOM is commonly visualized as two layers of information: an input layer and an output layer. The input layer consists of a series of nodes, each of which represents an input vector (e.g. a single multivariate time sample of a movement trial). The output layer consists of a grid of nodes, which are each associated with a respective weight vector. The weight vectors in the output layer compete to best represent nodes in the input layer and, as a result, collectively model the input layer. Because of the competitive learning algorithm, SOMs are able to model high-dimensional, time-series data with a simple low-dimensional, visualizable mapping, while maintaining the original topology of the input. Therefore, similar to PCA, SOMs provide an opportunity to study complex coordinated movement. Additionally, SOMs are also able to model nonlinear relationships in the input – a prevalent feature of neurobiological systems. The nonlinear input-output mapping is possible, owing to the competitive learning strategy and the neighbourhood function (see Kohonen 2001), which together tend to cluster similar data to similar map regions.

In the two-layer SOMs, the output layer represents postures or coordination states during the movement. By connecting the sequence of best-matching nodes for a single movement trial and superimposing the trajectory on a mapping of the output layer, the time-series change in coordination can be visualized. SOMs have been used to identify changes in coordination for trials of gait (e.g. Barton *et al.* 2006; Lamb *et al.* 2011a) and various sports actions, including discus throwing (Bauer and Schöllhorn 1997), football kicking (Lees and Barton 2005) and golf chipping (Lamb *et al.* 2011b).

Several authors have employed a second SOM or a third layer, which is trained on the output of the original SOM (e.g. Barton 1999; Lamb *et al.* 2011b). The sequence of the best-matching nodes is used as input for the second SOM, which represents the movement pattern as a whole, rather than the various states of coordination during the movement. Classifying the movement as a whole can often be used to complement the findings of the original SOM, especially when the coordination patterns underlying the classification are of interest. In particular, and relevant to the coordination dynamics framework, Lamb *et al.* (2011b) used the SOM trajectory of best-matching nodes to study the coordination dynamics of the golf chip. Since the SOM trajectory represents the evolution of coordination throughout the movement, the authors used the trajectory as a collective variable, which they then used to train a second SOM and subsequently to identify coordination stability and transitions to new stable patterns.

SOMs represent a powerful tool for studying human movement, particularly from a coordination dynamics perspective. Some issues that remain contentious are whether to train one SOM on the data of several subjects, at the risk of masking intra-individual changes in coordination, or to introduce several SOMs unique to each subject, at the risk of generalizing between subjects; how to determine the training parameters and which normalization procedures are most appropriate. General solutions to these issues are difficult and should instead be considered with respect to the specific research question. For example, data normalization should be treated as Hamill *et al.* (2000) outline for the continuous relative phase. Training parameters should be data driven, the principal components of the input data give an objective method for determining the number of nodes, the dimensions of the map and the training length (both rough and fine tuning; Vesanto *et al.* 2000). With continued use by researchers, SOM analyses should become more familiar and their use more uniform across different working groups.

Why coordination dynamics are relevant for sports performance

Having introduced some of the key concepts underpinning coordination dynamics and the various techniques used to examine these characteristics, we finally consider what this field of study can offer for our understanding of sport performance. Athletes in sports exemplify self-organizing, complex systems, using specific information sources to coordinate their actions with respect to important environmental objects, surfaces, and events (Turvey 1990). As they train, athletes educate their attention by becoming better at detecting key information variables that specify movements from the myriad variables that do not (see Chapter 4). In addition, learners calibrate actions by tuning existing coordination patterns to critical information sources and, through practice, establish and sustain functional information–movement couplings to regulate coordinated activity with the environment (see Chapter 18). Coordination dynamics may be conceived as the manifestation of these processes, whereby athletes match their intrinsic dynamics to the requirements of a task (i.e. behavioural information).

Performance enhancement

With knowledge of the coordination dynamics of a system, it is theoretically possible to model a task space and to determine potential solution spaces ('hot spots') within that area in which high levels of performance are most likely to surface (Cohen and Sternad 2009). Furthermore, manipulation of control parameters that move a system towards these hot spots would enable sports practitioners to systematically improve an athlete's performance (McGinnis and Newell 1982). In other words, understanding the stability attributes of the athlete–environment system allows one to identify potential strengths and weaknesses and, hence, these can be used to develop strategies and tactics in an objective fashion (as opposed to relying on the intuition of a coach). For instance, in team sports such as soccer and basketball, the dynamics of the team centroid (including its position and stretch index) can be used to predict and potentially influence critical moments in a game such as shots or turnovers in possession (see Chapter 19).

A number of applied studies exemplify these practical suggestions. In association football (soccer), Duarte *et al.* (2012b) demonstrate how the stability of a defending group of players is upset by the collective movements of attacking players as they converge toward the goal. Moreover, a series of studies in futsal have recently shown how key parameters such as interpersonal distance, phase angle between attacker and defender relative to goal and the distance from goal influence the likelihood of success in attacking scenarios (for an overview see Button *et al.* 2012). Switching to individual sports, Barbosa *et al.* (2010) identified a number of critical factors related to optimizing swimming performance. They noted that a swimmer's segmental mechanics and centre of mass kinematics are strongly related to energetics and ultimately to optimal performance. Cignetti *et al.* (2009) examined how the coordination dynamics of cross-country skiing were adapted under varying degrees of slope steepness (e.g. 0–7°). Common to many other studies of bimanual coordination, a number of stable modes of coordination were revealed and transitions between them were marked by temporary losses in stability.

Technique modification, rehabilitation and injury prevention

During training, coordinative structures form a kind of 'task-specific device' suited for specific performance circumstances. Neurobiological systems 'soft assemble' the coordination solutions into movement problems. These ideas suggest that the inclusion of movement pattern variability is a useful strategy for training of coordination and control processes in sport. Movement system variability is an important part of learning design in sport and rehabilitation. The abundance of mechanical degrees of freedom available in the degenerate human movement system can be configured in different ways by athletes to perform a diverse range of tasks. In appropriately designed training environments, athletes can learn how to utilize different system degrees of freedom to stabilize a functional coordination pattern. The implication is that coordination training should not be aimed at reproduction of a putative common optimal movement pattern by all learners but that each individual performer needs to learn how to exploit variability within the movement system in different ways to adapt to changing task constraints over time (see Chapter 19).

The functional role of coordination variability in helping to prevent injury and also rehabilitating from disease or injury has been recognized for over a decade now (Hamill *et al.* 1999; Davids *et al.* 2003). It has been proposed that movement variability is necessary to encourage injured and rehabilitating individuals to adapt to the new, changing constraints imposed upon them, in contrast to the traditional medical model, in which deviation from ideal patterns is viewed as abnormal. For example, athletes recovering from anterior cruciate ligament injuries show reduced centre of pressure variability in comparison to healthy, control athletes (Davids *et al.* 1999). Hence, higher variability in sway should not be associated with increased instability but instead is indicative of normal exploratory behaviour.

The key question for practitioners is how to use this information in diagnosing and treating injuries and/or disease. It is possible that knowledge of the coordination dynamics of a system can be used to identify, monitor and treat for the influence of pain amongst injured athletes. For example, van Ryckeghem *et al.* (2012) propose that a multi-task switching paradigm can be used to investigate how pain interferes with the ability of an individual to carry out multiple tasks in complex environments. Neilsen and Cohen (2008) remind us that corticospinal plasticity plays an important role in the acquisition of athletic skills to a high standard. In particular, they suggest that neurorehabilitation clinics should explore the use of emerging therapies that simultaneously stimulate sensory inputs whilst also activating the motor cortex, which may lead to enhanced cortical representations of motor skills, as well as the excitability of the specific muscles engaged in those skills. Finally, as Tessitore *et al.* (2011) demonstrate it is possible that monitoring the coordination of athletes at various phases in their periodization cycle (such as during preseason training in soccer) can lead to more effective, targeted injury prevention strategies.

In summary, we have briefly explained some of the key concepts underpinning the emerging field of coordination dynamics. This chapter overviewed a number of studies using sports performance as vehicles to reveal the coordination dynamics of athletes. Coordination dynamics exist across multiple timescales and as such a range of analysis tools may be required to uncover their characteristics. Sports scientists have begun to reveal that coordination dynamics has the potential to unlock new enhancements in performance in a range of different sports. Modifications to athletic techniques can be brought about through coordination training as performers develop metastable characteristics. Finally, coordination dynamics may also play an important role in sports medicine, as clinicians seek to prevent injury and rehabilitate athletes who must balance heavy training demands with the need to optimize performance in competition.

References

Barbosa, T. M., Bragada, J. A., Reis, V. M., Marinho, D. A., Carvalho, C. and Silva, A. J. (2010) Energetics and biomechanics as determining factors of swimming performance: updating the state of the art. *Journal of Science and Medicine in Sport*, 13: 262–9.

Barton, G. (1999) Interpretation of gait data using Kohonen neural networks. *Gait and Posture*, 10: 85–6.

Barton, G., Lees, A., Lisboa, P. and Attfield, S. (2006) Visualisation of gait data with Kohonen self-organising neural maps. *Gait and Posture*, 24: 46–53.

Batschelet, E. (1981) *Circular Statistics in Biology*. London: Academic Press.

Bauer, H. and Schöllhorn, W. I. (1997) Self-organizing maps for the analysis of complex movement patterns. *Neural Processing Letters*, 5: 193–7.

Bernstein, N. A. (1967) *The Coordination and Regulation of Movements*. London: Pergamon Press.

Brétigny, P., Leroy, D., Button, C., Chollet, D. and Seifert L. (2011) Coordination profiles of the expert field hockey drive according to field roles. *Sports Biomechanics*, 10 (4): 339–50.

Brisson, T. A. and Alain, C. (1996) Should common optimal movement patterns be identified as the criterion to be achieved? *Journal of Motor Behavior*, 28: 211–23.

Button, C. and Farrow, D. (2012) Working in the field (Southern Hemisphere), in N. Hodges and M. Williams. (eds) *Skill Acquisition in Sport*, 2nd edn. Abingdon: Routledge, pp. 367–80.

Button, C., Chow, J-Y., Travassos, B., Vilar, L., Duarte, R., Passos, P., Araujo, D. and Davids, K. (2012) A nonlinear pedagogy for sports teams as social neurobiological systems: how teams can harness self-organization tendencies, in A. Ovens, T. Hopper and J. Butler. (eds) *Complexity Thinking in Physical Education: Reframing Curriculum, Pedagogy and Research*. Abingdon: Routledge, pp. 135–50.

Chang, R., Emmerik, R. Van and Hamill, J. (2008) Quantifying rearfoot-forefoot coordination in human walking. *Journal of Biomechanics*, 41 (14): 3101–5.

Chen, H. H., Liu, Y. T., Mayer-Kress, G. and Newell, K. M. 2005. Learning the pedalo locomotion task. *Journal of Motor Behavior*, 37: 247–56.

Cignetti, F., Schena, F., Zanone, P. G. and Rouard, A. (2009) Dynamics of coordination in cross-country skiing. *Human Movement Science*, 28: 204–17.

Cohen, R. and Sternad, D. (2009) Variability in motor learning: relocating, channeling and reducing noise. *Experimental Brain Research*, 193 (1): 69–83.

Daffertshofer, A., Lamoth, J. C., Meijer, O. and Beek, P. J. (2004) PCA in studying coordination and variability: A tutorial. *Clinical Biomechanics*, 19: 415–28.

Davids, K., Kingsbury, D., George, K., O'Connell, M., and Stock, D. (1999) Interacting constraints and the emergence of postural behavior in ACL-deficient subjects. *Journal of Motor Behavior*, 31: 358–66.

Davids, K., Glazier, P., Araújo, D. and Bartlett, R. M. (2003) Movement systems as dynamical systems: the role of functional variability and its implications for sports medicine. *Sports Medicine*, 33: 245–60.

Davids, K., Button, C., Araújo, D., Renshaw, I. and Hristovski, R. (2006) Movement models from sports provide representative task constraints for studying adaptive behavior in human movement systems. *Adaptive Behavior*, 14: 73–95.

Derrick, T. R. and Thomas, J. M. (2004) Time series analysis: the cross-correlation function, in N. Stergious (ed.) *Innovative Analyses of Human Movement*. Champaign, IL: Human Kinetics, pp. 189–205.

Duarte, R., Araújo, D., Correia, V. and Davids, K. (2012a) Sports teams as superorganisms: implications of sociobiological models of behaviour for research and practice in team sports performance analysis. *Sports Medicine*, 42 (8): 633–42.

Duarte, R., Araújo, D., Freire, L., Folgado, H., Fernandes, O. and Davids, K. (2012b) Intra- and inter-group coordination patterns reveal collective behaviors of football players near the scoring zone. *Human Movement Science*, 31 (6): 1639–51.

Ferber, R., Davis, I. M. and Williams, D. S. (2005) Effect of foot orthotics on rearfoot and tibia joint coupling patterns and variability. *Journal of Biomechanics*, 38 (3): 477–83.

Field-Fote, E. C and Tepavac, D. (2002) Improved intralimb coordination in people with incomplete spinal cord injury following training with body weight support and electrical stimulation. *Physical Therapy*, 82: 707–15.

Forner-Cordero, A., Levin, O., Li, Y. and Swinnen, S. P. (2005) Principal component analysis of complex multijoint coordinative movements. *Biological Cybernetics*, 93 (1): 63–78.

Forner-Cordero, A., Levin, O., Li, Y. and Swinnen, S. P. (2007) Posture control and complex arm coordination: analysis of multijoint coordinative movements. *Journal of Motor Behavior*, 39: 215–26.

Freeman, H. (1961) On the encoding of arbitrary geometric configurations. *IEEE Transactions on Electronic Computers*, EC-10: 321–31.

Glazier, P. S. (2010) Game, set and match? Substantive issues and future directions in performance analysis. *Sports Medicine*, 40: 625–34.

Glazier, P. S. and Davids, K. (2009) Constraints on the complete optimization of human motion. *Sports Medicine*, 39: 15–28.

Haken, H., Kelso, J. A. S. and Bunz, H. (1985) A theoretical model of phase transitions in human hand movements. *Biological Cybernetics*, 51: 347–56.

Hamill, J., van Emmerik, R. E. A., Heidersheit, B. C. and Li, L. (1999) A dynamical systems approach to lower extremity injury. *Clinical Biomechanics*, 14: 297–308.

Hamill, J., Haddad, J. and McDermott, W. (2000) Issues in quantifying variability from a dynamical systems perspective. *Journal of Applied Biomechanics*, 16: 407–18.

Haykin, S. (1999) *Neural Networks: A Comprehensive Foundation*, 2nd edn. Englewood Cliffs, NJ: Prentice-Hall.

Hershler, C. and Milner, M. (1980) Angle-angle diagrams in the assessment of locomotion. *American Journal of Physical Medicine*, 59: 109–25.

Irwin, G. and Kerwin, D. G. (2007) Inter-segmental coordination in progressions for the longswing on high bar. *Sports Biomechanics*, 6 (2): 131–44.

Jantzen, K. J., Oullier, O. and Kelso, J. A. S. (2008) Neuroimaging coordination dynamics in the sport sciences. *Methods*, 45: 325–35.

Jeka, J. J. and Kelso, J. A. (1995) Manipulating symmetry in the coordination dynamics of human movement. *Journal of Experimental Psychology Human Perception and Performance*, 21: 360–74.

Kelso, J. A. S. (1981) On the oscillatory basis of movement. *Bulletin of the Psychonomic Society*, 18: 63.

Kelso, J. A. S. (1984) Phase transitions and critical behavior in human bimanual coordination. *American Journal of Physiology: Regulatory, Integrative and Comparative Physiology*, 15: R1000–4.

Kelso, J. A. S. (1995) *Dynamic Patterns: The self-organisation of Brain and Behaviour*. Cambridge, MA: MIT Press.

Kelso, J. A. S. (2009) Coordination dynamics, in R. A. Meyers (ed.) *Encyclopedia of Complexity and Systems Science*. New York: Springer, pp. 1537–64.

Kohonen, T. 2001. *Self-organizing Maps*, 3rd edn. Berlin: Springer.

Krasovsky, T. and Levin, M. F. (2010) Review: toward a better understanding of coordination in healthy and poststroke gait. *Neurorehabilitation and Neural Repair*, 24 (3): 213–24.

Lamb, P. F., Mündermann, A., Bartlett, R. M. and Robins, A. (2011a) Visualizing changes in lower body coordination with different types of foot orthoses using self-organizing maps (SOM). *Gait and Posture*, 34: 485–9.

Lamb, P. F., Bartlett, R. M. and Robins, A. (2011b) Artificial neural networks for analyzing inter-limb coordination: the golf chip shot. *Human Movement Science*, 30: 1129–43.

Lamoth, C. J. C., Beek, P. J. and Meijer, O. G. (2002) Pelvis-thorax coordination in the transverse plane during gait. *Gait and posture*, 16 (2): 101–14.

Lamoth, C.J., Daffertshofer, A., Meijer, O. G. and Beek, P. J. (2006) How do persons with chronic low back pain speed up and slow down? Trunk-pelvis coordination and lumbar erector spinae activity during gait. *Gait and Posture*, 23 (2): 230–9.

Lee, M., Roan, M. and Smith, B. (2009) An application of principal component analysis for lower body kinematics between loaded and unloaded walking. *Journal of Biomechanics*, 42 (14): 2226–30.

Lees, A. and Barton, G. (2005) A characterisation of technique in the soccer kick using a Kohonen neural network analysis, in T. Reilly, J. Cabri, and D. Araújo (eds) *Science and Football V: Proceedings of the Fifth World Congress on Science and Football*. London: Routledge, pp. 83–8.

McGarry, T. I. M., Khan, M. A. and Franks, I. A. N. M. (1999) On the presence and absence of behavioral traits in sport: an example from championship squash match-play. *Journal of Sports Sciences*, 17: 297–311.

McGinnis, P. and Newell, K. (1982) Topological dynamics: a framework for describing movement and its constraints. *Human Movement Science*, 1 (4): 289–305.

Mullineaux, D. R., Bartlett, R. M. and Bennett, S. (2001) Research design and statistics in biomechanics and motor control: research design and statistics in biomechanics and motor control. *Journal of Sports Sciences*, 19: 37–41.

Nielsen, J. B. and Cohen, L. G. (2008) The Olympic brain: does corticospinal plasticity play a role in acquisition of skills required for high□performance sports? *Journal of Physiology*, 586 (1): 65–70.

O'Halloran, J., Hamill, J., McDermott, W. J., Remelius, J. G. and Van Emmerik, R. E. (2012) Locomotor-respiratory coupling patterns and oxygen consumption during walking above and below preferred stride frequency. *European Journal of Applied Physiology*, 112 (3): 929–40.

Olney, S. J., Griffin, M. P., and McBride, I. D. (1998) Multivariate examination of data from gait analysis of persons with stroke. *Physical Therapy*, 78 (8), 814–28.

Ong, A., Koh, M. and Hamill, J. (2011) Quantifying lower limb gait coordination in of-the-shelf orthotic shoes. *Footwear Science*, 3: 83–90.

Palut, Y. and Zanone, P.-G. (2005) A dynamical analysis of tennis: concepts and data. *Journal of Sports Sciences*, 23 (10): 1021–32.

Peters, B. T., Haddad, J. M., Heiderscheit, B. C., Van Emmerik, R. E. and Hamill J. (2003) Limitations in the use and interpretation of continuous relative phase. *Journal of Biomechanics*, 36 (2): 271–4.

Pinder, R. A., Davids, K., Renshaw, I. and Araujo, D. (2011) Representative learning design and functionality of research and practice in sport. *Journal of Sport and Exercise Psychology*, 33: 146–55.

Pohl, M. B. and Buckley, J. G. (2008) Changes in foot and shank coupling due to alterations in foot strike pattern during running. *Clinical Biomechanics*, 23 (3): 334–41.

Rosenblum, M. and Kurths, J. (1998) Analysing synchronization phenomena from bivariate data by means of the Hilbert transform, in H. Kantz, J. Kurths and G. Mayer-Kress (eds) *Nonlinear Analysis of Physiological Data*. Berlin: Springer, pp. 91–9.

Schöner, G. and Kelso, J. A. S. (1988) A dynamic pattern theory of behavioral change. *Journal of Theoretical Biology*, 135: 501–24.

Schöner, G., Haken, H. and Kelso, J. A. S. (1986) A stochastic theory of phase transitions in human hand movement. *Biological Cybernetics*, 53: 247–57.

Sidaway, B., Heise, G. and Schonfelder-Zohdi, B. (1995) Quantifying the variability of angle-angle plots. *Journal of Human Movement Studies*, 29: 181–97.

Silfies, S. P., Bhattacharya, A., Biely, S., Smith, S. S. and Giszter, S. (2009) Trunk control during standing reach: a dynamical system analysis of movement strategies in patients with mechanical low back pain. *Gait and Posture*, 29 (3): 370–6.

Sparrow, W. A., Donovan, E., Van Emmerik, R. E. A. and Barry, E. B. (1987) Using relative motion plots to measure changes in intra-limb and inter-limb coordination. *Journal of Motor Behavior*, 19: 115–29.

Temprado, J., Della-Grasta, M., Farrell, M., and Laurent, M. (1997) A novice-expert comparison of (intra-limb) coordination subserving the volleyball serve. *Human Movement Science*, 16 (5): 653–76.

Tepavac, D. and Field-Fote, E. C., (2001) Vector coding : a technique for quantification of intersegmental coupling in multicyclic behaviors. *Journal of Applied Biomechanics*, 17: 259–70.

Tessitore, A., Perroni, F., Cortis, C., Meeusen, R., Lupo, C. and Capranica, L. (2011) Coordination of soccer players during preseason training. *Journal of Strength and Conditioning Research*, 25: 3059–69.

Turvey, M. T. (1990) Coordination. *American Psychologist*, 45 (8): 938–53.

van Orden, G. C., Holden, J. G. and Turvey, M. T. (2003) Self-organization of cognitive performance. *Journal of Experimental Psychology: General*, 132: 331–50.

van Ryckeghem, D. M. L., Crombez, G., Eccleston, C., Liefooghe, B. and Van Damme, S. (2012) The interruptive effect of pain in a multitask environment: an experimental investigation. *Journal of Pain*, 13: 131–8.

Vesanto, J., Himberg, J., Alhoniemi, E. and Parkankangas, J. (2000) *SOM Toolbox for MATLAB 5*, Technical Report No. A57). Espoo, Finland: Neural Networks Centre, Helsinki University of Technology. Available from www.cis.hut.fi/projects/ somtool-box/ (accessed 15 July 2013).

Wheat, J. S. and Glazier, P. (2005) Measuring coordination and coordination variability, in K. Davids, S. Bennett and K.Newell (eds). *Movements Systems Variability*. Champaign, IL: Human Kinetics, pp. 167–81.

Whiting, W. C. and Zernicke, R. F. (1982) Correlation of movement patterns via pattern recognition. *Journal of Motor Behavior*, 14: 135–42.

Williams, A. M. and Ford, P. R. (2009) Promoting a skills-based agenda in Olympic sports: the role of skill-acquisition specialists. *Journal of Sports Sciences*, 27: 1381–92.

Williams, A. M. and Hodges, N. J. (2005) Practice, instruction and skill acquisition in soccer: challenging tradition. *Journal of Sports Sciences*, 23: 637–50.

Wilson, C., Simpson, S. and Hamill, J. (2009) Movement coordination patterns in triple jump training drills. *Journal of Sports Sciences*, 27 (3): 277–82.

4 Psychobiological integration during exercise

*Natàlia Balagué Serre, Robert Hristovski,
Alfonsas Vainoras, Pablo Vázquez and
Daniel Aragonés*

For over a century, physiologists have tried to find the limits of performance following a reductionist approach. Although this approach has provided a wealth of descriptive knowledge about acute and chronic changes of systemic components with different types of exercise, it has failed to supply a unified and clear explanation about the limits of exercise tolerance. Trying to find such limits in specific sites or processes, the initial and major focus of research has been the muscle and its metabolism, followed by the brain (McKenna and Hargreaves 2008). Owing to controversial findings (Cairns 2006; Enoka and Duchateau 2008; McKenna and Hargreaves 2008; St Clair Gibson and Noakes 2004; Nybo 2008; Weir *et al.* 2006), more recently, an increasing attention has been paid to integrative approaches (Lambert *et al.* 2005), with renewed emphasis being placed on the role of the brain in establishing the limits of exercise tolerance (Marcora and Staiano 2010, Noakes, St Clair Gibson and Lambert 2005; Taylor *et al.* 2006).

The extant integrative models highlight the function of variables such as perceived exertion in relation to the decision to terminate (Marcora 2008; Shephard 2009; Weir *et al.* 2006). With regard to the way in which this decision is made, there is now a lively debate about the respective roles of the brain and the muscle (Marcora and Staiano 2010). However, two basic questions need to be answered before engaging with this debate about the integrative aspects of effort tolerance. Firstly, what kind of integration is there between the different system components of the human organism: is it linear or nonlinear? Secondly, and linked to the first question: is the integration based on fixed, time-invariant and well-defined encapsulated modules or is it task dependent, context sensitive and, therefore, flexible? This chapter discusses these possibilities and proposes ways of resolving these questions in light of recent empirical findings.

From linear to nonlinear models of psychobiological integration

In exercise biology, what is known as the 'systems approach' still treats the human organism as a machine or technical device and therefore its integrative functions are studied within the framework of traditional control theory. Concepts such as homeostasis and explicit feedback loops, controllers and plants (i.e.

controlled subsystems) are usually evoked to describe the ongoing regulation and control of biological systems. This 'engineering' approach aims to apply adequate corrective solutions in order to obtain the desired stability and predictability of the subsystems under control. In doing so, the notion of proportionality between inputs and outputs is usually used to explain how the system adapts to internal (temperature, pH, gas concentration, etc.) or external changes (workload, type of muscle contraction, etc.; Kenney *et al.* 2011).

Descriptive block diagrams are commonly used to represent the way in which organic structures and processes interact to achieve and regulate different functions during exercise (such as voluntary movement; Figure 4.1). The basic assumption of these diagrams (formed by control loops and controllers) is that of time-invariant encapsulated modules, processes and regulation profiles.

As long as one deals with conceptual (i.e. verbal) descriptive modelling, this approach based on explicit feedback loops seems fine. Problems arise, however, when one tries to model mathematically more than a couple of interlinked components together (Kelso 1995). Then, the system rapidly becomes impossible to treat in terms of explicit feedback circuits.

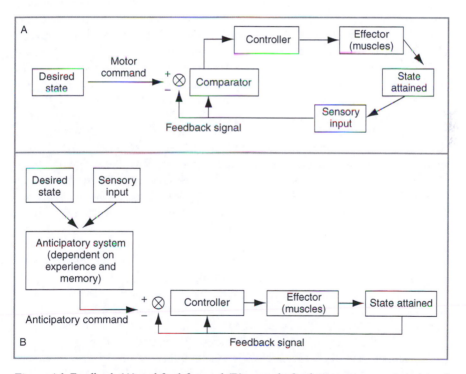

Figure 4.1 Feedback (A) and feed-forward (B) control of voluntary movement. A sign of correction is created in both mechanisms to change the action of the muscles according to the difference between the desired and achieved states

Another important problem is that, in contrast to what is claimed by models based on control theory, complex biological dynamical systems do not have simple and constant reference states with which feedback can be compared and no single locus where comparison operations are performed (see, for example, Thompson and Swanson 2010). Rather, steady states emerge from the nonlinear interactions between the system's components but without explicit and simple feedback-regulated set points or reference values, as in, for example, an engineered thermostatic device (Fox *et al.* 2005; Izhikevich *et al.* 2004). Linear models have also problems in predicting certain observations, such as critical behaviour. In fact, they have serious prediction problems because linearity and additivity are barely evident or nonexistent in the human organism (Van Orden and Paap 1997).

Two different models of exercise tolerance are currently being debated in the exercise physiology literature: the 'central governor' model (St Clair Gibson and Noakes 2004) and the psychobiological model of exercise tolerance (Marcora 2008; Marcora *et al.* 2008, 2009) based on motivational intensity theory (Wright 1996). The former uses the notion of a regulatory device or 'governor' that is able to integrate algorithmically the large number of changing variables during effort (Lambert *et al.* 2005; Noakes *et al.* 2005). Through a kind of activation threshold (i.e. a set point), this central device may produce cessation of activity in order to avoid systems failure (St Clair Gibson and Noakes 2004). The efficiency of such a programmer or regulatory unit is thought to be unconstrained, i.e. it functions as an encapsulated module that is able to control at any given time any peripheral change and it is unaffected by the fatigue process (as noted by Balagué and Hristovski 2010). Later authors mention two problems in relation to this psychobiological model: 1) an infinite regress problem, i.e. who programs the programmer?; and 2) is it possible for the programmer to remain unaffected by the changes occurring at all levels?

The psychobiological model of exercise tolerance does not consider the need for a subconscious 'entity' such as the central governor, because the decision as to when to terminate exercise is deemed to be made by the conscious brain (Marcora 2008). The end of exercise therefore arrives when exercise continuation is perceived as impossible. Perceived exertion, considered as the awareness of central motor commands to the locomotor and respiratory muscles, seems to be generated from efferent rather than afferent sensory inputs and it would fix the limits of exercise tolerance. Thus, the increase in central motor command required to exercise at the same workload with muscles weakened by locomotor muscle fatigue is perceived as increased effort.

Both models may find it difficult to explain the qualitative changes occurring during exercise in varied contexts (such as the above mentioned fatigue-induced termination point) unless they resort to specific ad hoc explanations. In fact, neither of them specifically explains the onset of exercise termination. Even if performers are conscious of exercise termination, this does not necessarily mean that the termination is consciously produced. Moreover, the processes that under-pin this event are not explained at all by saying that the termination is consciously produced.

The fact that every new context (such as a different type of exercise) requires a different mechanism or adaptation process leads, in general, to fragmented knowledge (this being the current state of affairs in the majority of sciences dealing with the biological order). This, in turn, brings about the above-mentioned controversial findings and fosters the idea that there may not be general principles for the psychological and biological domains. At first glance, these considerations seem to suggest that complex biological systems are unable to satisfy the aims of general scientific theories. However, before rejecting this possibility, it is worth considering that any macroscopic behaviour of a complex adaptive system, such as performance in sport, is the result of an immense number of highly coordinated spatiotemporal processes. In other words, macroscopic behaviour is a collective effect of sets of highly interdependent components within the system, i.e. a result of their synergy in space and time. Research showed some time ago (Haken 1983) that these collective (or cooperative) effects can be successfully studied by searching for collective variables which capture the coherent, coordinated behaviour of a system's component processes. These collective variables or order parameters (since they represent the macroscopic state of biological order) are the most adequate for studying the behaviour of complex systems because they capture the approximately linear and also nonlinear regimen of operation of such systems. These variables are best determined close to the points of qualitative, discontinuous change, where a large set of other variables become subservient to them and the behaviour of the system becomes low dimensional. As they contain compressed information about all subservient variables, the collective variables also become the most informative quantities, i.e. to external observers (e.g. researchers) they are 'informators' about the macroscopic behaviour of complex systems (Haken 2000).

Testing the behaviour of such collective variables under the change of constraints, i.e. applying a coordination dynamics approach (Kelso 1995), would seem to be a viable way of investigating the type of integration shown by a complex system. Complex adaptive systems may exhibit different kinds of collective behaviour, such as stationary or nonstationary, i.e. metastable, periodic or chaotic behaviour. The mode of behaviour depends basically on the configuration of constraints or control parameters, i.e. on variables that do not specifically prescribe or impose the behaviour of the system but which constrain it. In short, the control of dynamical systems is constraints based. For a certain configuration of constraints, nonlinear systems undergo a qualitative change in their behaviour, a partial or complete rearrangement of their component interactions and, hence, a discontinuous change in the order parameter. These events are referred to as bifurcation phenomena. One reason why these phenomena arise is because there is more than one possible stable state, and this property, i.e. multistability, stems from the nonlinear interactions between the system's components.

Exercise-induced fatigue experiments

In order to study the psychobiological integration during exercise performed until failure from the perspective of coordination dynamics we performed a set of experiments (Table 4.1). The accumulated effort was the control parameter in all experiments.

The behaviour of four different potential collective variables providing information about the state of the system as a whole during constant static and dynamic exercises performed until the fatigue-induced spontaneous termination point (FISTP) were continuously monitored and analyzed (Hristovski and Balagué 2010). Two variables were kinematic (elbow angle and pedalling frequency) and two psychological (attention focus and volition state). Changes in these variables over time provide information about the state of performer/task interactions. In complex systems, these states may exist in different modes as pointed out before. These modes reveal the type of interactions that occur between the different components and processes in the system. Thus, they may help to get a clearer picture of the kind of system we are dealing with, i.e. the type of integration between components in the system.

Variables that capture the biological or psychological state of collective order are classically studied either separately or through a hierarchy of encapsulated general purpose modules, as illustrated by the recent debate regarding 'mind over muscle' (Marcora and Staiano 2010). However, the interaction between variables and, more importantly, their task dependence are almost completely ignored when trying to separate their effect from the general context.

As is well known, accumulated effort is accompanied by continuous changes in both peripheral constraints (lactic acid accumulates, muscle substrates change

Table 4.1 Summary of the four experiments performed until the fatigue-induced spontaneous termination point

Experiment	Exercise	Order parameter	Nonlinear change
1. How fatigue constrains quasi-isometric exercise	Isometric arm-curl flexion 90°	Elbow angle (0°)	From 90° to 0° (gravity alignment)
2. How fatigue constrains volition states		Volition state (UP/DOWN)	From metastable to stable 'down' state
3. How fatigue constrains dynamic exercise	Cycling at 70 RPM	Cycling frequency (RPM)	From 70 RPM to close to 0 RPM
4. Attention focus with effort accumulation	Running while having dissociative thoughts	Attention focus	From imposed dissociative thoughts to associative

RPM = revolutions per minute

their concentration, etc.) and central constraints (rate of perceived exertion increases, attention focus change, etc.). In our research, we hypothesized that, for a certain configuration of constraints, nonlinear or qualitative change in the behaviour might occur and, therefore, there would be a discontinuous change in the order parameter (as described in the fourth column of Table 4.1). As the termination point is understood here, as a result of a bifurcation phenomenon (FISTP), it must be manifested as an abrupt shift in the activity towards lower energy expenditure levels or rest (Hristovski and Balagué 2010).

A second and equally important aspect of our research was that we sought to find the dynamical hallmarks of these transitions, such as the enhancement of fluctuations and change in the dimensionality of fluctuation dynamics as the termination point approached. These effects would corroborate the hypothesis that the termination point is a dynamical product, an effect of self-organizing processes. Note that such effects are not at all predicted by extant theories of fatigue. Conversely, they are a generic prediction of formal theories of self-organizing systems (e.g. Haken 1983). Therefore, the finding of these effects provided strong support for the hypothesis that the termination point is a self-organizing dynamic event, which in turn poses a serious challenge to theories which, assuming a linear integration, do not predict these effects.

How fatigue constrains quasi-isometric exercise performance

On five alternating days over a period of two weeks, six well-trained participants, who were familiar with the task, performed a quasi-isometric arm-curl exercise holding an Olympic bar (weight: 80% of the one-repetition maximum) with an initial elbow flexion of 90° until the FISTP. Participants were encouraged to persist, even if the initial 90°-angle was lost finalizing when the spontaneous disengagement from the task was produced. Changes in both elbow angles during the trial were registered at a rate of 50 Hz by an electrogoniometer (Biometrics, software by Ebiom; Figure 4.2).

As shown in Figure 4.3A (for details, see Hristovski and Balagué 2010) the elbow angle starts fluctuating weakly and continuously around 90°, owing to the initial fine adjustments. These adjustments are produced by the intentionally sustained cooperation among the higher control loops (presumably responsible for task specific perception, attention, motivation), down to spinal reflexes and muscular processes. As fatigue develops, the continuous changes occurring in the neuromuscular system progressively destabilize the elbow angle, producing an increase in its variability. The competition between the intention to sustain the task and the progressive loss of neuromuscular tension is illustrated by the sudden increases in angle values (above 90°) during the second third of the exercise. Finally, the enhancement of elbow angle (i.e. order parameter) fluctuations precedes the sudden reduction in the angle which coincides with the FISTP. It is interesting to note that the participants' loss of ability to return to and remain at the initial elbow-angle values after some accumulated effort may be interpreted as a loss of stability of that initial attractor. The system was unable to relax back

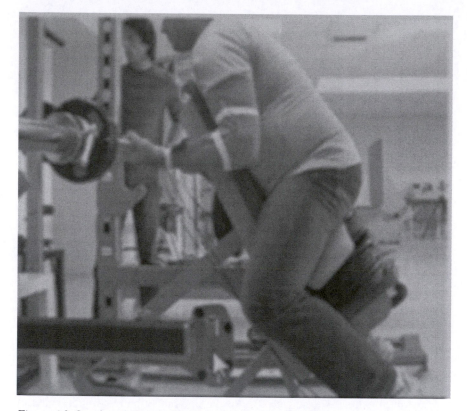

Figure 4.2 Quasi-static arm-curl exercise holding an Olympic bar with an elbow flexion
of 90° at 80% of the one-repetition maximum until the fatigue-induced
spontaneous termination point

to the previous attractor, which means that the relaxation time became infinite for
that state. The fact that performers were able to sustain other smaller angles for
some time suggests that the intentionally sustained state of exertion may dwell in
a metastable, rugged energy landscape, trapping the system in transient basins of
attraction far from the final termination point.

An additional analysis using spectral degrees of freedom (Blackman and
Tuckey 1958; Vaillancourt and Newell 2003) revealed a highly significant reduction in the degrees of freedom as the FISTP approached (Figure 4.4).

In other words, the dynamics within the system became increasingly low
dimensional, which points to the enhanced cooperative, i.e. mutually aligned, as
well as competitive behaviour of component processes within the neuromuscular
axis of performers. In the first third of the exercise, the combination of weak fluctuations and the higher value of spectral degrees of freedom signify a potential for
more flexible control of the task goal. By contrast, the combination of enhanced,
bursting fluctuations (Figure 4.3A) and the low value of spectral degrees of

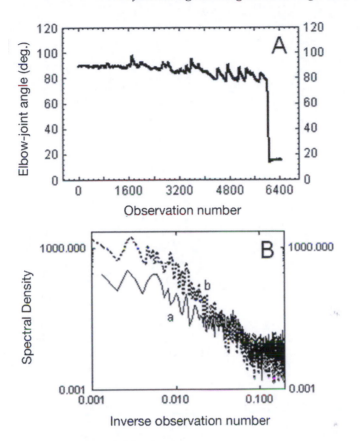

Figure 4.3 A) Time series of the elbow-angle data for participant 1; B) A typical difference in the power spectral density values for the online fluctuations of the elbow angle in the first (a) and the last (b) third of the quasi-static exercise. The difference of the elbow angle variability between the first and the third phase spans over sub-second and seconds time scale. This signifies a correlated instability of the system under fatigue (Hristovski *et al.* 2010)

freedom signifies an increasingly coherent and, therefore, more rigid control of the activity. Similar results are routinely found at the level of the timing coordination dynamics of electrocardiographic signals (see Hristovski *et al.* 2010) where an enhanced coherence (lost of complexity) is emerging as the termination point approaches.

At the behavioural level, these dynamics of order parameter variability may be explained in terms of fatigue-induced dynamic competition between two global processes at the neuromuscular level: the increasingly cooperative protective inhibition and the goal-directed, intermittent bursting excitation, the aim of which is to match more closely the task constraints, i.e. to keep elbow flexion closer to the task-goal value of 90°. Under task constraints, the increasingly cooperative

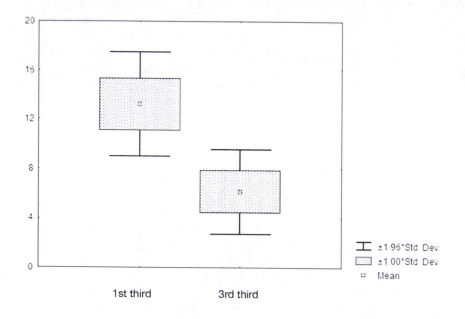

20

16

12

8

4

0

⊥ ±1.96*Std Dev.
▭ ±1.00*Std Dev.
▫ Mean

1st third   3rd third

Figure 4.4 Differences in means for the spectral degrees of freedom; horizontal axis: the first and third part of exercise; vertical axis: spectral degrees of freedom

protective inhibitory component processes, acting in compliance with the pull of gravity, have to be counteracted by increasingly cooperative excitatory component processes. Whereas in the initial phase of exercise these processes compete over shorter time scales, resulting in a stabilizing effect (small fluctuations) on the goal variable (elbow angle) as exercise proceeds, they begin to compete over longer time scales, i.e. seconds (Figure 4.3A), leading to larger fluctuations.

These increasingly coherent yet competitive processes seem to be responsible for the impending low dimensionality of order parameter variability close to the termination point. Such processes closely resemble the nucleation event of new-phase formation in first-order phase transitions (e.g. water phase and newly formed ice nuclei phase coexist close to the transition). The first small nuclei of the new inhibition phase, i.e. small areas within the neuromuscular system, may emerge simultaneously or with a short lapse of time in several distant places of the system (some muscle metabolic pathways, some synapses, etc.). The metabolic inhibition might be reflected, for example, by the lower contractile ability of some muscle fibres and provoke a larger inhibition effect. The increased GABA levels (Yakovlev 1979) in some central nervous system synapses can also enlarge the inhibitory effects at this level. The accumulated effort enhances the growth of this phase and it becomes increasingly macroscopic. On the other hand, owing to task-goal constraints the excitatory phase also segregates, becoming more coherent in order to counteract the increasing inhibition. Thus, what emerges is a formation of two macroscopic competing coalitions. However, the increasing accumulated effort makes the excitatory coalition increasingly unstable. Eventually, at the behavioural level, only the downwards movement mode survives as a result of the cooperation between the macroscopic neuromuscular inhibition and the gravitational pull under anatomical constraints, stabilizing as the new global minimum of dynamics is reached (alignment of the arm with gravity).

The power spectrum data (Figure 4.3B) show a globally correlated enhancement of variability in the elbow angle. This enhanced variability was simultaneously present on a sub-second scale to a tens-of-seconds scale, indicating that all control loops along the neuromuscular axis were destabilized by the accumulated effort. One can also see that the linear slope of the spectrum differs, with the one derived from the third part of the effort being steeper than the one derived from the first part. Together with the results of the spectral degrees of freedom analysis, this points to the increased rigidity of control under increasing accumulated effort. Hence, from the coordination dynamics point of view, the exercise-induced fatigue represents an ever-increasing destabilization of the previous configurations of the psychobiological network and their continual reconfiguration under immediate organismic, task and environmental constraints. In other words, fatigue, seen dynamically, may be viewed as a typical example of constraints-induced self-organization of metastable, soft-assembled configurations of action system components, which eventually finds its global energetic minimum aligning with the gravitational potential well.

Note how the reductionist approach, i.e. focusing only on the muscle or central processes and their isolated changes, would barely be able to give an account of how exercise termination emerges. By contrast, even a simple macroscopic approach within the framework of coordination dynamics is able to integrate gross psychological and physiological processes into a single language and capture the dynamic features of the impending exercise termination. In other words, exercise termination seems to be a dynamical event and it is increasingly clear that it should be studied and modelled as such. In the future, more elaborate models may be developed, taking into account well-defined control and dynamical variables.

How fatigue constrains volition states (quasi-static exercise)

A common general experience during a constant exercise (whether static or dynamic) that is performed until the termination point is struggling with the urge to cancel in the final moments. The aim of this experiment was to investigate the dynamics of conscious states of volition during the same arm-curl quasi static exercise described before.

On five alternating days (over a period of two weeks), six student volunteers who were familiar with resistance training performed an isometric arm-curl exercise – holding an Olympic bar (25 kg men, 17 kg women) with an initial 90° elbow flexion. Motivational strategies were applied to ensure that the participants continued exercising until their FISTP. During the effort they were asked to

verbalize their state of volition, simplifying its content to 'up' (continue) and
'down' (urge to cancel). Each one of the five trials was divided into ten non-
overlapping windows and the probabilities of 'up' and 'down' volition states were
calculated for each window. Probabilities of these states were interpreted as signs
of their relative attractiveness, i.e. stability. The evolution of the probabilities of
experienced and reported 'up/down' volition states across the trials showed the
existence of three phases: the first was dominated by an 'up' state, the second by
a meta-stable 'up-down' state, indicating competition between the two volition
states, and the third was dominated by a 'down' state (see Figure 4.5).

These results indicate that fatigue-induced conscious states of volition are
subject to nonlinear dynamical effects and give support to the hypothesis that the
state of will is a dynamical product of complex body-brain interactions.

It is tempting to associate the increased probability of finding the 'down' state,
as termination was approaching, with the increasing macroscopic inhibition
revealed in the first experiment. Indeed, it can be hypothesized that the enhanced
'down' urge is a conscious manifestation of this growing inhibition under the
accumulated effort. Hence, the termination of effort could be explained as a spontaneous dissolution, i.e. a loss of stability of the intention to act in a certain way.
From this perspective the role of the 'up' intentions is to keep the action stable.
In this sense, every 'up' collaborates on finding a new coordination to continue
the task. The final 'down' urge stabilizes as a consequence of the loss of stability
of excitatory 'up' intention. This leads to a spontaneous dissolution of the
conscious intention that emerges as a dynamical product and terminates the exertion. Note the difference between the current proposals of extant psychobiological

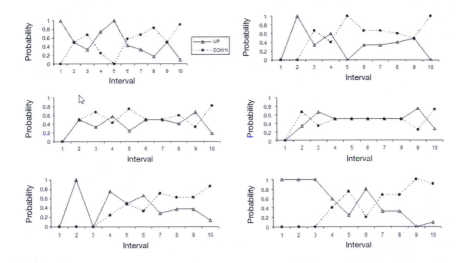

Figure 4.5 Volition-state dynamics in six participants during the quasi-static elbow angle
exercise

models supporting that termination is a conscious decision (Marcora 2008) or mediated by a central programmer (Lambert *et al*. 2005) and the claim of nonlinear models that the termination is a spontaneous dissolution of the conscious intention to act (Balagué *et al*. 2011; Hristovski and Balagué 2010). In this experiment, it was the 'up' intention as part of the task goal which stabilized the order parameter (elbow angle), creating an attracting basin around the goal value (elbow flexion under 90°) other than the resting state. The dissolution of this attractor through a dynamic loss of stability mechanism implied the dissolution of the intention to act. Hence, within this framework the termination is not consciously produced but, rather, spontaneously emerges at a psychological and action level as dissolution of the intentional act.

How fatigue constrains dynamic exercise performance

To test for the correlated properties of action variability during a continuous dynamic task performed until exhaustion the following experiment was conducted (Hristovski *et al*. 2010). Twelve triathletes performed a continuous cycle ergometer exercise at 80% of their maximum workload, the task goal being to maintain a pace of 70 revolutions per minute (RPM) until their FISTP. The cycling frequency was treated as a potential collective variable and its values were recorded continuously by a cycle ergometer system (Sport Excalibur 925900; Figure 4.6).

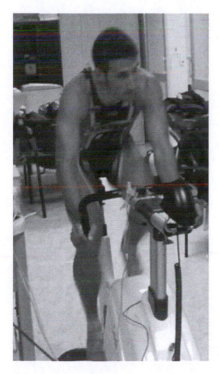

Figure 4.6 Cycle ergometer exercise

The time series of the RPM variable were analyzed by time and frequency domain methods (autocorrelation and spectral analysis). The spectral indexes were calculated by estimating the linear fit slope of the power spectrum with respect to frequency in logarithmic coordinates (Figure 4.7).

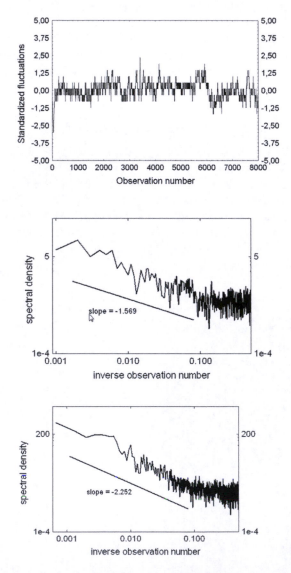

Figure 4.7 (Upper panel): standardized fluctuations from the data on revolutions per minute; (middle panel): power spectrum for the first half of the exercise with its slope of −1.5 showing anti-persistent fractional Brownian motion (fBm); (lower panel): power spectrum for the second half of the exercise with a slope of −2.2 showing persistent fBm

A scale-invariant relationship was found between the spectral power of RPM variability and the frequency. The values of the spectral indexes were in the intervals between −1 and −2.5, pointing to the presence of a fractal time structure for RPM variability (from anti-persistent to persistent fractional Brownian motion (fBm) as fatigue develops. The results of this experiment corroborate the results presented in experiment one for a dynamic type of exercise. The scale invariance in the power spectra suggests that there may be no specific site and associated timescale of their dynamics that would dominate the cycling frequency *variability*. In other words, the system seems to be dominated not by the components but rather by interactions between processes, e.g. control loops dwelling in different time scales.

The power spectra slopes showed a dominantly anti-persistent profile (between −2 and −1) for the RPM variable in the first half of the exercise (right upper panel). In the second half, there was a clearly persistent or super-diffusive fBm profile (spectral slope between −2 and −3) in participants who performed to exhaustion and whose time series at the end were dominated by high-amplitude non-stationary fluctuations of the RPM variable (lower panel). Performers who cancelled at accumulated effort values which did not produce such a fluctuation profile attained fBm values of around −2 and less.

These results are consistent with those of the previously discussed quasi-static exercise study from a different perspective. Anti-persistent fBm is characterized by dynamics in which increments are anticorrelated, meaning that the present trend is more likely to be followed by an opposite trend. This characteristic points to a stabilizing synergy for constant continuous tasks, such as maintaining cycling frequency at 70 RPM. On the other hand, persistent fBm is characterized by increments which are positively correlated in time; in other words, the present trend is more likely to be followed by the same trend rather than the opposite. This tendency puts the system in a state that is dominated by inappropriately low frequency variability at the expense of high-frequency, shorter timescale corrections, as well as by the inability to maintain the mean value constant around 70 RPM. Such a profile clearly points to a system whose stability is disrupted. These findings show that when highly motivated performers are close to the termination point the fluctuation profile closely resembles the one discussed earlier and points to a change in the neuromuscular cooperative processes prior to stop.

Attention focus during a dynamic accumulated effort

To investigate the emergent nature and dynamics of task-related thoughts (TRT) during accumulated effort, 11 participants ran twice on a treadmill at an intensity of 80% of their maximum heart rate until voluntary exhaustion, while self-monitoring and reporting through signs the changes in their thoughts (Figure 4.8). During the first run, the intrinsic dynamics of their thought processes was established. As no participant reported an emergence of task-unrelated thoughts (TUT), only TRT, they were asked during the second run to intentionally maintain TUT and to report back about spontaneous switches from TUT to TRT and

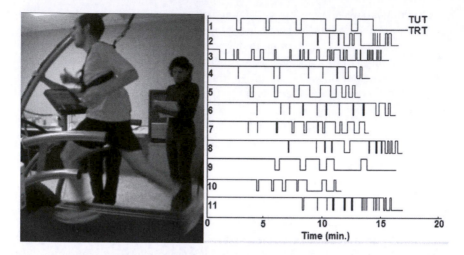

Figure 4.8 A: Treadmill exercise with a participant reporting through signs; B: sample
of 11 individual time series of task-unrelated–task-related thought dynamics.
Starting with the task-unrelated thoughts (TUT) state, one can observe the
switches between TUT and task-related thoughts (TRT). Eventually, the TRT
state becomes the one that precedes the exhaustion point. Numbers on the
left signify participants

vice versa (for more details, see Balagué *et al.* 2012). As can be seen in Figure
4.8B, the results revealed that the intentionally imposed TUT was stable at the
beginning of the exercise but switched spontaneously to TRT with accumulated
effort. Close to voluntary exhaustion the TUT and TRT competed, showing a fully
developed metastability until the final TRT state prevails. In summary, a nonlinear dynamic effect of thought processes (loss of stability of TUT, spontaneous
emergence of TRT, spontaneous switches from TUT to TRT (a metastable dynamical regimen) and, finally, an absolute destabilization of TUT and spontaneous
transition to TRT) during the dynamic exercise was noted until the termination of
effort. This is a further demonstration that intentional systems are subject to
different constellations of peripheral and central constraints (like attention focus)
as exertion and fatigue accumulates.

This results illustrate that performers were not able to impose TUT deliberately
with equal efficiency during the exercise. Rather, the thought states were constrained
by the accumulated effort. The intention and attention focus spontaneously self-
organized into a different, more stable solution, i.e. the TRT state of mind.

Phases of psychobiological integration

In summary, some general traits of nonlinear psychobiological integration during
exercise performed until exhaustion may be discerned from the findings
discussed above. These traits give raise to three effort phases:

- The initial part of the effort is characterized by greater flexibility and stability of the psychobiological integration, as revealed through the dynamics of the kinematic and psychological studied variables. Smaller values of the elbow angle and the RPM fluctuations and their dominantly anti-persistent profile, as well as the higher values of spectral degrees of freedom are noticed on the kinematic level. The ability of performers to maintain the intentionally imposed TUT, which are intrinsically unstable under high exertion rates, and the low probability of finding urges to terminate the exercise illustrate the stability and flexibility that are present on the psychological level.
- The second effort phase is characterized by relative stability at the kinematic level, although the spontaneous, i.e. involuntary, emergence of TRT (such as body monitoring) constitutes the first sign of destabilizing effects of the accumulated effort. Within this interval there is a metastable regimen characterized by switching from TRT to TUT and vice versa, as well as balanced probabilities of urges to terminate and volition to continue the exercise.
- The third phase is characterized on the kinematic level by a reduction in the spectral degrees of freedom of the collective variable (elbow angle in the quasi-static exercise) or by persistent or super-diffusive fBm (RPM in the dynamic exercise) and enhanced fluctuations in both. This profile signifies the formation of low-dimensional competition between two increasingly coherent processes of inhibition and excitation, correlated across the whole neuromuscular axis of performers. On a psychological level these processes are associated with dominance of the urge to terminate, the loss of stability of TUT and stabilization of TRT. The stabilization of TRT points to the loss of flexibility and a lowering of the dimensionality of attentional/thought processes, which corresponds to the lowering of the spectral degrees of freedom on the kinematic level. Eventually, the urge to cancel, being itself a TRT, becomes stabilized close to and at the termination point. Taken together, all this suggests a psychobiological integration that is not fixed, and only at some points creates an association between psychological and biological spaces. Especially when close to the termination point their mutual coupling results in lower dimensionality and a dominant more rigid dynamics.

Implications for the future

As has been shown in the different experiments, the psychobiological integration is highly likely to be nonlinear, soft-assembled and metastable. In this context, exercise-induced effects and control may be explained through the 'self-organization under constraints' paradigm. This generic mechanism would enable biological systems, through their immense behavioural flexibility and constant striving, to adapt to task and environmental demands. The experimental results suggest that a viable way of investigating psychobiological adaptation during exercise would be to study collective variables, which are products of the cooperative, coordinated interactions among component processes. As has been shown, these potential collective variables may be observed at different levels of the human psychobiological continuum. Thus, it would be especially important to study the ways in which these coordinated dynamics are reconfigured on different time scales and also to carry out more elaborate studies of key control parameters, i.e. configurations of constraints that act upon the stability properties of coordinated states.

In this regard, the findings described in this chapter present a challenge for future research and might have important implications for cognitive and physical interventions used to improve performance. Dynamical concepts such as stability, metastability and loss of stability may prove to be important in resolving the extant controversies concerning such interventions and could help to identify suitable strategies for improving performance. While intentions may change the peripheral states (e.g. pacing, etc.), the periphery also seems to constrain the intentions and stability properties of the mind (Balagué *et al.* 2011). Hence, the idea of circular causality, which captures not only interaction but also interdependence, rather than a simple, linear top-down cause–effect relationship between the mind and peripheral systems, seems more plausible and provides further evidence of nonlinearity.

From the perspective developed here it would seem unfruitful to pose the debate in terms of the 'mind over muscle' hypothesis (Marcora and Staiano 2010) or 'muscle over mind'. As has been shown, there appears to be no unique site or process that is responsible for exercise termination. Rather, this event seems to be produced by the destabilization of interactions between a number of components belonging to both central and peripheral subsystems. This interaction is not fixed (as occurs when invariant set points are in charge) but, rather, is task-specific, soft-assembled and therefore flexible, thereby enabling adaptation to the different conditions created in the organism and the environment during the development of fatigue.

A further point of note is that, since the system prior to termination dwells close to the instability point, many contingent and also emergent accidental events (a small increment of discomfort or pain, onset of nausea, dizziness, and so forth), may sufficiently perturb the organization of the already destabilized action system. This, in turn, could trigger exercise termination, i.e. the switch toward the low-activity, resting state, a global minimum of the rugged metastable energy landscape. In this sense, exercise termination is an emergent phenomenon, a consequence of fatigue-induced instability/dissolution of the couplings within the distributed control loops that are responsible for the maintenance of the intended activity. This means that the system flows through its dynamical states controlled by immediate constraints and there is no need for specific peripheral site impairment or a specialized exercise-termination module within the brain that would be fully responsible for controlling and switching off the activity by issuing strict commands to the periphery. Rather, it is sufficient for there to be a distributed neuromuscular network of components that self-organize under constraints into local, transient or, eventually, global energy minimum states. This nonlinear, constraints-based control of exercise flow and termination is also experimentally demonstrable in the hysteresis behaviour of the collective variable with respect to certain physiological constraints (Balagué and Hristovski 2010). Future research emphasizing the task-dependent dynamic formation and dissolution of functional structures within physiological variables may prove to be a viable way of capturing soft-assembling coordination dynamics on that level. Integration of these findings with psychological processes, such as those mentioned in this chapter, could lead to more detailed, formal models of psychobiological integration during exercise.

Questions for students

1. Identify and compare the main characteristics of the linear and nonlinear psychobiological integration models that are mentioned in the text.
2. Name some of the variables included in each of the order parameters studied in the different experiments.
3. Describe, using four different graphs, the nonlinear change produced by the control parameter in the four different order parameters as fatigue develops (Table 4.1).
4. Explain why there is a change in the slope of the spectral density of elbow angle between the first and third part of the quasi-static exercise (Figure 4.3B) and a change in the slope of the spectral density of the RPM between the first and second half of the dynamic exercise (Figure 4.5).
5. Describe and define using the same graph (with exertion time on the horizontal axis), the three phases found in each of the four sets of experimental results.
6. Explain the dynamics of order-parameter variability in the first two experiments (static and dynamic exercise) in terms of psychobiological inhibition/excitation processes. How gravitational pull cooperates with inhibition?
7. Describe the differences between the currently debated models of psychobiological integration and the nonlinear approach to explain fatigue-induced exercise termination.

References

Balagué, N. and Hristovski, R. (2010) Modeling physiological complexity: dynamic integration of the neuromuscular system during quasi-static exercise performed until failure, in J. Wiemayer, A. Baca and M. Lames (eds) *Sportinformatik Gestern, Heute, Morgen: Festschrift zu Ehren von Prof. Dr Jürgen Perl*. Hamburg: Feldhaus, pp. 163–71.

Balagué, N., Hristovski, R. and Aragonés, D. (2011) Rol de la intención en la terminación del ejercicio inducida por la fatiga. Aproximación no-lineal [Role of intention in the fatigue induced exercise termination; nonlinear approach]. *Revista de Psicologia del Deporte*, 20 (2): 505–21 [Spanish].

Balagué, N., Hristovski, R., Aragonés, D. and Tenenbaum, G. (2012) Nonlinear model of attention focus during accumulated effort. *Psychology of Sport and Exercise*, 13: 591–7.

Blackman, R. B. and Tukey, J. W. (1958) *The Measurement of Power Spectra: From the Point of View of Communications Engineering*. New York: Dover.

Cairns, S. P. (2006) Lactic acid and exercise performance. Culprit or friend? *Sports Medicine*, 36: 279–91.

Enoka, R. M. and Duchateau, J. (2008) Muscle fatigue: what, why and how it influences muscle function. *Journal of Physiology*, 586: 11–23.

Fox, M. D., Snyder, A. Z., Vincent, J. L., Corbetta, M., Van Essen, D. C. and Raichle, M. E. (2005) The human brain is intrinsically organized into dynamic, anticorrelated functional networks. *PNAS: Proceedings of the National Academy of Sciences of the USA*, 27: 9673–8.

Gandevia, S. C. (2001) Spinal and supraspinal factors in human muscle fatigue. *Physiological Reviews*, 81: 1725–89.

Haken, H. (1983) *Synergetics. An Introduction*. Heidelberg: Springer.

Haken, H. (2000) *Information and Self-organization. A Macroscopic Approach to Complex Systems*. Heidelberg: Springer.

Hristovski, R. and Balagué, N. (2010) Fatigue-induced spontaneous termination point: nonequilibrium phase transitions and critical behavior in quasi-isometric exertion. *Human Movement Science*, 29: 483–93.

Hristovski, R., Venskaityte, E., Vainoras, A., Balagué, N. and Vázquez, P. (2010) Constraints controlled metastable dynamics of exercise-induced psychobiological adaptation. *Medicina*, 46: 447–53.

Izhikevich, E., Gally, J. A. and Edelman, G. (2004) Spike-timing dynamics of neuronal groups. *Cerebral Cortex*, 14: 933–44.

Kelso, J. A. S. (1995) *Dynamic Patterns. The Self-organisation of Brain and Behavior*. Cambridge, MA: MIT Press.

Kenney, W. L. Wilmore, J. H. and Costill, D. L. (2011) *Physiology of Sport and Exercise* (5th ed.). Champaign, IL: Human Kinetics.

Lambert, E. V., St Clair Gibson, A. and Noakes, T. D. (2005) Complex systems model of fatigue: integrative homeostatic control of peripheral physiological systems during exercise in humans. *British Journal of Sports Medicine*, 39: 52–62.

McKenna, M. J. and Hargreaves, M. (2008) Resolving fatigue mechanisms determining exercise performance: integrative physiology at its finest! *Journal of Applied Physiology*, 104: 286–7.

Marcora, S. (2008) Do we really need a central governor to explain brain regulation of exercise performance? *European Journal of Applied Physiology*, 104: 929–31.

Marcora, S., Staiano, W. and Manning, V. (2009) Mental fatigue impairs physical performance in humans. *Journal of Applied Phisiology*, 106: 857–64.

Marcora, S. M. and Staiano, W. (2010) The limit to exercise tolerance in humans: mind over muscle? *European Journal of Applied Physiology*, 109: 763–70.

Marcora, S. M., Bosio, A. and de Morree, H. M. (2008) Locomotor muscle fatigue increases cardiorespiratory responses and reduces performance during intense cycling exercise independently from metabolic stress. *American Journal of Physiology Regulatory Integrative and Comparative Physiology*, 294: R874–83.

Noakes, T. D., St Clair Gibson, A. and Lambert, E. V. (2005) From catastrophe to complexity: a novel model of integrative central neural regulation of effort and fatigue during exercise in humans. *British Journal of Sports Medicine*, 38: 511–14.

Nybo, L. (2008) Hyperthermia and fatigue. *Journal of Applied Physiology*, 104: 871–8.

Shephard, R. J. (2009) Is it time to retire the 'central governor'? *Sports Medicine*, 39: 709–21.

St Clair Gibson, A. and Noakes, T. D. (2004) Evidence for complex system integration and dynamic neural regulation of skeletal muscle recruitment during exercise in humans. *British Journal of Sports Medicine,* 38, 797–806.

Taylor, J. L., Todd, G. and Gandevia, C. (2006) Evidence for a supraspinal contribution to human muscle fatigue. *Clinical and Experimental Pharmacology and Physiology*, 33: 400–5.

Thompson, R. H., and Swanson, L. W. (2010) Hypothesis-driven structural connectivity analysis supports network over hierarchical model of brain architecture. *Proceedings of the National Academy of Sciences*, 107: 15235–9.

Vaillancourt, D. E. and Newell, K. M. (2003) Aging and the time and frequency structure of force output variability. *Journal of Applied Physiology*, 94: 903–12.

Van Orden, G. C. and Paap, K. R. (1997) Functional neuroimages fail to discover pieces of mind in the parts of the brain. *Philosophy of Science*, 64: 85–94.

Weir, J. P., Beck, T. W., Cramer, J. T. and Housh, T. J. (2006) Is fatigue all in your head? A critical review of the central governor model. *British Journal of Sports Medicine*, 40: 573–86.

Westerblad, H., Allen, D. G. and Lannergren, D. J. (2002) Muscle fatigue: lactic acid or inorganic phosphate the major cause? *News in Physiological Sciences*, 17: 17–21.

Wright R. A. (1996) Brehm's theory of motivation as a model of effort and cardiovascular response, in P. M. Gollwitzer and J. A. Bargh (eds) *The Psychology of Action: Linking Cognition and Motivation to Behavior*. New York: Guilford, pp. 424–53.

Yakovlev, N. N. (1979) *Biochemistry of Sport*. Moscow: Fiskultura i Sport [Russian].

Part 2

Methodologies and techniques for data analyses in investigating complex systems in sport

5 Nonlinear time series methods for analyzing behavioural sequences

Nikita Kuznetsov, Scott Bonnette and Michael A. Riley

This chapter provides an overview of nonlinear analysis methods that quantify the time-dependent characteristics of behavioural sequences. We review the fundamental notions useful for an understanding of these analyses and briefly summarize several frequently used methods. We then describe *sample entropy* (SampEn) in more detail and provide a tutorial example of calculating it. Finally, some relevant factors for the interpretation and design of experiments employing sample entropy are discussed.

The analyses discussed in this chapter quantify the structure of variability in time series. While the utility of using a time series approach is determined by the motivating theoretical questions of a field of study, practically any observable phenomenon can be recorded as a time series. Many disciplines use time series to gain insights into their phenomena of interest. Stock price fluctuations have for a long time puzzled economists (Scheinkman and LeBaron 1989). In psychiatry and psychology, variations in mood over time can provide useful clinical insights into mood disorders (Pincus 2006) and time series methods have led to a conceptualization of self-perception as an emergent property (Delignières *et al.* 2004). Similar analyses provide clues about the structure of the cognitive system by quantifying response time variability (Van Orden *et al.* 2003). Perceptual-motor control has also benefited from the application of time series analyses (Riley and Turvey 2002). We believe that the methods described in this chapter (together with Chapter 7) provide similar insights for sport science.

Dynamics and time series

Sequential dependence

In sport science, the time series we capture will usually have *sequential dependence* – the order of the data points matters. This occurs when the underlying process that generated the data is not random. The position of a player on the pitch at one point in time is influenced by that player's position at some earlier time or by the position of the ball, for example. These dependencies can be strong or weak. Sometimes, when the dependency is strong, we can discern a highly specific, deterministic rule that describes how our measured quantity (the 'output' of the behavioural system under study) varies over time as a function of some inputs and some parameters. This is often not possible, however, and more often we can identify some general properties about how the measurements change over time but not an exact rule. In either case, though, pinpointing the nature of sequential dependence in the data helps us to understand what kinds of laws or constraints shape the behaviour of the system we are studying.

Figure 5.1 shows two artificial time series. Both have means of about zero but they clearly differ visually. The bottom series is more structured, with upward and downward trends, while the top is more erratic and unpredictable. Typical measures of variability, like the standard deviation, just measure the spread of observations around the mean, and do not measure how the time sequence impacts the data. The series' means or standard deviations would not differ.

The more interesting differences between the time series in Figure 5.1 lie in the patterns of change over time (i.e. the *dynamics* of the behaviour). These dynamics are a consequence of the sequential dependence (or lack thereof) of the time series. If you randomly rearranged the order of data points in a time series, the mean and variance would not change but doing this would destroy any dependence among the data points and thus would alter the dynamics. Time-series analyses quantify the dynamics of behaviour. Using a method described later (detrended fluctuation analysis; DFA), it can be shown that the two series evolve over time very differently. The bottom series exhibits a type of sequential dependence termed *1/f scaling* and the data points are correlated with each other over time, whereas the top series lacks this temporal structure and evolves over time randomly (it lacks sequential dependence altogether).

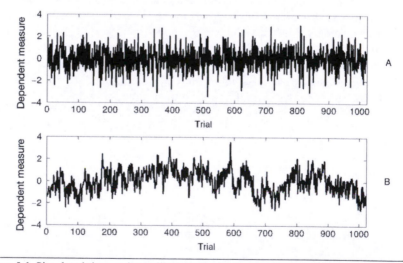

Figure 5.1 Simulated time series to illustrate the distinction between measures of central tendency and measures sensitive to the sequential properties of the time series. Panel A depicts random uncorrelated noise, while Panel B shows 'pink' or 1/f noise where each successive observation is positively correlated with the others

Nonlinearity

There are many kinds of sequential dependence. As noted, one distinction is strength. A system with weak dependence is impacted more strongly by random factors than one with stronger sequential dependence. Another basic distinction is whether the sequential dependence is linear or nonlinear. This is a fundamentally important distinction.[1]

Nonlinear is a term used to describe a type of physical system or mathematical equation for which the 'output' is not directly proportional to the 'input'. Any system, whether it is the movement of an entire football (soccer) team or repeated finger-tapping movements, is assumed to have components or mechanisms responsible for the process (see Carello and Moreno 2005). Linear and nonlinear analyses assume that the components of a system interact in fundamentally different ways. For a linear system, the components interact additively, so their behaviour adds up to the system's behaviour – the whole is the sum of its parts. For nonlinear systems, the components interact multiplicatively rather than just additively, which is why the output is disproportional to the input and the whole can differ from the sum of its parts. Nonlinearity is more general than linearity. A practical implication of this is that nonlinear time-series analyses can work if the system under study is linear but linear time series analyses may not work for studying nonlinear systems. This is a reason to strongly prefer nonlinear time series analyses over linear. (This does not imply, however, that linear methods are not useful or that they are never preferred. Many linear methods, such as spectral analysis, have well-developed mathematical foundations that are not yet available for some nonlinear methods, for example.)

Dynamical systems

Nonlinear time-series analyses stem from a field of mathematics known as *nonlinear dynamical systems*. For good introductions to the topic see Kaplan and Glass (1995) and Kantz and Schreiber (2004). Dynamical systems are simply those systems whose states change over time. To better appreciate nonlinear time-series methods, it is useful to understand a few basic concepts of dynamical systems.

The mathematical study of dynamical systems usually employs well-known equations rather than empirical data. An example is the *Lorenz system*, which is used to model processes of heat transfer known as thermal convection, given by:

$$\dot{x} = \sigma(y - x)$$
$$\dot{y} = x(\rho - z) - y \qquad (1)$$
$$\dot{z} = xy - \beta z.$$

The Lorenz system has three state variables (x, y and z) and three parameters (σ, ρ and β). The values of the state variables change over time according to equation 1. The dot over the variables on the left side of the equal sign signifies change over time in the variable (i.e. the derivative of the variable) and the terms on the right-hand side specify the exact rule according to which this change occurs. Although we have written three separate equations (one for each state variable), the Lorenz system is considered to be a unified system because the state variables are coupled to each other – the equation for each state variable contains at least one of the other state variables, meaning that the evolution of each state variable depends on that of the others. We can simulate these equations and plot time series of each state variable (Figure 5.2) but none of those individual time series fully characterizes the total behaviour of the system. The proper way to visualize the system is a plot of the phase space – a three-dimensional (in this case) space whose coordinates are the state variables *x*, *y* and *z*.

A graph of the phase space (Figure 5.2, left) shows that the Lorenz system gravitates toward certain regions and never enters others; the trajectory is drawn to a subset of the phase space. This subset is called an *attractor* and it is the solution to the underlying equations. The attractor is termed such because whatever the initial values of the state variables, the trajectory will eventually be drawn to the attractor. The Lorenz attractor is called a 'strange' attractor because the Lorenz system exhibits *deterministic chaos* – a small change in initial conditions or a small perturbation will become amplified so that the long-term behaviour of the system is unpredictable, even though there is no element of actual randomness (the system is completely deterministic but unstable). Trajectories in the phase space never actually cross each other, because of a mathematical rule known as the *uniqueness theorem* (differential equations must have unique solutions; if the trajectories crossed, it would mean two solutions existed at once).

How does this relate to using nonlinear time series analyses on behavioural sequences? Usually, we do not know the underlying equations that govern the behavioural sequences that we analyze. Nor do we usually even know what the

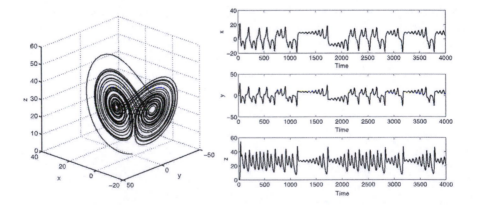

Figure 5.2 The phase space plot of the Lorenz attractor; we used the parameters $\rho = 10$, $\sigma = 28$ and $\beta = 8/3$ and initial conditions of $x = 1$, $y = 1$, $z = 1$

state variables are, or what the attractor may look like. Presumably, the variables that we can measure are relevant state variables but, even then, we are left with a one-dimensional view of a potentially high-dimensional system. This one-dimensional signal may contain distortions that result from projecting the data from a higher-dimensional space to the single dimension of the measured variable (just like a two-dimensional map of the three-dimensional Earth contains distortions in the shape and size of land masses). However, thanks to another mathematical theorem called the *embedding theorem* (Takens 1981; also see Webber and Zbilut 2005), it turns out that measuring a single-state variable (i.e. a single time series) is sufficient to allow us to understand the underlying dynamics of the system. Essentially, this theorem permits us to reconstruct a phase space that preserves the dynamical properties of the system and that is free of projection distortions, provided that the underlying system is nonlinear (a safe assumption in practice) and the state variables are coupled. *Phase-space reconstruction* (Abarbanel 1996) is a first step for several nonlinear methods, such as recurrence quantification analysis (RQA). Webber and Zbilut (2005) and Pellecchia and Shockley (2005) discuss phase-space reconstruction extensively in the context of RQA, so we do not go into more detail here.

Analyzing real-world data is very different than analyzing idealized mathematical signals. Real data usually contain measurement noise, can be non-stationary and are frequently measured over a brief time. Some consequences of these properties are discussed below.

Important properties of time series

There are several properties of a time series that influence how it should be analyzed. We discuss three of these in the following paragraphs. The experimenter has direct control over the first two, while the other sometimes can be manipulated by statistical procedures. All three properties entail special nuances in data treatment and analysis, because they can influence the results of nonlinear time-series analysis, sometimes considerably, depending on both the system and the particular analysis.

The first property is the *sampling rate*. This is simply the rate at which observations are recorded by the researcher. The sampling rate can be as many as thousands of observations per second or as few as a single observation per day or less. For most of the analyses discussed in this chapter, choosing an appropriate sample rate is critical for obtaining valid results. A sampling rate that is too low will not provide enough information about a behaviour. However, a sampling rate that is too high can lead to an oversaturation of data points (Abarbanel 1996); rather than providing new information about the system under study, an oversampled time series gives the illusion of greater sequential dependence than might be present. There are clear criteria for sampling frequency selection for linear systems (e.g. the Nyquist sampling theorem) but nonlinear systems do not necessarily follow the same guidelines. One should be careful to choose a sampling rate that does not oversample the phenomenon of interest and should tailor sampling frequency to the guiding questions of the study and pragmatic considerations (see Chapter 2 of Kantz and Schreiber 2004). For example, it is often not necessary to sample the position of a player in the game every 100 milliseconds but it may be necessary if a very detailed analysis of a single event is desired (e.g. attacker defender interaction during an attack in football).

A second property is the *time series length*. Generally, results are more accurate with a large number of data points (N). Typically the minimum N ranges from about 100 to 1,000, depending on the analysis. This requirement exists because many techniques are derived from methods that assume mathematically perfect time series of infinite length. Obviously, the challenge for the experimenter lies in balancing real-world practicality with the need to obtain as large an N as possible. A temptation is to simply increase the sampling rate to increase N; however, because of the oversaturation problem noted above, this is often not a valid solution.

A third property is *stationarity*. Stationarity is present when the moments of the distribution of the data are independent of time (Kaplan and Glass 1995). A more practical definition of stationarity is that the parameters of the measured system remain constant over the duration of the measurement (Kantz and Schreiber 2004). Most time-series analysis methods assume stationarity and will yield erroneous results if used on non-stationary data. It is often practically impossible to positively establish that a given time series is stationary with absolute certainty but, for most purposes, it is sufficient to check for stationarity of the mean (first moment) and variance (second moment) because these are assumed by many analyses. A stationary time series has a stable mean and variance, while those quantities change over time for a non-stationary time series (see Figure 7.2 in Chapter 7). An easy method to investigate a time series' stationarity is to divide the series into several non-overlapping windows. If the means and variances of each window are statistically different, it is likely the series is non-stationary. Sometimes it is possible to make a time series stationary by *differencing* (subtracting each data point from the subsequent value) or by fitting a line or polynomial function and subtracting the fitted trends from the data (Kantz and Schreiber 2004). However, this is often not advisable – you may discard important information. In the case of non-stationary data, it is advisable to use a method that does not assume stationarity, such as RQA (Riley *et al.* 1999; Webber and Zbilut 1994, 1996, 2005).

The variety of nonlinear measures

In the following sections we briefly review several methods that have been developed for examining the time-dependent properties of behavioural time series. Many other methods exist and the studies presented in each category merely scratch the surface of the current literature and do not constitute the full scope of the work done using these techniques.

Recurrence quantification analysis

Recurrence plots were developed by Eckmann *et al.* (1987). Recurrence plots capitalize on the property of dynamical systems to repeat over time (i.e. to recur). They allow you to visualize how the states of dynamical systems evolve using a two-dimensional plot and can reveal hidden patterns in complex and irregular-looking data sets (Marwan *et al.* 2007). Webber and Zbilut (Webber 1991; Webber and Zbilut 1994, 1996) developed RQA as a way of objectively quantifying the visual features of recurrence plots. RQA allows one to measure (with corresponding RQA measures in parentheses): how often the system visits the same state (recurrence rate); how often the same sequences of states repeat (determinism); how long are the repeating segments (meanline and maxline); how many different patterns of repeated sequences are there (entropy); how long the time series remains in the same state (laminarity and trapping time); and whether the time series is stationary (trend). RQA is often suitable for noisy, brief, and non-stationary time series, but presents the challenge of having to identify values of a number of input variables. Webber and Zbilut (2005) provided an excellent tutorial on RQA.

RQA has been successfully applied in a variety of settings from astrophysics to psychology. There are few applications in sport science so far. One study by Cotuk and Yavuz (2007) used RQA to examine the changes in the dynamics of successive passes in football games from the 2006 World Championship as an indication of play organization of the teams.

Fractal measures

Fractal methods have been widely used for investigating dynamical systems in physiology, movement science, psychology and other disciplines (e.g. Bassingthwaighte *et al.* 1994; Holden 2005; Liebovitch 1998). Most of these methods describe how a measure of variability scales with sample size (i.e. the amount of data over which the measure is computed). Many people are familiar with visual images of fractals that repeat geometric patterns (i.e. they are self-similar) across different spatial scales. Fractal signals are also self-similar across scales – this is what is meant by 'variability scales with sample size' – but, in this case, we refer to *time scales* rather than spatial scales and the self-similarity is statistical rather than exact. The various fractal analyses usually provide a single measure, the *scaling exponent*, which describes the relation between the measure of variability and time scale. Brown and Liebovitch (2010) provide a good introduction to practical uses of fractal methods and Chapter 7 discusses the closely related concept of long-range correlations.

There are many kinds of fractal analyses, each with unique procedures and assumptions about the data being analyzed (Eke *et al.* 2000; Gao *et al.* 2006). Spectral analysis (see Chapter 7) – a linear method – can be used to measure fractal scaling in a time series because fractals exhibit what is termed a $1/f$ power spectrum wherein spectral power scales inversely with frequency, f. In this case, the scaling exponent is the slope of a linear fit (in log–log coordinates) of the power spectrum. For certain types of data, spectral analysis can be a preferred method but it places limiting assumptions on the data (particularly stationarity).

A robust (especially with regard to non-stationarity) and widely used fractal method is DFA (Peng *et al.* 1994). DFA yields a scaling exponent, α, which describes how a variability measure called the *detrended fluctuation function* scales with the size of a time window over which it is computed. Like scaling exponents derived from other fractal analyses, α can be used to classify the type of sequential dependence in a time series. For α = 0.5, the time series lacks sequential dependence; the data are random white noise and each point is independent of the others. For α = 1.0, the time series possesses sequential dependence; the data are correlated. The particular sequential dependence indicated by this α value is *pink noise*, which is another term for $1/f$ noise. For α = 1.5, the data are more strongly structured *brown noise*.

DFA and related fractal methods have been frequently used to study motor control, where changes in α may indicate changes in neuromuscular control, such as those that result from learning. One recent study, for example, showed that people's hand movements become more pink (closer to ideal $1/f$ noise) with practice on a Fitts' law task (Wijnants *et al.* 2009).

Approximate entropy

Entropy is a measure of the amount of disorder in a system. To get an intuitive feel for the meaning of the original usage of the concept of entropy (from statistical mechanics), imagine a room with a bottle of perfume in the middle. There is no draft or exchange of air with the outside world – the room is a closed system. In the initial state, the molecules of the perfume are all concentrated in the bottle and therefore are in a state of low entropy (high order) with respect to the total positions that the room allows them to take. Low entropy reflects the fact that the distribution of perfume molecules is not uniform across the room such that one particular location contains a disproportionally large quantity of molecules. When the bottle is opened, the perfume molecules spread in the room and will fill the whole room uniformly given enough time. In this process, the perfume molecules reach a state of high entropy (high disorder), wherein all parts of the room have the same probability of housing perfume molecules.[2]

There are similar notions about the amount of 'disorder' in observed measurements. This sense of entropy is rooted in information theory (Schneider and Sagan 2005). The information-theoretical definition of entropy (Kolmogorov–Sinai entropy; KS) indexes the predictability of a time series (Gao *et al.* 2007). Entropy in this case is related to the following question: if we measure a value of a system (a value in a time series) at a particular moment in time, how much can we predict about the next state of the system (Kantz and Schreiber 1994) or how much information is generated about the system with each measurement? For deterministic periodic systems, prediction of future states is easy – we only need to know a few points to be able to perfectly predict their evolution; these systems have low entropy. For example, knowing only one cycle of a sine wave is enough to fully describe the underlying system that produced it (Gao *et al.* 2007). Things become more interesting when irregularity and randomness appear because the rate of information obtained about the system underlying these time series increases with each measurement. Such systems have higher entropy.

Pincus (1991) introduced *approximate entropy* (ApEn) with the intention of providing a practical method of calculating the regularity or repeatability of relatively short and noisy empirical time series. This measure is conceptually related to KS entropy but KS entropy requires really large N to be accurate. The logic of ApEn is simple: what is the average probability that a sequence of $m + 1$ data points finds a match in the time series given that it has already found a match for m data points? (see Pincus 1991, for a mathematical definition). Matches do not have to be exact; matching sequences are identified within a tolerance defined by r. The probability of finding matches is expressed as a negative logarithm to yield the ApEn value. If ApEn is closer to zero, the signal is very regular, predictable, and less complex – the next observation can be readily predicted from the previous m observations. If ApEn is high (closer to two), the signal is more unpredictable, random and, consequently, more complex. We suggest Pincus and Goldberger (1994) for a detailed step-by-step visual introduction to ApEn.

ApEn has been applied to cardiovascular dynamics (Pincus and Viscarello 1992; Tulppo *et al.* 2001), postural control (Cavanaugh *et al.* 2005), isometric force production (Slifkin and Newell 1999) and psychological time series (Bauer *et al.* 2011; Yeragani *et al.* 2003). A general finding from the application of this and other measures of complexity to the cardiovascular system is that less-healthy systems show more regular, less-complex dynamics (lower ApEn). In the context of cardiac physiology, Pincus (1994, 2006) hypothesized that a decrease in complexity corresponds to a breakdown of communication between the subsystems participating in cardiovascular control. Conversely, increased complexity (higher ApEn) suggests greater coupling between the subsystems and fast and efficient communication. This hypothesis has been supported using numerical simulations from a variety of different types of mathematical models (Pincus 1994). These and similar observations using DFA have led to a general perspective (Goldberger *et al.* 2002) that associates health with complex fluctuations in physiological systems and pathology with a loss of complexity. However, the pattern of changes in complexity with disease does not always follow this trend (Vaillancourt and Newell 2002).

ApEn has also been applied to behavioural time series. Cavanaugh *et al.* (2005) found that the regularity of centre of pressure (COP) fluctuations exhibited by healthy young adults decreased with the removal of sensory information. Following Pincus (1994), they interpreted the decrease in complexity as an indication of restriction of the interactions among components of the postural system. Cavanaugh *et al.* (2005) also reported that athletes, following concussion, have more regular sway compared with their own preinjury baseline values. In terms of recovery rates from concussion, Cavanaugh *et al.* (2006) found that, while the traditional measure of postural stability (equilibrium score) returned to preinjury levels within three to four days, ApEn remained lower than the baseline level beyond this period. The major implication is that the recovery is not as fast as has been previously thought and that these athletes should not be allowed to return to sport participation so soon.

Despite its success, ApEn is susceptible to some shortcomings related to the specifics of the calculation of the conditional probabilities of repeating patterns (Richman and Moorman 2000). The original ApEn algorithm requires that each pattern of length m and $m + 1$ (called template vectors) find at least one match in the time series, because the algorithm involves taking a logarithm and the log of 0 is undefined. The algorithm therefore counts self-matches in the estimates of conditional probability to make sure that at least one match is present. This means that ApEn is a biased statistic and does not estimate the population value of entropy well, especially for short time series. To alleviate the bias, Richman and Moorman introduced an improved algorithm called *sample entropy*, SampEn (described in detail below), which does not count self-matches and uses a slightly different procedure to quantify regularity of the time series. Additionally, ApEn is more affected by measurement noise and sampling frequency than SampEn (Rhea *et al.* 2011). Practically, this means that SampEn may be more reliable than ApEn when comparing across studies that use different equipment or sampling rates. Because of these limitations of ApEn, we focus on SampEn as a measure of complexity.

Sample entropy

SampEn also quantifies signal regularity and is conceptually similar to ApEn. Here, we demonstrate the SampEn calculations based on the description provided by Richman and Moorman (2000). It is possible to do these calculations using Microsoft Excel® but Matlab® (MathWorks Inc.) is better because it is well suited for working with vectors. The Excel and Matlab files used in the example are posted online at http://homepages.uc.edu/~rileym/pmdlab/nonlinear/index.html. The sample code is for illustration purposes only and we encourage you to use the more robust code by Lake, Moorman and Hanqing available on PhysioNet (www.physionet.org) for data analysis.

Assume that we continuously sampled a time series from a system of interest. A plot of these data (Figure 5.3A) shows that they are relatively stationary (the mean is about 5 and the variance does not change drastically over the measurement period). The presence of stationarity is an important requirement for SampEn (Govindan *et al.* 2007). Our example data series is [0, 4, 8, 0, 4, 2, 0, 10, 8, 10, 7, 2, 3, 6, 1, 6, 7, 9, 0, 10, 8, 7, 4, 1, 8, 5, 9, 8, 2].

We first define all possible vectors of length $m = 2$ from the original $N = 30$ time series. A vector in this case is simply an array of numbers taken from the original time series. We combine two consecutive measurements into a vector and then move ahead one point to define the next two-element vector until the last data point is reached. These vectors are fundamental to the algorithm because all other calculations are based on them. Following the algorithm for SampEn

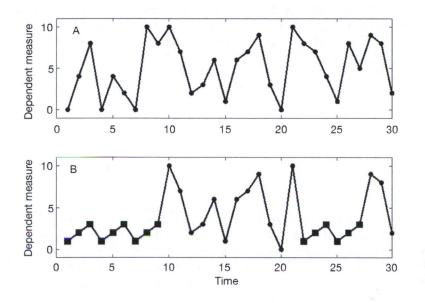

Figure 5.3 Panel A shows the simulated time series used in the tutorial calculation of SampEn; panel B shows the same time series with added patterns of [1, 2, 3] values (shown in squares) to increase the regularity of the time series (see text for details)

introduced by Richman and Moorman (2000), the total number of vectors will be equal to $N-m$; in this case, it is 28. The vectors are (where i stands for the vector number):

$$X_{m=2} (i = 1) = [0, 4],$$
$$X_{m=2} (i = 2) = [4, 8],$$
$$X_{m=2} (i = 3) = [8, 0],$$
$$X_{m=2} (i = 4) = [0, 4],$$
$$X_{m=2} (i = 5) = [4, 2],$$
$$X_{m=2} (i = 6) = [2, 0],$$
$$X_{m=2} (i = 7) = [0, 10],$$
$$\dots$$
$$X_{m=2} (i = 28) = [9, 8].$$

Now we designate one vector as a template with which all other vectors are compared. We will take $X_{m=2}$ ($i = 1$) as a template and find the number of other vectors whose respective elements (i.e. values in the time series) differ from the template by an amount less than the matching threshold parameter r. For this example, we set $r = 1$. We exclude self-matches; they do not add any new information about the regularity of the vectors extracted from the time series (self-matches are counted in ApEn). The calculation below applies to the first vector $X_{m=2}$ ($i = 1$) but the procedure is exactly identical for all other vectors:

$$X_{m=2} \ (i = 1) - X_{m=2} \ (i = 2) = [-4, -4],$$
$$X_{m=2} \ (i = 1) - X_{m=2} \ (i = 3) = [-8, 4],$$
$$X_{m=2} \ (i = 1) - X_{m=2} \ (i = 4) = [0, 0],$$
$$X_{m=2} \ (i = 1) - X_{m=2} \ (i = 5) = [-4, 2],$$
$$X_{m=2} \ (i = 1) - X_{m=2} \ (i = 6) = [-2, 4],$$
$$X_{m=2} \ (i = 1) - X_{m=2} \ (i = 7) = [0, -6],$$

$$\ldots$$

$$X_{m=2} \ (i = 1) - X_{m=2} \ (i = 28) = [-9, -4].$$

Out of all possible 27 comparisons, only one vector $X_{m=2}$ ($i = 4$) is within $r = 1$ from the template vector $X_{m=2}$ ($i = 1$). We record that fact as a match for this particular vector i of length $m = 2$:$\mathrm{MATCH}_{i=1}{}^{m=2} = 1$. We then calculate the probability of having a matching vector for our template by dividing the number of observed matches by the number of possible matches:

$$B_{i=1}{}^{m=2}(r) = \mathrm{MATCH}_{i=1}{}^{m=2}/(N-m-1) = 1/27 = 0.037.$$

We repeat these steps for all vectors (i from 1 to 28) and find the average probability of finding a matching vector $B^{m=2}(r)$ for vectors of length $m = 2$ in the whole time series:

$$B^m(r) = \mathrm{sum}(B_{i=1:27}{}^{m=2}(r))/(N-m).$$

For this particular time series, $B^{m=2}(r) = 0.00793651$ represents the probability of finding a vector of length $m = 2$ that matches the template vector within the radius r in the time series.

   We then repeat these steps for vector length $m+1$ to find the probability of finding matching vectors of length 3. This quantity is exactly equal to $B^{m=3}$ as defined above but, in the literature, it is sometimes referred to as $A^m(r)$. In the case of this time series, $A^m(r) = 0.00284903$.

   We then convert the probabilities of observing recurrences of vectors of length m and $m+1$ into the numbers of actual recurrences denoted by B and A for $B^m(r)$ and $A^m(r)$, respectively. Using the formula provided by Richman and Moorman (2000):

$$B = [((N-m-1) \times (N-m))/2] \times B^m(r)$$
$$A = [((N-m-1) \times (N-m))/2] \times A^m(r).$$

This calculation is also warranted because simply calculating all possible matches of between the vectors overestimates the number of real matches. For example, vector 1 may be recurrent with vector 2 and the algorithm would automatically count the match of vector 2 with vector 1, as well thus introducing redundancy. This formula removes the redundancy – it effectively forces only forward matches to be counted.

We then find the ratio between the number of matches of $m+1$ length ($A^m(r)$) and the number of matches of length m ($B^m(r)$). The ratio of A to B is the conditional probability that two sequences within a tolerance r for m points remain within r of each other at the next point (Richman and Moorman 2000, p. 2042). We take the negative natural logarithm (ln) of this ratio to make the final value positive, since number of matches of length $m+1$ will always be less than the number of matches of length m. If the A is exactly the same as B, then we have a limiting case in which the SampEn of the system is 0. As the time series becomes less predictable, the number of $m+1$ matches becomes smaller, making the ratio closer to 0 while the $-$ln of the ratio increases. The SampEn of our sample data time series is thus:

$$SampEn(m,r,N) = -\ln(A/B) = -\ln(1/15) = 1.0986$$

This rather high SampEn value suggests the time series has few repeatable patterns that remain close to one another. This is not surprising because these data were actually generated using uncorrelated samples from a Gaussian distribution. The lowest non-zero SampEn value is $[(N-m-1)*(N-m)]/2$ and the maximum value is $\ln(N-m)+\ln(N-m-1)-\ln(2)$ (Richman and Moorman 2000).

To gain additional intuitions about what SampEn measures, we deliberately increased the degree of predictability of the measurements by introducing sequences of values [1, 2, 3] in the early and late parts of the time series (Figure 5.3B). After performing the calculation described above, we find that SampEn is 0.559 – a lower value than one for the original time series.

It is always possible to get a number for SampEn. It is up to the researcher to make sense of the results. In general, the interpretation is easier if one has a good intuitive feel for the structure in the data, which can be enhanced by always inspecting a plot of the data.

Empirical considerations for using SampEn

Parameter selection

Typical parameter settings are $m = 1$ or 2 and r between 0.1 and 0.25 of the standard deviation of the time series (Pincus and Goldberger 1994). However, there are more involved selection criteria that rely on the calculation of autoregression parameters of the time series (Lake *et al.* 2002). Alternatively, Ramdani *et al.* (2009) proposed to estimate m by plotting median SampEn values for the time series as a function of different values of r. The m value at which the SampEn-r curves become similar should be selected. They also recommended selecting r based on estimates of SampEn relative error in entropy estimation (Richman and Moorman 2000). The r value at which relative error is minimal should be chosen for the analysis. One thing to keep in mind is that these parameters should be kept constant between all compared conditions once they are selected (Pincus 1991). A practical piece of advice is to perform the analysis with a range of different r values to make sure that the results are not just an artefact of parameter selection.

Data length

The appropriate length of the time series for regularity classification depends on the quality of the measurements. In some cases, signals as short as 60 points may work (Pincus 2006). Richman and Moorman (2000) suggested using time series of the order of 100 to 20,000 data points.

There are situations when the experimenter expects that the lengths of time series will naturally differ across conditions because of natural differences in the durations of measured behaviour. For example, one may be interested in the complexity of the attacker's movement trajectory between successful and unsuccessful attacker–defender situations. The duration of the measured time series will differ from one behavioural sequence to another, owing to a host of factors. Despite the fact that length of the time series may distort the results of SampEn, it is still possible to compare the regularity across these qualitatively similar conditions. But to minimize the effects of data length it is advisable to standardize the length of the time series to some reasonable value (e.g. average length of all recorded time series).[3] In other situations, it may not be possible to use the same strategy, especially when the behaviour of interest qualitatively changes as a function of measurement length. For example, comparing the complexity of heart rate between a four-minute and a ten-minute practice period is not appropriate because the players may be using different strategies for conserving energy between the two.

Outliers

SampEn is not very susceptible to singular outliers. However, one way outliers may affect estimation of SampEn is by biasing the value of r. A typical suggestion is to set r as a percentage of the standard deviation of the series (e.g. 10–25%). However, the standard deviation (SD) is likely to be inflated owing to outliers, leading to an increase in r and a consequent decrease in SampEn. One can remove outliers if appropriate or use the median instead of the mean for the SD calculation.

Non-stationarity

SampEn is designed to work with stationary data and it is likely to malfunction when strong non-stationarity is present. Positively establishing stationarity is tricky in nonlinear systems (Kantz and Schreiber 2004). One practical solution is to use RQA to check for stationarity prior to SampEn analysis using the trend parameter. As an example of poor applicability of SampEn to non-stationary signals, we take the results of Rhea *et al.* (2011), who showed that SampEn of non-differenced COP position data decreased with faster sampling rate whereas differenced, stationary COP signals were not subject to this artefact. Ramdani *et al.* (2009) showed that SampEn discriminated between standing with eyes open compared with closed only when analyzing the differenced (stationary) COP. Of course, differencing removes non-stationarity but it should only be done if the differenced signal is theoretically meaningful as in the case of postural control (Delignières *et al.* 2011).

Long-range correlations

A time series has long-range correlations when the autocorrelation function decays exponentially slowly as a function of time lag (Diniz *et al.* 2011). This is typical of fractal processes described earlier and in Chapter 7. The presence of long-range correlations reduces estimates of system complexity provided by SampEn, potentially biasing the estimate (Govindan *et al.* 2007; Richman and Moorman 2000). SampEn assumes that there are only significant lag-1 autocorrelations because the template vectors are created from consecutive values from the time series. If there are correlations, then the template vectors need to be defined from non-consecutive values (e.g. take every fifth value) to minimize the correlations between the template vectors (Govindan *et al.* 2007). However, for truly long-range correlated signals it is impossible to find an appropriate lag for creating the vectors, so Govindan *et al.* (2007) also suggested differencing the time series and conducting the analysis on the increments.

Periodic data

The method proposed by Govindan *et al.* (2007) will be useful for periodic, continuously sampled data such as breathing and gait kinematics. In such cases, it is still possible to use SampEn but now we need to introduce a delay into the definition of the template vectors. Another possibility is to difference the data as suggested above (Bruce 1996) or define the events of interest and do the analysis on the differences between these events along the time or magnitude dimensions. One apparent disadvantage of increasing the delay time for vector embedding is a reduction in the number of template vectors.

Sampling rate

Time series collected using *A/D* converters are digitized versions of the recorded continuous processes. When the resolution of the *A/D* converter (or any other measurement procedure) is not fine enough to capture the continuous dynamics of the phenomenon of interest, SampEn of the system will become an ordinal variable (Stevens 1946). Consider the time series of COP velocity presented in the left panel of Figure 5.4. This time series was obtained by differencing the COP recorded from a person standing on a force plate sampled at 100 Hz for three

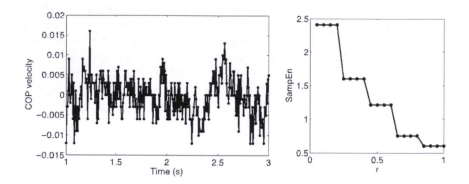

Figure 5.4 Illustration of the digitization (quantization) effect on the SampEn calculation

seconds. There is a clear discretization effect such that the values of the velocity vary between a limited number of states (especially –0.006, 0.003, 0.004, and 0) – this is also known as quantization error. In such cases, entropy does not change continuously with r. To illustrate this, we calculated SampEn as a function of r varying between 0.05 and 1 in steps of 0.05 and plotted the SampEn–r curve in the right-hand panel of Figure 5.4. As expected, increasing the radius decreases SampEn but there are also apparent plateaus of constant entropy. The effect of discretization seems to be more apparent in short time series. Plateaus and discontinuity in the entropy estimates on SampEn–r plots make SampEn an ordinal-dependent variable, with the implication that only non-parametric statistics should be used for data analysis. Therefore, we recommend examining how SampEn changes as a function of r in a representative subset of the data before doing the statistical analysis to establish whether parametric or non-parametric statistics should be used. If SampEn changes continuously with r for all experimental time series, then parametric statistics are appropriate.

Filtering

Filtering usually makes the time series more regular so it will lower SampEn. As long as all conditions are filtered similarly, this should not affect the overall pattern of results within a study. But differences in the filtering procedures need to be considered when making comparisons across studies (Rhea *et al.* 2011). In general, a good practice is to filter the signal as little as possible because excessive filtering may remove the legitimate aspects of the dynamics in the time series instead of measurement artefacts (Abarbanel 1996).

Implications for sport science and conclusions

The dynamical systems approach and the time-series analyses described in this chapter can potentially provide useful information about the phenomena of interest to sport scientists beyond that of the standard measures of central tendency and variability. Time-series measures take into consideration time-dependent properties of the data and therefore are sensitive to changes in evolution of the time series. Our hope is that this will allow researchers to develop more sensitive measures of performance, more efficient methods of learning new skills and more effective treatment evaluation protocols for injuries. Measures of signal complexity such as SampEn are especially promising because they can be readily applied to short and noisy sequences of data that are typical of sport science.

Questions for students

1. How can nonlinear measures be applied in such a way so as provide supplemental information to the questions previously addressed by traditional measures (mean, SD)?
2. What kinds of questions do you wish to ask about your system of interest? This will constrain the choice of analysis method.
3. Does your measurement protocol permit collection of a sufficiently long time series?
4. Can you ground the results of nonlinear time series analysis in some mechanistic understanding or model of your system of interest?
5. Do your data meet the assumptions of your preferred analysis method?
6. How do you make empirical predictions based on dynamical system models or time series methods?

Acknowledgements

Supported by NSF grant BCS 0926662.

Notes

1   Standard statistical quantities such as mean and variance derive from a linear perspective on how the natural world works. For this reason these are sometimes (e.g. Harbourne and Stergiou 2009) referred to as 'linear measures' and this term is used to distinguish them from other methods of analysis. This is a valid distinction when comparing those quantities to the kinds of nonlinear methods featured later in this chapter. A more accurate and fundamental distinction is that only time series methods are sensitive to sequential dependence. Moreover, there are both linear (e.g. autocorrelation and spectral analysis; see Chapter 7) and nonlinear (e.g. DFA and many others described later) time-series analyses; thus, labelling those statistical quantities as 'linear' does not accurately distinguish them.

2   Note that 'order' and 'disorder' have somewhat counterintuitive meanings in this context provided by statistical mechanics. Disorder is tantamount to uniformity and order to non-uniformity. When the perfume is in the bottle, the molecules are all concentrated in that location rather than dispersed evenly across the room, as is the case after the bottle has been opened and the perfume has uniformly filled the room.

In the latter case, individual perfume molecules could swap locations in the room without creating a change in the overall system, while that is not true when the molecules are enclosed in the bottle.

3   For example, in Matlab 'normData = spline(1:length(data),data,linspace(1,length (data),100))'; will turn a time series of any N into one with a length of 100 points while preserving the overall pattern of the observations.

References

Abarbanel, H. D. I. (1996) *Analysis of Observed Chaotic Data*. New York: Springer.

Bassingthwaighte, J. B., Liebovitch, L. S. and West, B. J. (1994) *Fractal Physiology*. New York: Oxford University Press.

Bauer, M., Glenn, T., Alda, M., Grof, P., Sagduyu, K., Bauer, R., Lewitzka, U. and Whybrow, P. C. (2011) Comparison of pre-episode and pre-remission states using mood ratings from patients with bipolar disorder. *Pharmacopsychiatry*, 44: S49–53.

Brown, C. and Liebovitch, L. (2010) *Fractal Analysis*. Los Angeles, CA: Sage.

Bruce, E. N. (1996) Measures of respiratory pattern variability, in M. C. K. Khoo (ed.) *Bioengineering Approaches to Pulmonary Physiology and Medicine*. New York: Plenum, pp. 149–59.

Carello, C. and Moreno, M. (2005) Why nonlinear methods? in M. A. Riley and G. C. Van Orden (eds) *Tutorials in Contemporary Nonlinear Methods for Behavioral Scientists Web Book*. Arlington, VA: National Science Foundation, pp. 1–25. Available online at www.nsf.gov/sbe/bcs/pac/nmbs/nmbs.jsp (accessed 6 June 2013).

Cavanaugh, J. T., Guskiewicz, K. M. and Stergiou, N. (2005) A nonlinear dynamic approach for evaluating postural control: new directions for the management of sport-related cerebral concussion. *Sports Medicine*, 35: 935–50.

Cavanaugh, J. T., Guskiewicz, K. M., Giuliani, C., Marshall, S., Mercer, V. S. and Stergiou, N. (2006) Recovery of postural control after cerebral concussion: new insights using approximate entropy. *Journal of Athletic Training*, 41: 305–13.

Cotuk, B. and Yavuz, E. (2007) Recurrence plot analysis of successive passing sequences in 2006 World Championship. *Journal of Sports Science and Medicine*, 6 (Suppl 10): 4. Available online at www.aemef.org/turquia_2007.pdf (accessed 6 June 2013).

Delignières, D., Fortes, M. and Ninot, G. (2004) The fractal dynamics of self-esteem and physical self. *Nonlinear Dynamics in Psychology and Life Sciences*, 8: 479–510.

Delignières, D., Torre, K. and Bernard, P. L. (2011) Interest of velocity variability and maximal velocity for characterizing center-of-pressure fluctuations. *Science and Motricité*, 74: 31–7.

Diniz, A., Wijnants, M. L., Torre, K., Barreiros, J., Crato, N., Bosman, A. M. T., Hasselman, F., Cox, R. F. A., Van Orden, G. C. and Delignières, D. (2011) Contemporary theories of $1/f$ noise in motor control. *Human Movement Science*, 30: 889–905.

Eckmann, J.-P., Kamphorst, S. O., and Ruelle, D. (1987) Recurrence plots of dynamical systems. *Europhysics Letters*, 4: 973–7.

Eke, A., Herman, P., Bassingthwaighte, J. B., Raymound, G. M., Percival, D. B., Cannon, M., Balla, I. and Ikrenyi, C. (2000) Physiological time series: distinguishing fractal noises from motions. *European Journal of Physiology*, 439: 403–15.

Gao, J., Hu, J., Tung, W.-W., Cao, Y., Sarshar, N., and Roychowdhury, V. P. (2006) Assessment of long-range correlation in time series: how to avoid pitfalls. *Physical Review E, Statistical, Nonlinear, and Soft Matter Physics*, 73 (1 Pt 2): 016117.

Gao, J., Cao, Y., Tung, W-.W. and Hu, J. (2007) *Multiscale Analysis of Complex Time Series*. Hoboken, NJ: John Wiley and Sons.

Goldberger, A. L., Peng, C.-K., and Lipsitz, L. A. (2002) What is physiologic complexity and how does it change with aging and disease? *Neurobiology of Aging*, 23: 23–6.

Govindan, R. B., Wilson, J. D., Eswaran, H., Lowery, C. L. and Preißl, H. (2007) Revisiting sample entropy analysis. *Physica A Statistical Mechanics and its Applications*, 376: 158–64.

Harbourne, R.T. and Stergiou, N. (2009) Movement variability and the use of nonlinear tools: principles to guide physical therapist practice. *Physical Therapy*, 89: 267–82.

Holden, J. G. (2005) Gauging the fractal dimension of response times from cognitive tasks, in M. A. Riley and G. C. Van Orden (eds) *Tutorials in Contemporary Nonlinear Methods for Behavioral Scientists Web Book*. Arlington, VA: National Science Foundation, pp. 267–318. Available online at www.nsf.gov/sbe/bcs/pac/nmbs/nmbs.jsp (accessed 6 June 2013).

Kantz, H. and Schreiber, T. (2004) *Nonlinear Time Series Analysis*. Cambridge: Cambridge University Press.

Kaplan, D. and Glass, L. (1995) *Understanding Nonlinear Dynamics*. New York: Springer.

Lake, D. E., Richman, J. S., Griffin, M. P. and Moorman, J. R. (2002) Sample entropy analysis of neonatal heart rate variability. *American Journal of Physiology Regulatory, Integrative and Comparative Physiology*, 283: R789–97.

Liebovich, L. S. (1998) *Fractals and Chaos Simplified for the Life Sciences*. New York: Oxford University Press.

Marwan. N., Romano, M.C., Thiel, M. and Kurths, J. (2007) Recurrence plots for the analysis of complex systems. *Physics Reports*, 438: 237–9.

Pellecchia, G. L. and Shockley, K. (2005) Application of recurrence quantification analysis: Influence of cognitive activity on postural fluctuations, in M. A. Riley and G. C. Van Orden (eds) *Tutorials in Contemporary Nonlinear Methods for Behavioral Scientists Web Book*. Arlington, VA: National Science Foundation, pp. 95–141. Available online at www.nsf.gov/sbe/bcs/pac/nmbs/nmbs.jsp (accessed 6 June 2013).

Peng, C.-K., Buldyrev, S. V., Havlin, S., Simons, M., Stanley, H. E. and Goldberger, A. L. (1994) Mosaic organization of DNA nucleotides. *Physical Review E*, 49: 1685–9.

Pincus, S. and Viscarello, R. (1992) Approximate entropy: a regularity measure for fetal heart rate analysis. *Obstetrics and Gynecology*, 79: 249–55.

Pincus, S. M. (1991) Approximate entropy as a measure of system complexity. *Proceedings of the National Academy of Sciences*, 88: 2297–301.

Pincus, S. M. (1994) Greater signal regularity may indicate increased system isolation. *Mathematical Biosciences*, 122: 161–81.

Pincus, S. M. (2006) Approximate entropy as a measure of irregularity for psychiatric serial metrics. *Bipolar Disorders*, 8: 430–40.

Pincus, S. M. and Goldberger, A. L. (1994) Physiological time-series analysis: what does regularity quantify? *American Journal of Physiology Heart and Circulatory Physiology*, 266: H1643–56.

Ramdani, S., Seigle, B., Lagarde, J., Bouchara, F. and Bernard, P. L. (2009) On the use of sample entropy to analyze human postural sway data. *Medical Engineering and Physics*, 31: 1023–31.

Rhea, C. K., Silver, T. A., Hong, S. L., Ryu, J. H., Studenka, B. E., Hughes, C. M. L. and Haddad, J. M. (2011) Noise and complexity in human postural control: interpreting the different estimations of entropy. *PLoS One*, 6 (3): e17696; doi:10.1371/journal.pone.0017696

Richman, J. S. and Moorman, J. R. (2000) Physiological time-series analysis using approximate entropy and sample entropy. *American Journal of Physiology Heart and Circulatory Physiology*, 278: H2039–49.

Riley, M. A. and Turvey, M. T. (2002) Variability and determinism in motor behavior. *Journal of Motor Behavior*, 34: 99–125.

Riley, M. A., Balasubramaniam, R. and Turvey, M. T. (1999) Recurrence quantification analysis of postural fluctuations. *Gait and Posture*, 9: 65–78.

Scheinkman, J. A. and LeBaron, B. (1989) Nonlinear dynamics and stock returns. *Journal of Business*, 62: 311–37.

Schneider, E. D. and Sagan, D. (2005) *Into the Cool: Energy Flow, Thermodynamics, and Life*. Chicago, IL: University of Chicago Press.

Slifkin, A. B. and Newell, K. M. (1999) Noise, information transmission, and force variability. *Journal of Experimental Psychology: Human Perception and Performance*, 25: 837–51.

Stevens, S. S. (1946) On the theory of scales of measurement. *Science*, 103: 677–80.

Takens, F. (1981) Detecting strange attractors in turbulence, in D. Rand, and L.-S. Young (eds) *Lecture Notes in Mathematics, Vol. 898, Dynamical Systems and Turbulence, Warwick 1980*. Berlin: Springer, pp. 366–81.

Tulppo, M. P., Hughson, R. L., Mäkikallio, T. H., Airaksinen, K. E. J., Seppänen, T. and Huikuri, H. V. (2001) Effects of exercise and passive head-up tilt on fractal and complexity properties of heart rate dynamics. *American Journal of Physiology Heart and Circulatory Physiology*, 280: 1081–7.

Vaillancourt, D. E. and Newell, K. M. (2002) Changing complexity in human behavior and physiology through aging and disease. *Neurobiology of Aging*, 23: 1–11.

Van Orden, G. C., Holden, J. G. and Turvey, M. T. (2003) Self-organization of cognitive performance. *Journal of Experimental Psychology: General*, 132: 331–50.

Webber, C.L. (1991) Rhythmogenesis of deterministic breathing patterns. In H. P. Koepchen and H. Haken (eds) *Rhythms in Physiological Systems*, pp. 177–91. Berlin: Springer-Verlag.

Webber, C. L. and Zbilut, J. P. (1994) Dynamical assessment of physiological systems and states using recurrence plot strategies. *Journal of Applies Physiology*, 76: 965–73.

Webber, C. L. and Zbilut, J. P. (1996) Assessing deterministic structures in physiological systems using recurrence plot strategies, in M. C. K. Khoo (ed.) *Bioengineering Approaches to Pulmonary Physiology and Medicine*. NewYork: Plenum Press, pp. 137–48.

Webber, C. L. and Zbilut, J. P. (2005) Recurrence quantification analysis of nonlinear dynamical systems, in M. A. Riley and G. C. Van Orden (eds) *Tutorials in Contemporary Nonlinear Methods for Behavioral Scientists Web Book*. Arlington, VA: National Science Foundation, pp. 26–94. Available online at www.nsf.gov/sbe/bcs/pac/nmbs/nmbs.jsp (accessed 6 June 2013).

Wijnants, M. L., Bosman, A. M. T., Hasselman, F., Cox, R. F. A. and Van Orden, G. C. (2009) 1/f scaling in movement time changes with practice in precision aiming. *Nonlinear Dynamics, Psychology, and Life Sciences*, 13: 75–94.

Yeragani, V. K., Pohl, R., Mallavarapu, M. and Balon, R. (2003) Approximate entropy of symptoms of mood: an effective technique to quantify regularity of mood. *Bipolar Disorders*, 5: 279–86.

6 Interpersonal coordination tendencies induce functional synergies through co-adaptation processes in team sports

Pedro Passos, Duarte Araújo, Bruno Travassos, Luis Vilar and Ricardo Duarte

The use of measures that capture coordination in different levels of team sports, such as geometrical centres, inter- and intrateam interpersonal distances, relative velocities and angles between opponent players, as well as the network analysis, have been increasingly used to describe and explain coordination between performers in sport. This chapter summarizes the developments in this area of work.

During the last decade, there was an increase in research on interpersonal coordination in team sports. At the first stage, the main issue of researchers was to found variables that accurately describe the behaviour of a set of players in interaction, in other words, how to capture how several players coordinate with each other. These interactions prompt the emergence of collective behaviours that attain levels of performance that are different from the sum of individual performances (Duarte *et al.* 2012; Sumpter 2010). This led us to the notion of functional synergies (i.e. coordinative structures), which are groupings of structural elements (e.g. players) that temporally are constrained to function as a single coherent unit (Kelso 2009).

Coordinated collective behaviours demand the existence of co-adaptation (Kauffman 1993) among system components, a concept that was originally used to characterize how agents cooperate within complex biological systems. The existence of co-adaptation means that each agent within a system acts accordingly with the nearest neighbour. For instance, when the ball carrier of a sport team change his running line trajectory the players in his neighbourhood aiming to maintain the support to the ball carrier also adjust their running line trajectories accordingly. Thus, a continuous co-adaptation is a key issue for intrateam coordination in team sports. The same interpretation is lawful for interteam coordination since defenders continuously co-adapt to the attackers' actions which in turn co-adapt to defenders' behaviours. But do the players have the need (even if that was possible) to continuously co-adapt to all other players within the pitch?

Co-adaptation demands that players within a performance field must be informationally coupled. Some data have been supporting the expectations that the strength of coupling increases with decreasing of interpersonal distances among opponent players (Passos *et al.* 2011a). Players' behaviours are constrained by their intentions, goals and roles that decrease the randomness in their movement displacement trajectories in the field. However, the decreasing of interpersonal distances increases players' contextual dependency, meaning that each player's behaviour is mutually dependent from the behaviour of the other players in the neighbourhood. When this behavioural dependency occurs the players enter in a critical region where candidates to control parameters (e.g. players' relative velocities) might increase or decrease values moving the system towards an eventual performance outcome. When these candidates to control parameters values equalized transition values the attacker–defender system enter in a state of criticality (Jensen 1998), where something is about to occur and one player (or team) will gain advantage over the other.

In this chapter, we focus on the most frequently used methods for behavioural data analysis, mainly the tools and variables employed. Special attention will be directed to the coordinative variables that were used in different levels of analysis of team sports. Some studies go further and present candidates to control parameters, which aim to explain how an attacker–defender system moves from one stable state to another.

The last decade assisted to a considerable increase in the number of studies dedicated to interpersonal coordination in team games. Several researchers all over the world invest a lot of work aiming to describe how individuals interact on ongoing team sports performance. From Australia, New Zealand, Singapore to Portugal, France, Canada and Netherlands, issues regarding how players interact within a competitive performance environment were under analysis with a common feature: the focus of analysis was on the interaction that a performer has within a given context (e.g. the interaction between two or more players) rather than on the player as a single unit. As a result researchers found or create new variables to describe players' interactions with opponents and teammates and also candidates to control parameters that explain how the attacker–defender balance was broken. Associated with these investigations, some innovative methods of analysis appeared to better help sports scientists and practitioners to enhance their analyses, some of them being adopted from other areas of research. This is what we describe in the following sections of this chapter.

Uncovering interpersonal coordination in team sports

Players' behaviours are continuously constrained by a huge number of variables, which implies that attacker–defender systems are constrained by multiple causes that produce multiple effects, a general feature of complex systems.

In order to increase the understanding concerning the complex nature of interactive behaviours in team sports, researchers have been making an effort to identify relevant *coordinative variables*, which are single variables that capture and synthesise the interactive behaviours between the individual parts of a system. These compound variables aim to accurately describe the system states of coordination and its time-evolving dynamics (Duarte *et al.* 2012; Kelso 2009). To explain why the system transit from one state of coordination to another, researchers need also to explore the role of potential candidates to control parameters.

Interpersonal distances and player velocities have been considered relevant variables to analyze interpersonal coordination in team sports. The work of Araújo *et al.* (2002) in basketball investigated whether the distance of the attacker–defender dyad from the basket became less stable as the interpersonal distance between the attacker and defender decreased. For that purpose, the authors examined one-on-one attacker–defender dyadic behaviour proposing the medium point between attacker and defender to the basket as a coordinative variable that accurately describes dyadic system behaviours. Aiming to explain when the attacker–defender balance was broken, the authors proposed as candidates to control parameters the interpersonal distance between an attacker and his immediate defender, which when achieving a critical value, drove the dyadic system towards a specific performance outcome, such as a defender interception or a shot to the basket by the attacker. Candidates to control parameters sought to explain whether the balance of the attacker–defender dyad was disturbed or even broken at specific critical values of the players' interpersonal distance. The data revealed that the attacker–defender dyad distance to the basket as a coordinative variable was able to accurately describe two different states of the dyadic system: i) when the defender counterbalance the attackers' movements, the dyadic system stability remains unchanged, which is considered an advantageous situation for the defender; or ii) when the attacker was able to dribble past the defender and move closer to the basket. The former system state was consistent with a breaking in the spatiotemporal symmetry of the attacker-defender relations. Araújo *et al.* (2002) identified this sudden change in the dyadic system balance as evidence of a 'phase transition', which is a general feature of a non-linear dynamical system.

Also aiming to accurately describe the attacker–defender dyadic interactions, the works of Passos *et al.* (2006, 2008, 2009a) proposed a coordinative variable which was the angle formed between a vector linking the defender to the attacker and an imaginary horizontal line parallel to the try line (Figure 6.1).

The data from this coordinative variable displayed the intermittency between stability and volatility periods that characterize attacker–defender interactions. These volatility periods occur because of a marked decrease in players' interpersonal distances. Thus, interpersonal distances are candidates for controlling parameters that tend to move attacker–defender systems towards critical regions where opponent players become mutually dependent and some control parameters gain influence over another. For instance, the increase in the relative velocity (i.e. the difference between attacker and defender velocity) increases its influence on the performance outcome (i.e. a try or a tackle) but only within certain regions. An increase in the difference of players velocities led the system for try outcomes whereas similar velocities between players led it to tackle outcomes. Interestingly, outside specific values of interpersonal distances (i.e. around 4 metres in the studied sample), relative velocity had little or no influence on the performance outcome. This is why Passos *et al.* (2008) suggested the notion of

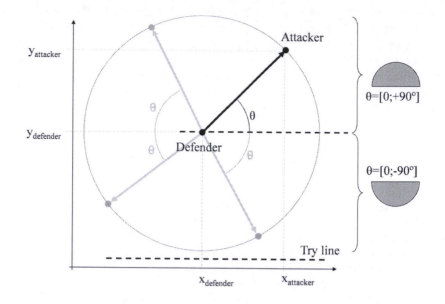

Figure 6.1 The calculation of the coordinative variable (reprinted with permission of the
Journal of Motor Behaviour)

nested control parameters to explain that the attacker–defender balance was
broken and a new state of coordination has emerged. The candidates for nested
control parameters that we identified (i.e. interpersonal distance and
attacker–defender relative velocity) are emergent system constraints because they
became spontaneously coupled without interference from an external agent.

A different approach to analyzing potential control parameters is shown in the
studies from Correia *et al.* (2011) in rugby union and Cordovil *et al.* (2009) in
basketball. Both manipulated task constraints, aiming to test potential system
parameters. The work of Correia *et al.* (2011) examined whether manipulating the
initial starting locations of two defenders near the try line influence the performance outcome (i.e. try or tackle). Data revealed important changes in the
displacement trajectories of defenders as a function of initial starting distance.
When defending participants started the task positioned further apart from each
other, they tended to move closer together (possibly acquiring an 'optimal' interpersonal distance that help them to face as a collective unit) and wait for the
attacker close to the try line (i.e. defenders tended to move laterally across the try
line instead of going forward, decreasing the distance to the attacker). On the
other hand, as the initial starting distance between defenders was decreased, they
tended to run forward in the direction of the attacker (i.e. decreasing the distance
to contact the attacker). The data revealed that when the defender's initial starting

distance was between 20 and 10 metres, a try results as the performance outcome. Below four metres of the defender's initial distance, the tackle was the preferred outcome. However, between eight and six metres of the defender's starting interpersonal distance, both system outcomes coexist with similar frequencies. We suggest that Correia *et al.* (2011) identified a critical region with plenty of uncertainty concerning the outcome. Owing to the manipulated task constraints, this study indicated that defenders' starting distances between eight and six metres exponentially augmented uncertainty to the agents involved on this triadic system. Thus, the decisions and actions must be sustained by information that is locally created owing to the players' contextual dependency. These findings add relevant insights for practice designs creating learning environments where players must deal with the uncertainty and the dynamics of the information that emerges locally.

Other types of task-constraint manipulation are illustrated in the work of Cordovil *et al.* (2009). Aiming to analyze potential control parameters, they sought to understand whether the patterns of coordination in the attacker–defender–basket system could be disturbed under the influence of common task constraints, such as coaching instructions and players' height. In a first experiment, different performance instructions (neutral, playing conservatively and risk taking) were given to the attacking players. The data revealed that coaching instructions disturbed the attacker–defender interactive behaviours (i.e. the conservative instructions led to an increase in the variability of attackers running-line trajectories; also, the attackers took more time to cross the mid-line court) but do not lead to differences in the frequency of phase transitions (i.e. the number of times that the attackers dribbled past the defender). Therefore, differences in coaching instructions failed as a candidate for control parameter. In a second experiment, the authors created dyads with different height relations, aiming to analyze whether this individual structural constraint might work as a potential control parameter. Contrary to the findings of the previous experiment, the data revealed significant differences in the frequency of phase-transition occurrences whenever the attackers were shorter in height than the defenders (Cordovil *et al.* 2009). These findings implied that a different height relation between players in the team sport of basketball may be interpreted as a candidate for control parameter that influences the balance in attacker–defender dyadic systems, providing a strong advantage for the attackers.

Another example of task-constraint manipulation was the work of Headrick *et al.* (2012) in one-on-one dyadic behaviour in association football. The aim of this investigation was to analyze whether the proximity to the goal area constrained the spatiotemporal interactions within attacker–defender dyads plus the ball. The results revealed that the defender-to-ball distance stabilized at significantly higher values (approximately 1.7 metres apart) when the interaction among attacker and defender occurred close to the defender's goal (which was consistent with a lower risk-taking behaviour from the defender) than when occurred far from the defender's goal area (defender-to-ball distance was approximately 1.2 metres; Headrick *et al.* 2012). When stabilizing the defender-to-ball distances, the authors suggested that attacker and defender became contextually dependent and the dyadic system entered a critical region. These critical regions displayed different characteristics depending on the attacker–defender distance to the goal area.

In summary, results from studies in dyadic and triadic behaviours in team sports revealed that players' behaviours are highly sensitive both to changes in initial task constraints (e.g. distance to the goal, initial distance between defenders, differences in players' height) and also to small changes in interpersonal interactions within critical regions demarcated by close interpersonal distances (e.g. changes in relative velocity). This signifies that opponent players interact differently, depending on performer and task constraints that shape the perceptual–motor landscape (the system region) for action. The information that emerges from player interactions within the critical regions implies that players' behaviours are context dependent and small changes in relevant candidates to control parameters (e.g. relative velocity) often lead to transitions in the attacker–defender system's structural organization (e.g. characterized by the relative positioning of each player to the goal). These transitions can be captured by abrupt and nonlinear changes in the coordinative variables. In the next section, we describe how these concepts are useful and explain collective behaviours observed in team sports.

Beyond dyadic behaviour in team ball sports

According to Oullier and Kelso (2009), one of the major problems that persists when investigating interpersonal coordination is the difficulty in manipulating or measuring the intensity/strength of coupling between agents. Following what was described for dyadic behaviours, the step further is to study collective behaviours in team sports. Based on studies in biological systems, Passos and colleagues developed research aiming to analyze pattern-forming dynamics and the strength of connection among players within the team sport of rugby union (Passos *et al.* 2011a). The analysis of collective behaviours in team sports requires two levels of analysis: i) intrateam couplings, aiming to characterize how players co-adapt to the teammates behaviour; and ii) interteam couplings, aiming to analyze attacker–defender co-adaptive behaviours.

Concerning the intra-team analyses, Passos *et al.* (2011a) explored interpersonal distances as a relevant variable that bounded teammates' behaviours. Similar to other biological systems (e.g. schools of fish, flock of birds), the results display that, in team sports, players' behaviours are ruled by functional interpersonal distances, which are sensitive to specific task constraints such as the opponents' proximity. The results revealed that players within an attacker subunit tend to remain close to each other when playing before the first defensive line and augment their interpersonal distances when playing between the first and the second defensive line. An issue that Passos *et al.* (2011a) aimed to solve was how to measure the strength of connection between players within an attacker subunit. Running correlation analyses were successfully used for that purpose on a four versus two plus two situations in rugby union.

An interteam analysis requires testing for a coordinative variable that accurately synthesizes and captures the behaviour of a set of players. Milho *et al.* (2010) suggested the use of geometrical centres (or centroids) calculated from the mean values for interpersonal distance between players within the subunit over time. This measure was later used in association football by Frencken *et al.* (2011) and Lames *et al.* (2010). The authors proposed that a centroid position and surface area (i.e. the space covered by the outfield players of a team) may provide meaningful system variables that capture the collective behaviours and the interactions between attacking and defending teams. The use of these sorts of coordinative variables might help to solve a problem raised by Oullier and Kelso (2009) concerning the large number of agents that were under analysis to describe social collective behaviours. Data from Milho *et al.* (2010) confirmed that the centroids trajectory emerging due to systemic couplings between players allowed a description of the teams' collective behaviours as a whole rather than as standalone entities or a sum of individual performances. This interteam coordinative variable was imported from the study of attacker–defender dyads and again calculated from the angle of vector-linked centroids (from the defence to the attack subunit) with an imaginary horizontal line parallel to the try line. When plotted on time data it was revealed that this interteam coordinative variable described different states of attacker–defender coordination: i) when the defenders were the players closer to the try line; ii) the moment that attackers overpass the defenders; and iii) when the attackers become the players closest the try line. Moreover, owing to a continuous decrease in attacker–defender interpersonal distances, an increase in the variability of the interteam coordinative occurred, highlighting when the attacker–defender balance is disturbed and the system undergoes a phase transition. The intermittency between stability and volatility periods on attacker–defender systems can be observed if we calculate the first derivative of the interteam coordinative variable. The volatility period characterized when attackers and defenders become mutually dependent and defined the entry in critical regions (Passos *et al.* 2009b).

Within these critical regions, some parameters might gain influence over the others, which moves the attacker–defender system to a performance outcome. The work of Rodrigues and Passos (2011) described and explained successful performance outcomes in attacker and defender subunits of rugby union. This research was developed in situ during rugby union matches. The first issue under investigation was which were the players under analysis? In other words, what are the attackers that are functionally coordinated forming a subunit evolving towards the score line? To solve this issue, the authors used running correlations (calculated based on players' distance from the goal line) as a tool that allowed measurement of the degree of coordination among all the players involved in each attacking situation. Positive values meant that both players were running in the same direction (presumably towards the goal line); negative values meant that one player was running towards goal line but the other was running apart; values close to zero meant weak correlation between player movement displacement trajectories. The data revealed that the behaviour of supporting players was strongly correlated with the ball carrier's behaviour. But correlation values decreased with the proximity to defenders, which sustains previous results from Passos *et al.* (2011a). The coordination patterns among players within an attacker subunit seem to be disturbed, owing to the influence of task constraints such as the approach of defenders. Based on the running correlation values, Rodrigues and Passos also identified three sorts of attacker–defender interactions that led to different performance outcomes: i) a strong correlation among attackers and a weak correlation among defenders usually led the attackers to succeed; ii) a strong correlation among defenders and a weak correlation among attackers often led the defenders to succeed; iii) when both attackers and defenders displayed similar levels of correlation, it was not possible to identify an outcome tendency (Rodrigues and Passos 2011).

The first conclusion from Rodrigues and Passos' research was that the functional synergies (i.e. subunits of attacking and defending players) that are formed within rugby union sub-phases of play could be captured through running correlation analyses (Rodrigues and Passos 2011). Despite this achievement, the use of running correlations requires some caution. In some situations, the players could be running laterally in the same direction (for a brief period of time), with a relatively stable distance to the try line, or one player could be running laterally and the other running forward; for both cases we might have weak correlations values. These data do not necessarily mean that players are not coordinated but only that they are not achieving symmetrical coordination tendencies (i.e. synchronously moving in the same direction at the same time). However, because of the nature and laws of the game, we reinforce that in almost all of the analyzed situations the running correlations allowed the uncovering of the attacking and defending subunits and explained their relative success in the match.

The second conclusion was that when a set of attacking players formed a functional synergy, this could be disturbed by the approach of defenders (i.e. a decrease in interpersonal distances between attackers and defenders), which is captured by the oscillation in the running correlation values. This research sustains the notion that forming functional synergies is an important advantage in success during team sport performance and the co-adaptive behaviour that is required by each player led to the emergence of functional synergies within each subunit of play, which reciprocally bounded player co-adaptive behaviour. We suggest that the work of Rodrigues and Passos supports the notion of circular causality of co-adaptive behaviour and functional synergies, as a general feature of performing in rugby union which could be tested in other team ball sports (Rodrigues and Passos 2011).

How can these attacking and defending functional synergies (i.e. the game subunits) break the initial stability featured by their relative positioning in relation to the try line? Rodrigues and Passos (2011) found that what moves the attacker–defender system to a phase transition was the increase in relative velocity. The relative velocity was revealed as a relevant candidate for control parameter that could explain the attacker subunit's success (Rodrigues and Passos 2011). This result is consistent with the previous work of Passos *et al.* (2008)

presented earlier in this chapter. Similar to the previous work in one-on-one dyads in rugby union, in this study, the relative velocity only gained influence on the performance outcome within regions of short interpersonal distance between attackers and defenders. These results supported once again the argument that important changes in team sport behaviours evolve within critical regions formed by the emergence of contextual dependency in players' interactions. It was only 'inside' these regions (i.e. regions of contextual dependency) that the attacker–defender balance might be broken, presenting an advantage to the attackers. Outside these regions, the game remains stable and without much change in attacker–defender structural organization.

In summary, from the studies presented in this section, it is possible to highlight the relevance of variables such as players' interpersonal distances to describe collective functional behaviours in team sports. It is based on the dynamics of interpersonal distances (i.e. the continuous adjustments towards suitable interpersonal distances) that we sustain the existence of contextual dependency among players within game sub-phases, which leads to the emergence of functional synergies based on processes of co-adaptation. This implies that a set of players often coordinates their behaviours to perform collectively as a single unit. Also, interpersonal distances poised attacker–defender systems within critical regions where contextual dependency governs and is governed by players' interactive behaviours. The circular causality between co-adaptive behaviour and functional synergies is based on local informational rules (e.g. interpersonal distances and players relative velocity) suggesting that attacker–defender interactions are self-organized.

Nonlinear analysis of team-game coordination

Research in intrapersonal coordination (e.g. on dual-limb or hand movements) has demonstrated that patterns of coordination can be captured in terms of cycling frequency and phase relations (Haken *et al.* 1985; Schmidt *et al.* 1990; Schmidt 1997). Phase attractors, i.e. stable and strong patterns of coordination, emerge by a coupling of limb or hand phase relations and frequencies. To measure such coordination, Haken *et al.* (1985) used the relative phase, which was demonstrated to be acting as a collective variable capturing the spatiotemporal relations between two oscillating agents by considering their amplitudes and frequencies (Oullier and Kelso 2009). An oscillating agent can be considered to be a cyclical behaviour that occurs in space and time such as a pendulum, the body sway or the heart rate measured over time. The phase angle corresponds to the amount of time in which the signal of the two oscillating agents is delayed or shifted (Rosenblum *et al.* 2001). For example, if two fingers or two players are moving to the left and to the right at the same time, there is no delay registered in the coordination of the agents and 0° of phase angle (i.e. an in-phase mode of coordination) may be observed. On the contrary, if one finger or player is moving to the left and the other is moving to the right at the same time, the phase angle values display a delay of 180° (i.e. an anti-phase mode of coordination). Intermediate values, such as −60°, indicates that the second oscillating agent is leading the relation by one-sixth of a cycle. The advantage of using relative phase to capture nonlinear behaviours in comparison with other linear measures (e.g. running correlations) is that relative phase measures the amplitude and frequency of two signals to calculate the phase relation whilst linear measures just consider the frequency of the signals. Disregarding the amplitude of oscillation may mask the dynamical coupling of agents (Rosenblum *et al.* 2001), which may make the complete analysis of the time-evolving dynamics of a system difficult.

More recently, relative phase applications to intrapersonal coordination have been extended to interpersonal coordination, namely in sports. Considering that sport contests tend to exhibit forward–backward and left–right behaviours (i.e. oscillating behaviours on the field) McGarry *et al.* (2002) proposed that the emergent patterns of behaviour between players or teams could also be captured using relative phase. This would allow researchers to explain how the interaction between players constrains the emergence of patterns of stability (i.e. high attraction to few coordination modes between performers), variability (i.e. high attraction to larger number of coordination modes between performers) and symmetry breaking in systems organizational states (i.e. when new patterns of coordination emerge during performance; Vilar *et al.* 2012a). This is a relevant issue that sport scientists and coaches need to pursue and understand in analyses of team-game performances (Araújo *et al.* 2006; Davids *et al.* 1994; Handford *et al.* 1997).

The first research in sport contests using relative phase analyses was conducted in tennis and squash (Lames 2006; McGarry *et al.* 1999; Palut and Zanone 2005). These studies showed that relative phase is a pertinent collective variable that captured different modes of coordination between players over time. In addition, the authors suggested self-organization as the process through which the coordinated behaviours between players emerged. Following the suggestion of McGarry *et al.* (2002) that game dynamics might emerge from the coupling within players of the same team (i.e. intrateam relations) and between players of opposite teams (i.e. interteam relations), research was extended to team sports settings, such as basketball and futsal. With the goal of understanding the intra- and interteam couplings of players in basketball, two studies were conducted by Bourbousson *et al.* (2010a,b). Considering the interteam relations (i.e. coordination between all possible attacking–defending dyads), data revealed strong in-phase attractions in the longitudinal (basket-to-basket) displacements, especially between direct opponents for attacker–defender relations (e.g. right wing of team A and left wing of team B). In futsal (the five-a-side indoor association football) Travassos *et al.* (2011) used relative phase to examine not only intra- and interteam player relations but also the relation that each player developed with ball trajectory. Results were expected to highlight how the location of the ball is an important constraint on game behaviour, since players seek to gain ball possession to score goals and prevent the opponents from doing the same. The movement trajectories of the ball and players were recorded in both lateral and longitudinal directions and investigated using relative phase as a collective variable. Travassos *et al.* (2011) observed stronger in-phase attractions between players and ball (specifically between defenders and ball with a lag of 30°) than just between players. A lag of 30° means that the ball led the spatiotemporal relation with players by one-twelfth of a cycle, suggesting that players adjusted their positions according to and just after the movement of the ball. Indeed, this finding demonstrates that ball dynamics are an important constraint on behaviour that needs to be further considered to analyze performance in team games. The analysis of intrateam dyadic relations revealed stronger coordination patterns between defenders than between attackers. Therefore, it was suggested that defenders tried to couple their displacements in relation to the ball closing the paths to the goal, whilst attackers explored high-variable spatiotemporal relations among each other to disrupt the defensive structure. For interteam couplings, stronger in-phase modes of coordination were observed between the attacker and the closest direct opponent. Similarly to a previous study of basketball (Bourbousson *et al.* 2010a), these results demonstrated different modes of coordination for different phases of the game (i.e. while attacking or defending). Finally, the authors reported stronger in-phase modes of coordination for lateral displacements than for longitudinal ones. These findings are opposite to the results obtained by Bourbousson *et al.* (2010a) in basketball and may be explained by the differences on the task constraints that bound the playing conditions (five-versus-five in basketball and five-versus-four plus goalkeeper in futsal). The numerical advantage of the attacking team in the futsal task is suggested as having constrained the defending team to use a zone-marking strategy, whilst players' numerical equivalence in basketball afforded the possibility of using a 'man-to-man' marking strategy. The numerical relation between players was shown to constrain players' interactions and the strength of coupling between them. Changing the numerical relations is then proposed to be a major task constraint that coaches may manipulate during practice tasks to promote specific adaptations of interpersonal relations sustaining the use of zone and man-to-man defensive playing strategies. In addition, in a second study also conducted in futsal (Travassos *et al.* 2012) examined interpersonal coordination between teams. The authors advanced the study of Bourbousson *et al.* (2010a) by measuring the phase relations between the geometrical centre of each team with regard to its location on the field of play referenced to the goal position. Measuring variations in the angle between the geometrical centre of each team and the goal position, Travassos *et al.* (2012) observed higher tendencies towards specific modes of coordination than when using lateral and longitudinal displacements (Figure 6.2). These results demonstrated game behaviours anchored on the goal location. For example, the defending team seeks to close the paths to the goal in relation to changes in ball positioning, attacking player behaviours and goal location and not just based on abstract lateral and longitudinal displacements. Measuring team relations with regard to their location on the field of play referenced to the goal position takes into account the key goal of the game and allows a functional understanding of emergent patterns of coordination.

Also in futsal, Vilar *et al.* (2012b) investigated how the goal and ball locations

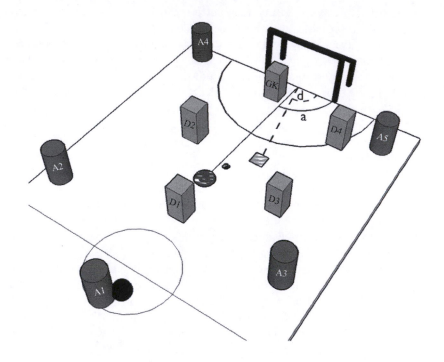

Figure 6.2 Angle between geometrical centre of each team and the goal position

constrain interpersonal patterns of coordination between inter-team (i.e. attacker-defender) dyads. The authors sought to capture dyadic relations using relative phase analyses between the distances and the angles of each player to the ball and to the centre of the goal. The distances captured the dynamics of proximity between players to the ball or to the goal while the angle measured the alignment between them. Vilar *et al.* (2012b) reported predominant in-phase modes of coordination between attackers and defenders for angles as well as for distances regarding the ball and the goal. However, stronger in-phase modes of coordination were reported between attacker and defenders when related to the goal than between players and the ball. These data revealed that the location of the goal exerts a larger constraining influence on dyadic coordination than the location of the ball. Finally, when a goal was scored similar distances between attackers and defenders to the goal were observed and instability in the players' angular relations to the goal was registered, suggesting that the angular relations between attackers and defenders may be candidates for control parameters that move this dyadic system to a phase transition. At this point, the attacker and defender stability was broken, emerging an advantageous situation for the attacker to kick at goal without the defender being able to intercept its trajectory.

Summarizing, relative phase was showed to capture attacker and defender interpersonal interactions relative to locations of the goal and the ball. Understanding the spatiotemporal relations among players and key performance constraints that bound players' dyadic and collective behaviours within competitive settings provides coaches with updated information for manipulating task constraints, allowing them to create representative practice designs to promote functional adaptations in players' performances.

Social networks as tools for describing player interactions

How teams perform collectively in competition is an issue that is highly topical in sports sciences. Practitioners have been analyzing performance with the goal of providing information that may improve team performance and to create awareness among players and coaches of how individual players can influence team patterns (McGarry 2009). One of such methods recently proposed for analyzing performance in team ball sports is social networks analysis (Duch *et al.* 2010; Passos *et al.* 2011b). These tools consider teams as complex social systems, recognizing their 'degeneracy' (i.e. inherent adaptive flexibility in the way in which teams achieve successful performance outcomes; Edelman and Gally 2001). Next, we introduce the instruments for network analysis supported on small-world networks and by graph theory and discuss their application in the investigation of interpersonal relations in team sports.

In team sports, the structure of the web of interpersonal interactions between players constrains the organization and functioning of teams. Players coordinate their actions to achieve patterns of collective behaviour that allow them to satisfy game demands. Often, two players can become interconnected for performing through a path of only a few passes between few players. This allows different sets of players to become linked to form a subunit in a team to perform successfully. The myriad of interactions that emerge among team players during competitive performance might lead to the emergence of distinct but functional equivalent patterns of play (Passos *et al.* 2011b). Therefore, team sports may be conceptualized as a small-world social system, in which system behaviour might evolve from the interpersonal interactions among system agents (Barabasi and Oltvai 2004). The term *small-world effect* was originally observed in studies of collective networks. A small-world network is a connected simple graph in which each node is linked to a relatively well-connected set of neighbouring nodes with short-cut connections between some nodes (Watts and Strogatz 1998).

Recently, the small-world effect was shown to capture the rich interactions among players in team sports (Duch *et al.* 2010; Passos *et al.* 2011b). One of the main tools that have been used for the quantitative study of networks is graph theory. Its concepts have been applied to discuss network issues in complex social (e.g. traffic jams), biological (e.g. cells, schools of fish, flocks of pigeons) or communication systems (e.g. the worldwide web). A graph consists of a set of nodes (or vertices) together with a set of links (or edges) that connect various pairs of nodes (Batten 2000). Nodes may have states and links may have directions and weights. For example, recent research in water polo (Passos *et al.* 2011b) examined the intrateam pattern-forming in attacking sub-phases of water polo (i.e. from the moment a team gained ball possession to the moment that ball possession was recovered by the opponent). Each node corresponded to each one of the six offensive players and two linkage levels were established: (i) when a player passed the ball to a teammate; or (ii) when players changed position in the performance area due to displacement of a teammate.

There are different ways to structure data relative to a graph in a computer system. For example, an adjacency list consists on a list of links whose element $i \rightarrow j$ shows a link going from node i to node j. Passos *et al.* (2011b) build an adjacency matrix for each unit of attack to identify the proximity of interacting players. The adjacency matrix is used to build a finite $n \times n$ network where the entries represent the linkages between players (e.g. when player A passes the ball to player B). Finally, graphs are frequently drawn as node-link diagrams in which the vertices are represented as disks and the edges are represented as line segments (Di Battista *et al.* 1994). Graphs may be displayed as different shapes (complete graph, regular graphs, planar graph, directed graph, weighted graph, etc.), depending on the nature of problem that the graph is intended to illustrate. In the exemplar research in water polo, the authors used a combination between a weighted graph, with an associated number indicating the strength of the edge, and a directed graph, displaying edges that were directional (Figure 6.3). The direction of the arrows indicates the pass direction, i.e. the origin of the arrow represents the player who passed the ball and the arrowhead represents the player

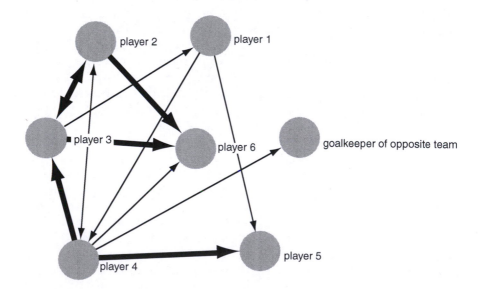

Figure 6.3 Exemplar data of a network in water polo (reprinted with permission of the *Journal of Science and Medicine in Sport*)

who received the ball. The width of the black arrows denoted the quantity of passes from one player to another during performance (i.e. thicker arrows illustrated more passes occurring between specific players and thinner arrows represented fewer passes taking place among players; Passos *et al.* 2011b).

One of the main potentials of network analysis tools is to provide understanding of the strengths and weaknesses in specific performance situations in a range of sports. By using different measurements of the topological properties of networks in several 'units of attack', researchers may describe the structural organization of the attacking performance of players and teams (Passos *et al.* 2011b). For example, the order of the graph informs about the number of nodes (i.e. players) acting on the network, whilst the number of links (e.g. passes performed between players) is referred to as the size of the graph. This analysis may inform about the number of different players typically engaging in the offensive plays, as well how many passes do teams perform until loosing or shooting the ball on goal. This is expected to shed some light on the style of play adopted (e.g. 'direct play' or 'possession play'), that is, if teams seek to use shorter or longer passing sequences as a means of scoring goals.

Using the same type of approach, Duch *et al.* (2010) analyzed the performance of players in the association football European Cup 2008. The representation of the 'flow network' of successful passing balls in different matches, allowed comparison of the performance of the two teams and identification of the most relevant players (i.e. the players who successfully passed and received more balls to and from different teammates) of each team when different team strategies were used. The most common analysis in networks framework concerns the centrality measures of each node. For example, the degree centrality of node n is the number of links connected to n; that is, how many connections the player has. However, in a directed graph, such as the ones typically considered in team sports, the in-degree of each node corresponds to the number of nodes n' of the system that are directly linked to n by an inward-pointing link to n. Conversely, the number of nodes n' of the system that are directly linked to n by a link pointing outward from n is called out-degree of n. These data may inform practitioners about how many passes each player receives and how often he passes the ball efficiently. Other different measures of centrality may also be considered, such as: (i) the betweenness centrality, which refers to how many shortest paths go through each player; and (ii) the closeness centrality, which informs about how close the player is to other players. This measurement can be a very useful way of accurately identifying the key 'decision makers' or 'emergent leaders' during important phases of competitive performance. Similarly, the degree distribution gives a rough profile of how the connectivity is distributed within the team, by displaying the total number of players with degree k.

The connectivity of the network may be also a relevant topological measure of a team, informing about the degree to which players interact with each other (Batten 2000). A connectivity measure would generally take into account two aspects of this interaction pattern: (i) which players are interacting with one another; and (ii) what is the strength (frequency, regularity, impact, etc.) of these interactions. For example, the shortest path length (or distance) between node n and n' refers to the minimum number of links that must be traversed to travel from a node n to another node n'. This may inform about how many passes typically occur for the ball to arrive from a given player to a different one. Moreover, this technique may also provide a collective measurement of team closeness. The characteristic path length of a network is the median of the means of the shortest path lengths connecting each node to all other nodes (Watts 1999).

Finally, the clustering coefficient is also suggested as a relevant topological property that measures the degree to which players in a team tended to be linked. To calculate the clustering coefficient of a node n, one should first consider the number of nodes in the neighbourhood (k); that is, how many nodes n' are linked to n. Since, in team sports, the direction of the pass is important (directed graph), for each neighbourhood there are $k(k-1)$ links that could exist among the vertices within the neighbourhood (k is the total [in plus out] degree of the vertex). Thus, the clustering coefficient of a given node is equal to the proportion of links between the nodes within its neighbourhood divided by the number of links that could possibly exist between them. The clustering coefficient of a specific node may inform practitioners about subgroups of players who may coordinate their actions very well among each other (e.g. left back, central midfielder and left forward in association football). In addition, one may also calculate the clustering coefficient of the network by averaging the clustering coefficient of all nodes in a network. A large clustering coefficient implies that the team is well connected locally to form a cluster.

In summary, we suggest that networks tools are able to provide understanding about how players (i.e. nodes) may interact to form a team (i.e. network). They can explain how the structure and specific topology of a team might constrain the emergence of collective behaviours in team sports, which can be used in tactical and strategic decision making for competition. The possibility of plotting a pattern of play with an observable network structure and topology allows us to identify the players engaged in more and less frequent interactions within a team and to compare outcomes of successful and less successful patterns of play during performance.

Concluding remarks and applications

This chapter has presented an overview of the conceptual and methodological developments in the recent study of interpersonal coordination in team sports. From the analysis of dyadic system interactions to the understanding of group behaviours in subunits of play, interactions within sport teams seem to assemble into functional synergies. The emergence of these functional grouping tendencies are governed by locally generated information sources from the relative positioning of other team players, motion directions and changes in motion, which attest the significant meaning of inter- and intrateam co-adaptation processes (Passos *et al.* 2011b).

The findings presented in this chapter might have some important implications concerning performance analysis, as well as for learning and training design. For example, social networks can help performance analysts to enhance their analyses using simple notation data, such as passing actions and switching positions. Moreover, other coordinative variables discussed in this chapter can be used to evaluate the interactive performance behaviours of team players in different sub-phases and levels of analysis. The recent technological advances in player tracking systems, such as electronic portable devices (Carling *et al.* 2008) and multi-player video-based systems (Barris and Button 2008) offer a novel opportunity to develop evaluations of the coordination tendencies emerging within sport teams during performance (competition and training settings). For example: is the distance between the three midfielders of a football team presenting similar values during competition and practice sessions? The variables and measurement tools presented here might support the innovative approaches to performance analysis, which allow answering this type of relevant questions about performance.

Regarding learning and training design, by changing the local available information that guides player behaviour, coaches can manipulate the local rules governing interactions between neighbour teammates and opponents, inducing the emergence of new patterns of collective movement solutions. For example, increasing the regular ratio of area per player could create larger areas of influence which promote the need for players to fine tune their positioning and their interpersonal distances to efficiently cover the spaces during the defensive phases. A constraints-led approach has been suggested as a practical and meaningful tool to promote the emergence of movement patterns under constraints (Davids *et al.* 2008; Glazier 2010) which can be used to enhance learning and performance.

References

Araújo, D., Davids, K. and Hristovski, R. (2006) The ecological dynamics of decision making in sport. *Psychology of Sport and Exercise*, 7: 653–76.

Araújo, D., K., D., Sainhas, J. and Fernandes, O. (2002) Emergent decision-making in sport: a constraints-led approach, in L. Toussaint and P. Boulinguez (eds) *International Congress on 'Movement, Attention and Perception'*. Poitiers, France: Université de Poitiers, p. 77.

Barabasi, A. L. and Oltvai, Z. N. (2004) Network biology: understanding the cell's functional organization. *Nature Reviews Genetics*, 5 (2): 101–13.

Barris, S. and Button, C. (2008) A review of vision-based motion analysis in sport. *Sports Medicine*, 38 (12): 1025–43.

Batten, D. (2000) Sheep, explorers, and phase transitions, in D. Batten (ed.) *Discovering Artificial Economics: How Agents Learn and Economies Evolve*. Boulder, CO: Westview Press, pp. 81–115.

Bourbousson, J., Sève, C. and McGarry, T. (2010a) Space-time coordination patterns in basketball: Part 1 Intra- and inter-couplings amongst player dyads. *Journal of Sport Sciences*, 28 (3): 339–47.

Bourbousson, J., Sève, C. and McGarry, T. (2010b) Space-time coordination patterns in basketball: Part 2 Investigating the interaction between the two teams. *Journal of Sport Sciences*, 28 (3): 349–58.

Carling, C., Bloomfield, J., Nelsen, L. and Reilly, T. (2008) The role of motion analysis in elite soccer: contemporary performance measurement techniques and work rate data. *Sports Medicine*, 38 (10): 839–62.

Cordovil, R., Araújo, D., Davids, K., Gouveia, L., Barreiros, J., Fernandes, O. and Serpa, S. (2009) The influence of instructions and body-scaling as constraints on decision-making processes in team sports. *European Journal of Sport Science*, 9 (3): 169–79.

Correia, V., Araújo, A., Duarte, R., Travassos, B., Passos, P. and Davids, K. (2011) Changes in practice task constraints shape decision-making behaviours of team games players. *Journal of Science and Medicine in Sport*, 15 (3): 244–9.

Davids, K., Button, C. and Bennett, S. (2008) *Dynamics of Skill Acquisition. A Constraints-led Approach*. Champaign: Human Kinetics.

Davids, K., Handford, C. and Williams, M. (1994) The natural physical alternative to cognitive theories of motor behaviour: an invitation for interdisciplinary research in sports science? *Journal of Sports Sciences*, 12 (6): 495–528.

Di Battista, G., Eades, P., Tamassia, R. and Tollis, I. G. (1994) Algorithms for drawing graphs: an annotated bibliography. *Computational Geometry: Theory and Applications*, 4 (5): 235–82.

Duarte, R., Araújo, D., Correia, V. and Davids, K. (2012) Sport teams as superorganisms: implications of sociobiological models of behaviour for research and practice in team sports performance analysis. *Sports Medicine*, 42 (8): 1–10.

Duch, J., Waitzman, J. S. and Nunes Amaral, L. A. (2010) Quantifying the performance of individual players in a team activity. *PloS One*, 5 (6): e10937; doi:10.1371/journal.pone.0010937

Edelman, G. M. and Gally, J. A. (2001) Degeneracy and complexity in biological systems. *Procedings of the National Academy of Sciences of the U S A*, 98 (24): 13763–8.

Frencken, W., Lemmink, K., Delleman, N. and Visscher, C. (2011) Oscillations of centroid position and surface area of soccer teams in small-sided games. *European Journal of Sport Science*, 11: 215–23.

Glazier, P. S. (2010) Game, set and match? Substantive issues and future directions in performance analysis. *Sports Medicine*, 40 (8): 625–34.

Haken, H., Kelso, J. A. S. and Bunz, H. (1985) A theoretical-model of phase-transitions in human hand movements. *Biological Cybernetics*, 51 (5): 347–56.

Handford, C., Davids, K., Bennett, S. and Button, C. (1997) Skill acquisition in sport: some applications of an evolving practice ecology. *Journal of Sports Sciences*, 15: 621–40.

Headrick, J., Davids, K., Renshaw, I., Araújo, D., Passos, P. and Fernandes, O. (2012) Proximity-to-goal as a constraint on patterns of behaviour in attacker-defender dyads in team games. *Journal of Sport Sciences*, 30 (3): 247–53.

Jensen, H. (1998) *Self-Organized Criticality: Emergent Complex Behavior in Physical and Biological Systems*. Cambridge Lecture Notes in Physics, Vol. 10. Cambridge: Cambridge University Press.

Kauffman, S. (1993) *The Origins of Order: Self-organization and Selection in Evolution*. New York: Oxford University Press.

Kelso, S. (2009) Coordination dynamics, in R. A. Meyers (ed.) *Encyclopedia of Complexity and System Science*. Heidelberg: Springer, pp. 1537–64.

Lames, M. (2006) Modelling the interaction in game sports: relative phase and moving correlations. *Journal of Sports Science and Medicine*, 5: 556–60.

Lames, M., Erdmann, J. and Walter, F. (2010) Oscillations in football: order and disorder in spatial interactions between the two teams. *International Journal of Sport Psychology*, 41 (4): 85.

McGarry, T. (2009) Applied and theoretical perspectives of performance analysis in sport: scientific issues and challenges. *International Journal of Performance Analysis in Sport*, 9: 128–40.

McGarry, T., Anderson, D. I., Wallace, S. A., Hughes, M. D. and Franks, I. M. (2002) Sport competition as a dynamical self-organizing system. *Journal of Sports Sciences*, 20 (10): 771–81.

McGarry, T., Khan, M. A. and Franks, I. M. (1999) On the presence and absence of behavioural traits in sport: an example from championship squash match-play. *Journal of Sports Sciences*, 17 (4): 297–311.

Milho, J., Passos, P., Leandro, H., Borges, J., Araújo, D. and Davids, K. (2010) Collective decision making inter and intra-team analysis: new challenges to match analysis. *International Journal of Sport Psychology*, 41: 95–6.

Oullier, O. and Kelso, J. A. S. (2009) Coordination from the perspective of social coordination dynamics, in R. A. Meyers (ed.) *The Encyclopedia of Complexity and Systems Science*. Heidelberg: Springer, pp. 8198–213.

Palut, Y. and Zanone, P. (2005) A dynamical analysis of tennis: concepts and data. *Journal of Sports Sciences*, 23 (10): 1021–32.

Passos, P., Araújo, D., Davids, K., Gouveia, L., Milho, J., and Serpa, S. (2008) Information-governing dynamics of attacker–defender interactions in youth rugby union. *Journal of Sports Sciences*, 26 (13): 1421–9.

Passos, P., Araújo, D., Davids, K., Gouveia, L. and Serpa, S. (2006) Interpersonal dynamics in sport: the role of artificial neural networks and 3-D analysis. *Behavior Research Methods*, 38 (4): 683–91.

Passos, P., Araújo, D., Davids, K., Gouveia, L., Serpa, S., Milho, J. and Fonseca, S. (2009a) Interpersonal pattern dynamics and adaptive behavior in multiagent neurobiological systems: conceptual model and data. *Journal of Motor Behavior*, 41 (5): 445–59.

Passos, P., Araújo, D., Davids, K. W., Milho, J. and Gouveia, L. (2009b) Power law distributions in pattern dynamics of attacker-defender dyads in rugby union: phenomena in a region of self-organized criticality? *Emergence: Complexity and Organization*, 11 (2): 37–45.

Passos, P., Milho, J., Fonseca, S., Borges, J., Araujo, D. and Davids, K. (2011a) Interpersonal distance regulates functional grouping tendencies of agents in team sports. *Journal of Motor Behavior*, 43 (2): 155–63.

Passos, P., Davids, K., Araújo, D., Paz, N., Minguéns, J. and Mendes, J. (2011b) Networks as a novel tool for studying team ball sports as complex social systems. *Journal of Science and Medicine in Sport*, 14 (2): 170–6.

Rodrigues, M. and Passos, P. (2011) Padrões de coordenação interpessoal no rugby: análise de comportamentos colectivos em jogo. Paper presented at the XII Jornadas da Sociedade Portuguesa de Psicologia do Desporto, Portimão, Portugal.

Rosenblum, M., Pikovsky, A., Kurths, J., Schäfer, C. and Tass, P. A. (2001) Phase synchronization: from theory to data analysis, in F. Moss and S. Gielen (eds) *Handbook of Biological Physics, Volume 4, Neuro-informatics*. Amsterdam: Elsevier Science, pp. 279–321.

Schmidt, R., Carello, C. and Turvey, M. (1990) Phase transitions and critical fluctuations in the visual coordination of rhythmic movements between people. *Journal of Experimental Psychology: Human Perception and Performance*, 16 (2): 227–47.

Schmidt, R. C. (1997) Evaluating the dynamics of unintended interpersonal coordination. *Ecological Psychology*, 9 (3): 189–206.

Sumpter, D. J. (2010) *Collective Animal Behavior*. Princeton, NJ: Princeton University Press.

Travassos, B., Araújo, D., Vilar, L., and McGarry, T. (2011) Interpersonal coordination and ball dynamics in futsal (indoor football). *Human Movement Science*, 30: 1245–59.

Travassos, B., Araújo, D., Duarte, R. and McGarry, T. (2012) Spatiotemporal coordination patterns in futsal (indoor football) are guided by informational game constraints. *Human Movement Science*, 31 (4):932–45.

Vilar, L., Araújo, D., Davids, K. and Button, C. (2012a) The role of ecological dynamics in analysising performance in team sports. *Sports Medicine*, 42(1): 1–10.

Vilar, L., Araújo, D., Davids, K. and Travassos, B. (2012b) Constraints on competitive performance of attacker–defender dyads in team sports. *Journal of Sport Sciences*, 30 (5): 459–69.

Watts, D. (1999) Networks, Dynamics and the Small-world Phenomenon. *American Journal of Sociology*, 105, (2): 493–527.

Watts, D. and Strogatz, S. (1998) Collective dynamics of 'small-world' networks. *Nature*, 393 (6684): 440–2.

7 The measurement of space and time in evolving sport phenomena

Sofia Fonseca, Ana Diniz and Duarte Araújo

This chapter provides an introduction to methods for analyzing both space and time in behavioural data. An overview of methods for analyzing time and, in particular, some methodologies in the so-called time and frequency domains are presented to characterize dynamical behaviours across time. Some important functions, such as the autocorrelation function and the spectral density function, are presented and some illustrations are made. We also present and describe methods for extracting, from a system of interacting agents, spatial time-series data capable of describing underlying dynamic system behaviours. Particular attention is given to applications in team sports. Results from recent studies are considered to illustrate the models presented.

Efforts at player motion capture have traditionally involved a range of data collection techniques, from live observation to post-event video analysis, where players' movement patterns are manually recorded and categorized to determine performance effectiveness. A variety of systems and methods have been employed to analyze the motion of athletes during sports, where the movements vary in duration, field position and surface, speed, acceleration, direction technique and tactics (Barris and Button 2008).

Indeed, a large number of variables can be considered to describe and classify individual and collective performance, from physical to psychological and physiological markers. Of particular relevance to team ball sports are spatial markers and, more precisely, information on the spatial organization (i.e. space management) of the players, as members of a team and as opponents. Moreover, sport science research suggests that performance data in sports needs to be evaluated in a continuous manner, given the variability inherent in such multivariate processes, which implies a permanent update and adjustment of variables over time (Davids *et al.* 2003). However, the classical methods of analysis are based on descriptive statistics, such as the mean and the standard deviation, and tend to ignore the dimension of time. In contrast, time-series methods, in the so-called time and frequency domains, focus on the dynamical behaviours across time and allow for modelling and inference.

Time series analysis methods

A time series is a sequence of observations, typically measured at successive time instants spaced at uniform time intervals. Formally, a time series is often denoted by $\{Y_1,\ldots,Yn\}$, where n is the length of the series. Figure 7.1 displays a time series referent to the distance, in metres, from a given sailing boat to a fixed optimal starting position, before the start of the regatta, recorded at 25 Hz, i.e. every 0.04 seconds (Araújo 2006). This time series has a length of $n = 579$ points and duration of 23.12 seconds.

To assess the fundamental properties of a time series, it is assumed that they are realizations of stochastic processes. A stochastic process is one that evolves over time and whose evolution at each time step is governed, at least in part, by probability. More precisely, a stochastic process is a family of random variables $\{Yt, t \in T\}$, defined on a probability space. One can use the term stochastic to refer to a behaviour that is influenced, to some degree, by both deterministic and random processes. In the sailing example, the position of the sailing boat relative to the optimal starting position may be seen as a realization of a stochastic process, since the position of the boat at each time is dependent on its previous positions with a given probability.

For some situations but not all, time series have a kind of stability that can reasonably be modelled by stationary processes (see Chapter 5). A stationary process is a stochastic process whose joint probability distribution does not change when shifted in time or space. Consequently, parameters such as the mean and the variance, if they exist, do not change over time or position. In the sailing example, the distance from the sailing boat to the optimal starting position seems to fluctuate slowly around a nearly constant or slightly decreasing mean level and seems to have a cyclical component. This suggests that the sailing boat approaches and departs from the fixed starting position in a roughly cyclical manner.

When the mentioned characteristics (e.g. stability) are known, time series can be studied in two domains of analysis, the time domain and the frequency domain. These domains are presented in the next section and illustrated with real and simulated time series.

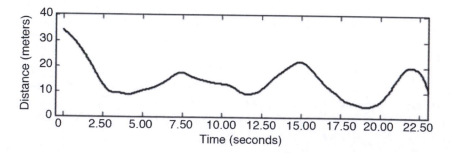

Figure 7.1 Exemplar data of the distance from a sailing boat to a fixed starting position before the start of the regatta; the length of this time series is 579 data points

Time domain analysis

In time domain analysis, the main goal is the evaluation of the behaviour of the process under study over time. In this domain, two central concepts are the mean and the autocorrelation function of the process. The latter function gives the correlation value of the process at different times. Formally, and in a wide sense, a stochastic process is said to be stationary if its mean is constant across time, its variance is constant across time and its autocorrelation function depends only on the time lag. Figure 7.2 illustrates realizations of length $n = 200$ of a stationary process and of two non-stationary processes. Note that the first time series (top panel) has a constant mean and a constant variance, the second has an increasing trend (middle panel) and the third has a growing variability (bottom panel).

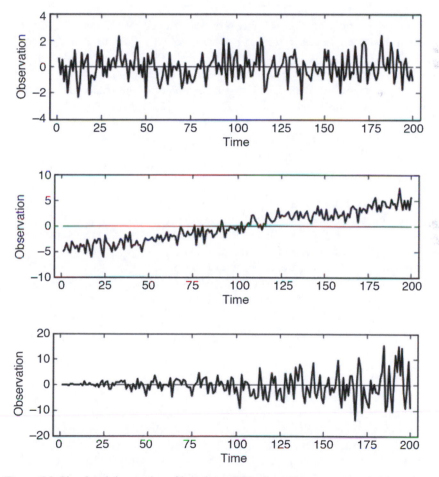

Figure 7.2 Simulated time series of length $n = 200$ of a stationary process (top), a non-stationary process with non-constant mean (middle) and a non-stationary process with non-constant variance (bottom)

When in the presence of non-stationary time series, the observed data points can usually be transformed into realizations of stationary processes by statistical techniques, such as differencing and others (e.g. Brockwell and Davis 1991, but see Chapter 5).

If the process $\{Yt, t \in T\}$ is stationary, then its autocorrelation function $\rho(.)$ is defined as:

$$\rho(k) = Corr(Y_t, Y_{t+k}), \text{ for all } t,k.$$

The function $\rho(.)$ has some important properties, such as:

$$-1 \leq \rho(k) \leq 1, \text{ for all } k,$$
$$\rho(-k) = \rho(k), \text{ for all } k.$$

The autocorrelation function $\rho(.)$ measures the strength of the statistical dependence of the process at each time lag. A value of $\rho(.)$ close to 1 at a given lag indicates strong positive correlation, while a value of $\rho(.)$ close to -1 at a given lag indicates strong negative correlation (or anti-correlation).

Given a time series $\{Y_1, \ldots, Yn\}$, an usual estimator of the autocorrelation function $\rho(.)$ is the sample autocorrelation function $\hat{\rho}(.)$ defined by:

$$\hat{\rho}(k) = \frac{\sum_{t=1}^{n-k} (Y_t - \bar{Y})(Y_{t+k} - \bar{Y})}{\sum_{t=1}^{n} (Y_t - \bar{Y})^2}, \ 0 \leq k \leq n - 1.$$

Notice that the sample autocorrelation function $\hat{\rho}(.)$ can be computed for any time series, even for series that are not realizations of stationary processes. Some works suggest that these sample autocorrelations $\hat{\rho}(.)$ should only be used if the series length n satisfies $n \geq 50$ and the time lag k satisfies $k \leq n/4$.

The simplest kind of stationary process is the white noise process. A stochastic process $\{Yt, t \in T\}$ is said to be white noise if the random variables have constant mean, usually equal to zero, constant variance and are uncorrelated (see also Chapter 5). This implies that the autocorrelation function $\rho(.)$ is zero everywhere, except at $k = 0$, and therefore is defined as:

$$\rho(k) = \begin{cases} 1, & k = 0, \\ 0, & |k| \geq 1. \end{cases}$$

Given a time series $\{Y_1, \ldots, Yn\}$, if the series is a realization of a white noise, then the sample autocorrelations $\hat{\rho}(.)$ should be relatively close to zero. More precisely, at a significance level of 5%, the sample autocorrelations $\hat{\rho}(.)$ should lie between the critical bounds $\pm 1.960/\sqrt{n}$. In contrast, one or more high values of the sample autocorrelations outside the critical bounds suggests that the time series is not a realization of a white noise.

Figure 7.3 illustrates a time series $\{Y_1, \ldots, Yn\}$ of length $n = 200$ generated from

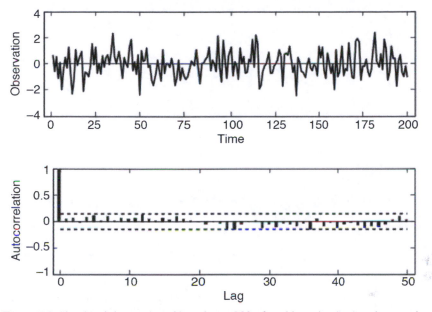

Figure 7.3 Simulated time series of length $n = 200$ of a white noise (top) and respective sample autocorrelation function at lags $k = 0, \ldots, 50$ (bottom) with critical bounds (dashed lines)

a white noise with mean zero and variance one. It also shows the sample autocorrelation function $\hat{\rho}(.)$ at lags $k = 0, \ldots, 50$ with the bounds $\pm 1.960/\sqrt{200} = \pm 0.139$.

Note that the time series fluctuates randomly around the mean and the sample autocorrelations are very close to zero lying between the critical bounds.

With respect to the sailing example shown earlier in this chapter, Figure 7.4 presents the time series $\{Y_1, \ldots, Y_n\}$ of length $n = 579$ relative to the distance from a sailing boat to a starting position. It also provides the sample autocorrelation function $\hat{\rho}(.)$ at lags $k = 0, \ldots, 350$ with the bounds $\pm 1.960/\sqrt{579} = \pm 0.081$.

Observe that the time series has a cyclical feature and the sample autocorrelations also exhibit a cyclical pattern lying outside the critical bounds. This implies that the sample autocorrelations are significant and take positive values at certain lags and negative values at other lags. Although it is unadvisable to compute the sample autocorrelations at lags larger than $n/4$, some of these values are represented here merely to show their periodicity.

Frequency domain analysis

In frequency domain analysis, the main objective is the decomposition of the process under study into a sum of sinusoidal components with fixed frequencies. A key concept is the spectral density function of the process. This function gives the amount of variance accounted for by each frequency in the process and

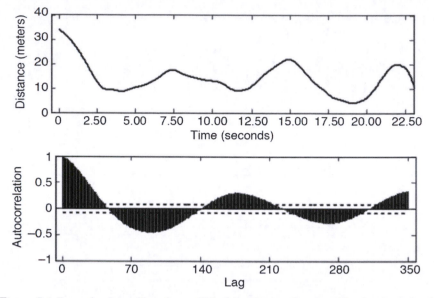

Figure 7.4 Exemplar data of length *n* = 579 of the distance from a sailing boat to a fixed starting position before the regatta starting (top) and respective sample autocorrelation function at lags *k* = 0, …, 350 (bottom) with critical bounds (dashed lines)

corresponds mathematically to the Fourier transform of the autocorrelation function. The Fourier transform is a mathematical operation that decomposes a function into its constituent frequencies. The spectral density function allows for identifying dominant frequencies in the process that may be associated to hidden periodicities. The frequency is the number of occurrences of a repeating process per unit of time and the SI unit for frequency is the Hertz (or cycles per second). Reciprocally, the period is the duration of one cycle in a repeating process and the SI unit for period is the second. The time domain analysis and the frequency domain analysis of time series are complementary and contribute, under different perspectives, to a better understanding of the observed phenomena.

If the process $\{Yt, t{\in}T\}$ is stationary, then its spectral density function $f(.)$ has some important properties, such as:

$$f(\lambda) \geq 0, \text{ for all } \lambda,$$
$$f(-\lambda) = f(\lambda), \text{ for all } \lambda,.$$

The spectral density function $f(.)$ measures the intensity of each frequency in the process over a range of frequencies. The larger the value of $f(.)$ at a given frequency, the larger the intensity (or power) of that frequency.

Given a time series $\{Y_1,…,Yn\}$, the usual estimator of the spectral density function $f(.)$ is the normalized periodogram $I_n(.)$ defined by:

$$I_n(\lambda_j) = \frac{1}{2\pi n} \left| \sum_{t=1}^{n} Y_t e^{-it\lambda_j} \right|^2, \quad \lambda_j = \frac{2\pi j}{n}, \quad j = 1,\dots, \left[\frac{n}{2}\right].$$

The normalized periodogram $I_n(.)$ is the modulus-squared of the discrete Fourier transform of the time series with a simple normalization and the λj are the frequencies.

If the process $\{Yt, t \in T\}$ is a white noise with mean zero and variance σ^2, then its spectral density function $f(.)$ is constant (flat) and is defined as:

$$f(\lambda) = \frac{\sigma^2}{2\pi}, \quad |\lambda| \le \pi.$$

Given a time series $\{Y_1,\dots,Yn\}$, if the series is a realization of a white noise, then the periodogram values $I_n(.)$ should be reasonably similar at all frequencies. In contrast, a high peak in the periodogram ordinates at a given frequency suggests that the time series is not a realization of a white noise and there is a preferred frequency. The significance of the largest peak in the periodogram ordinates can be tested using the Fisher's test (e.g. Brockwell and Davis 1991).

Figure 7.5 illustrates a time series $\{Y_1,\dots,Yn\}$ of length $n = 200$ generated from a white noise with mean zero and variance one. It also shows the normalized periodogram $I_n(.)$ at frequencies $\lambda_r = 2\pi r$ with $r = 0, \dots, 0.5$. Note that the time series fluctuates randomly around the mean and the periodogram values are reasonably similar at all frequencies.

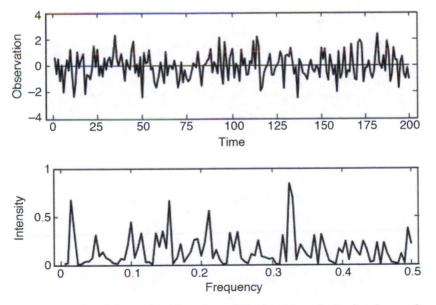

Figure 7.5 Simulated time series of length $n = 200$ of a white noise (top) and respective normalized periodogram at frequencies $\lambda_r = 2\pi r$ with $r = 0, \dots, 0.5$ (bottom)

For the sailing example, Figure 7.6 presents the time series $\{Y_1,...,Yn\}$ of length $n = 579$ relative to the distance from a sailing boat to a starting position. It also provides the normalized periodogram $I_n(.)$ at frequencies $\lambda_r = 2\pi r$ with $r = 0, ...,$ 0.5. Observe that the time series has a cyclical feature and the periodogram ordinates exhibit a high peak at a given frequency. The peak is significant and occurs at the frequency 0.00518, which implies a period of $1/0.00518 = 193$. This means that the series has indeed a cyclical pattern, repeating itself roughly every 193 time units, i.e. every 7.72 seconds.

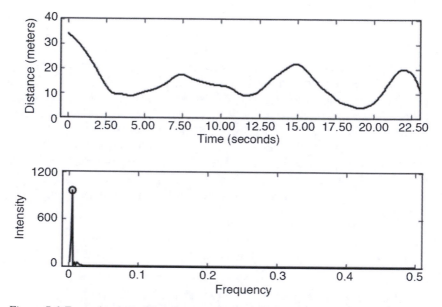

Figure 7.6 Exemplar data of length $n = 579$ of the distance from a sailing boat to a fixed starting position before the regatta starting (top) and respective normalized periodogram at frequencies $\lambda_r = 2\pi r$ with $r = 0, ..., 0.5$ (bottom)

In a stationary process, the autocorrelation function depends only on the time lag. In this case, the range of the correlation (or stochastic memory) of the process can be defined as the speed of the decay of the autocorrelation function.

Formally, a stationary process $\{Yt, t \in T\}$ is said to have short-range correlation (or short memory) if its autocorrelation function $\rho(.)$ satisfies the relation:

$$|\rho(k)| \leq c\, r^k, k = 0, 1, ...,$$

where c and r are two constants such that $c > 0$ and $0 < r < 1$ and k is the lag. This means that the function $\rho(.)$ decays to zero fast with a geometrically bounded decay.

Figure 7.7 represents a realization $\{Y_1,...,Yn\}$ of length $n = 200$ of a short-range correlation process. It also shows the sample autocorrelation function $\hat{\rho}(.)$

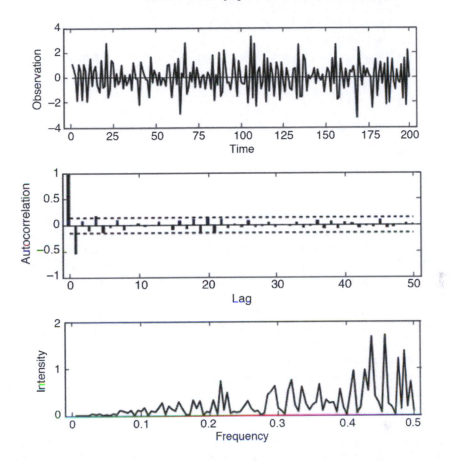

Figure 7.7 Simulated time series of length *n* = 200 of a short-range correlation process
(top), its sample autocorrelation function at lags *k* = 0, ..., 50 (middle) and
normalized periodogram at frequencies λ*r* = 2π*r* with *r* = 0, ..., 0.5 (bottom)

at lags *k* = 0, ..., 50 and the normalized periodogram $I_n(.)$ at frequencies λ*r* = 2π*r*
with *r* = 0, ..., 0.5. It is clear that the time series fluctuates rapidly around the
mean, the sample autocorrelation function has a large and negative value at lag
one with non-significant values after that, and the normalized periodogram has
larger values at high frequencies (which explains the series fluctuations).

Formally, a stationary process {*Yt*, *t*∈*T*} is said to have long-range correlation
(or long memory) if its autocorrelation function ρ(.) satisfies the power law:

$$\rho(k) \sim c \, k^{-(1-2d)}, \, k \to \infty,$$

where *c* and *d* are two constants such that *c* ≠ 0, *d* ≠ 0, and *d* < 0.5, and *k* is the
lag. This means that the function ρ(.) decays to zero very slowly with a hyperbolic
decay. Moreover, the process is said to have persistent long-range correlation if

$0 < d < 0.5$, so that $\Sigma k \; \rho(k) = \infty$, reflecting the fact that the remote past has an influence into the present.

In the frequency domain, a long-range correlation process can be defined as a process whose spectral density function $f(.)$ satisfies the power law:

$$f(\lambda) \sim c \; \lambda^{-2d}, \lambda \to 0,$$

where c and d are two constants such that $c \neq 0$, $d \neq 0$, and $d < 0.5$, and λ is the frequency. This means that the function $f(.)$ has a pole at zero if $0 < d < 0.5$, that is $f(0) = \infty$, signifying that the low frequencies predominate and therefore long-term oscillations are expected. These processes whose function $f(.)$ has the form $f(\lambda) \sim \lambda^{-\alpha}$, where α is a constant, are usually known as $1/f\,\alpha$ noise. This property of the spectral density function $f(.)$ can be used to distinguish different types of noise in terms of colour: $\alpha = 0$ (white noise) and $\alpha = 1$ (pink noise), amongst others. It is worth mentioning that pink noise has been found in a number of time series from human movement systems and some stochastic models have been proposed for explaining these phenomena (e.g. Diniz *et al.* 2010, 2011).

Figure 7.8 represents a realization $\{Y_1, \ldots, Yn\}$ of length $n = 400$ of a long-range correlation process. It also shows the sample autocorrelation function $\hat{\rho}(.)$ at lags $k = 0, \ldots, 50$ and the normalized periodogram $I_n(.)$ at frequencies $\lambda_r = 2\pi r$ with $r = 0, \ldots, 0.5$. It is clear that the time series exhibits long non-periodic oscillations around the mean, the sample autocorrelation function has large and positive values with hyperbolic decay and the normalized periodogram has larger values at low frequencies (which explains the series fluctuations).

For the distinction between short- and long-range correlations, the length of the time series is an important question. In fact, a realization of a stationary process with long-range correlation can easily be mistaken for a realization of a non-stationary process, if the series length is very small. The statistical discrimination between short- and long-range correlations can be done using several tests, such as the rescaled range method (R/S), the detrended fluctuation analysis (DFA) and others (e.g. Palma 2007; but see Chapter 5).

With the sailing example, the method of analysis of the distance between a sailing boat and an optimal point for the start of the regatta was illustrated in terms of its time structure. Somehow, space was analyzed as a function of time. It is also possible to analyze changes in the spatial structure across time. After presenting some bases for performing time series analysis, we then describe a method for performing spatial patterns analysis – Voronoi diagrams – which is starting to be used in sport sciences.

Voronoi-based models for team sports analysis

Studying spatial patterns formed by a group of individuals gives us some insight into the understanding of interactive behaviour, in both the individual and collective dimensions. For example, spatial patterns characterized by large distances between all individuals will indicate some source of inhibition, whereas small

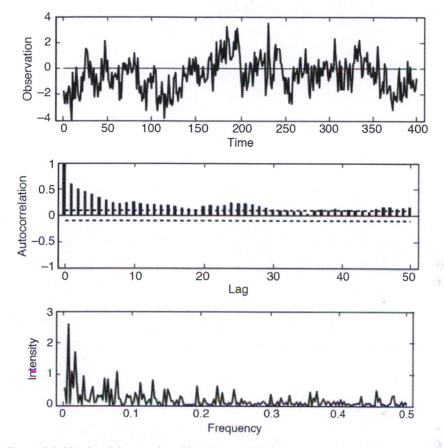

Figure 7.8 Simulated times series of length $n = 400$ of a long-range correlation process (top), its sample autocorrelation function at lags $k = 0, \ldots, 50$ (middle) and normalized periodogram at frequencies $\lambda_r = 2\pi r$ with $r = 0, \ldots, 0.5$ (bottom)

distances will indicate some source of attraction. In addition, larger interpersonal distances associated with a single individual may reflect some source of avoidance. In the sports context, spatial pattern analysis is thought to be a useful approach for characterizing and evaluating players' space management, which is associated with patterns of interacting behaviour.

The methods described below are based on a well-known two-dimensional spatial tessellation (or decomposition), the Voronoi diagrams. Given a set of n points distributed in a plane (Figure 7.9A), this spatial construction divides the plane into n cells (Figure 7.9B), each associated with one and only one point; in other words, each cell corresponds to a part of the plane that is closer to one of the points (see Okabe *et al.* 2000). For instance, in a soccer match, the points could be the position of the players, the plane the play area and the cells the regions associated to each player.

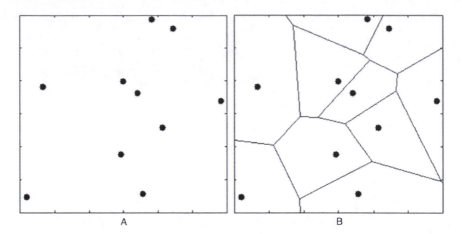

Figure 7.9 Example of a set of points in a plane (A) and corresponding Voronoi diagram
(B)

This spatial construction has already been suggested by other authors for studying players' spatial distribution in team sports, having been applied in variety of game settings, namely, electronic soccer games (Kim 2004), robotic soccer (Law 2005), on-field hockey games (Fujimura and Sugihara 2005) and on-field soccer games (Taki *et al.* 1996). The Voronoi cells that define the individual dominant region of each player (Taki *et al.* 1996; Fujimura and Sugihara 2005) change continuously over time, owing to continuous adjustments of the players' positions, which implies permanent changes in the global spatial configuration. Thus, for an adequate application of such markers in any team sports, these areas should be analyzed throughout the duration of the game or trial. For instance, in the work by Kim (2004), the spatial markers considered were area and number of vertices of each Voronoi region; however, these were averaged, eliminating the temporal component of the phenomenon, which in this particular study limits the understanding and explanation of players' spatial relation.

The models described here allow the study of performance at different levels of analysis: model 1 – player and team individual behaviour; and model 2 – intra- and interteam interaction behaviour. Here, we present some examples that, with some adaptations, can be applied to other sports. A particular aspect to be considered in such an adaptation is the number of players involved and the field dimensions. Codes are available upon request from the lead author of this chapter.

Model 1: player and team individual behaviour

In this model, we consider the Voronoi diagram generated to the set of points corresponding to the positions of players from two opponent teams during a game or trial.

When formally analyzing these regions across time, one can better understand player and team spatial interaction. For example, at a *team level* in football (soccer), the attacker team is expected to free up space, increasing its area of action, while the defender team tries to tie up space, decreasing its area of action (McGarry *et al.* 2002). At a *player level*, in soccer for example, players from the defender team are expected to maintain their space closed to prevent attacker players to score, keeping their net tight while in danger (Figure 7.10A); on the other hand, players from the attacker team are expected to keep greater dominant regions but some will try to disturb defenders' organization and create instability by changing their action (Passos *et al.* 2008), as entering the defence zone (Figure 7.10B).

A detailed description of the method is presented next. Given a game or trial of *f* frames (see Chapter 9), in a play area of dimension W × H metres, consider that the trajectory of each of the P players involved was captured and adequately converted to real coordinates, so that for each player a collection of coordinates $\{(x,y)^1,(x,y)^f\}$ is available.

The play area is mapped with a grid of W × H positions. At each frame (*f*), the area of the Voronoi cell of player k (VA(k), $k \in [1,P]$) is the sum of all grid positions (i,j) (where $i = 1,..,W$ and $j = 1,...,H$) that are closer to that player than they are to any other player. This can be mathematically defined as:

$$VA(k)^f = \sum_{i=1}^{W} \sum_{j=1}^{H} I_{(i,j)} \qquad k = 1,...,P$$

where $I(i,j)$ is a Boolean function that takes value 1 if player k is the closest player to the grid position (i,j) and 0 otherwise

$$I_{(i,j)} = \begin{cases} 1 & \text{if } \sqrt{(i - x_k^f)^2 + (j - y_k^f)^2} < \sqrt{(i - x_m^f)^2 + (j - y_m^f)^2}, \forall m \neq k, m = 1,...,P \\ 0 & \text{otherwise} \end{cases}$$

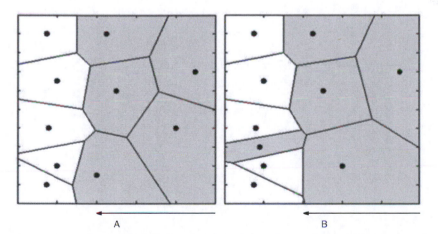

A   B

Figure 7.10 Spatial configurations: (A) attacker (grey areas) and defender (white areas) teams and; (B) attacker player breaking defence organization; the arrow indicates the direction of the attack

Grid points that are equidistant between two or more players constitute the boundaries of their respective regions and therefore are not added to the corresponding areas.

The calculated areas can be used to investigate how the size of the Voronoi cells changes over time for each team and/or for each player and related to specific phases, events and/or characteristics of the game.

The model described was applied to data from futsal (Fonseca *et al.* 2012b). We considered 19 trials from five versus four plus goalkeeper plays, all starting with similar conditions and each ending when the attack lost ball possession. On average, plays lasted 848 (± 374) frames (corresponding to approximately 0.57 (± 0.249) minutes), a minimum of 315 and maximum of 1558 frames (approximately 0.21 and 1.04 minutes, respectively). The main results are presented below.

With model 1, it was possible to verify the following: (1) on average and for all plays, the attacker team had Voronoi regions with larger areas in comparison with those defined by the defender team (Figure 7.11); (2) the area of these regions was more variable for the attacker team, which presented, in each frame and across the duration of all trials, a larger standard deviation of the Voronoi area (Figure 7.11). In addition, (3) the spatial behaviour of the attacking players was more stable during each trial, presenting Voronoi areas with smaller approximate entropy (see Chapter 5; see also Fonseca *et al.* (2012a) for criteria for normalizing time series for performing entropy analysis), as illustrated in Figure 7.12.

It is also interesting to study intra- and interteam behaviour, as we next describe.

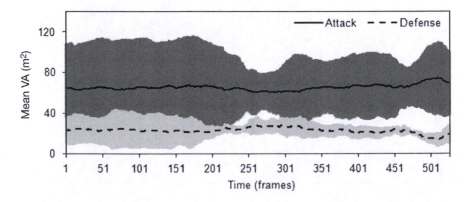

Figure 7.11 Example (one play) of the mean Voronoi area (VA) across time for each team; error bars represent the standard deviation (adapted from Fonseca *et al.* 2011a)

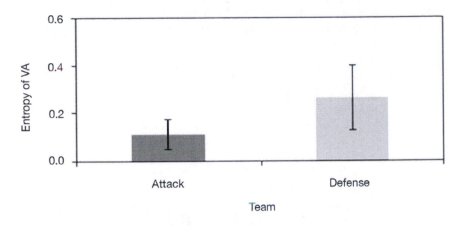

Figure 7.12 Comparison of the mean entropy of Voronoi area (VA) between teams in the
same trial; error bars represent the standard deviation (*** $P < 0.001$);
adapted from Fonseca *et al.* (2011a)

Model 2: intra- and interteam interaction behaviour

In this model, we consider Voronoi diagrams generated separately for the competing groups, e.g. in a sports application, these could be the attacker and defender
teams. The superimposition of these two diagrams, illustrated in Figure 7.13,
allows an interesting spatial analysis of individual and collective interaction
behaviour. This graphical construction can be considered as evaluating the similarity between the spatial distributions of two opponent groups. If each pair of

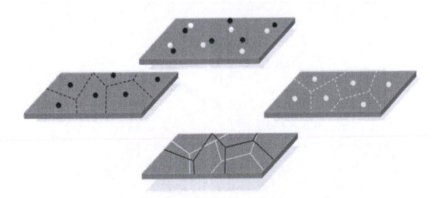

Figure 7.13 Construction of the superimposed Voronoi diagram (bottom) from
considering, separately, the Voronoi diagrams for team A (black dots) and
team B (white dots)

opponents is closely located, as illustrated in Figure 7.14A, the overlapped diagram will indicate an almost perfect fit between the two Voronoi diagrams. On the other hand, for spatially unrelated pairs, the described spatial composition will indicate the opposite, as in Figure 7.14B.

To quantify this spatial agreement, two variables were defined, one to measure the degree of coordination at an individual level and the other for measuring coordination at a team level. More precisely, the *maximum percentage of overlapped area* (max%OA) measures coordination at player level and the *percentage of free area* (%FA) measures coordination at team level.

The max%OA is calculated for each player and represents the maximum percentage of the Voronoi cell that is covered by the cell of an opponent; the smaller this measure the greater the number of opponents in the neighbourhood (Figure 7.15A). The %FA summarizes the degree of similarity between the

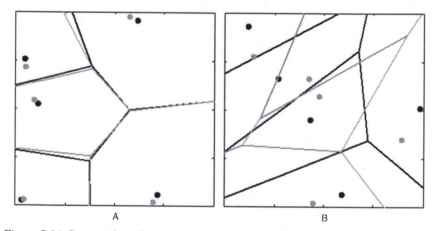

A   B

Figure 7.14 Construction of the superimposed Voronoi diagram for (A) exclusively paired opponents and (B) randomly located individuals

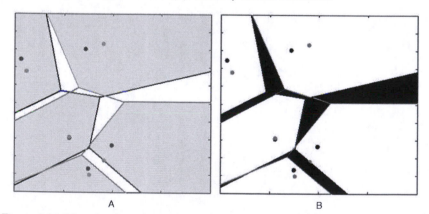

A   B

Figure 7.15 Measures from the superimposed Voronoi diagram: (A) maximum percentage of overlapped area for each individual of the group marked with black dots; and (B) percentage of free area (in black)

overlapped Voronoi diagrams, which is calculated by extracting from the plane the sum of the max%OA calculated for one of the groups (Figure 7.15B).

The %FA is inversely proportional to the degree of agreement between the spatial configurations of both groups and therefore can be used to analyze and characterize the interaction behaviour between them. This construction is of particular interest for studying interaction behaviour in team sports, where the two groups correspond to two competing teams.

Consequently, in team sports, when analyzing the spatial distribution of two opponent teams playing in a well-defined area of known dimensions, it is possible to consider reference values associated to two specific spatial relations: i) when each player of the defender team assumes an exclusive pairing with an opponent, which can be linked to a man-to-man defensive method; and ii) when players from both teams are randomly distributed in the playing area, which, while may not appear to be a reasonable assumption for players' behaviour, provides a reference for the interteam spatial arrangement when the location of each player is chosen, regardless of the location of the others. To exemplify this, model 2 was applied to data from futsal (Fonseca *et al.* 2011). We considered 19 trials from five versus four plus goalkeeper plays, all starting with similar conditions and each ending when the attack lost ball possession.

Reference values for this specific setting, ten players in a play area of 20 m², were generated for randomly distributed players and exclusively paired at different interpersonal (inter-pair) distances. For situations where players are exclusively paired with an opponent, the percentage of free area increases as the maximum distance allowed between the pairs increases. The lower and upper reference values obtained for complete spatial randomness (CSR), i.e. when all players are randomly allocated in space, were 0.22 and 0.50, corresponding to the upper and lower limits of a 95% confidence envelope for the %FA:

$$\begin{cases} \%FA_{CSR}^{lower} = \%FA_{25:1000} \\ \%FA_{CSR}^{upper} = \%FA_{95:1000} \end{cases}$$

where $\%FA_{25:1000}$ and $\%FA_{95:1000}$ represent the order, out of 1000, of the %FA obtained in simulated patterns of CSR.

Based on these reference values, it is possible to classify at each frame of a trial how players are spatially distributed; in particular, observed values below the lower limit of the 95% confidence envelopes for CSR suggest that the defender team is likely to be applying a man-to-man defence method (exclusive pairing). Figure 7.16 shows the %FA observed across the duration of one trial in this study.

A spatial approach of futsal players' collective behaviour in a five versus four plus one played in midfield suggests that players are not considering a man-to-man defence strategy, which is what was expected, given the setting of this study. It also indicates that the zone defence method spatially relates to an absence of interaction between players, as the observed value of %FA is, during most of each trial, within the corresponding bands, [0.22, 0.50].

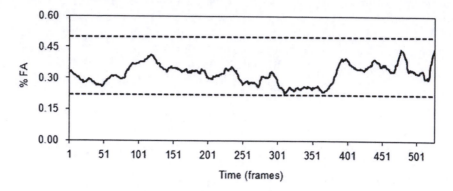

Figure 7.16 Example (one play) of the observed percentage of free area (%FA) across time (solid line) and the 95% confidence interval for spatial random distribution (dashed lines)

Conclusion

In sport, space and time are key parameters to consider if individual or collective behaviours are to be understood. However, space and time should not be considered in abstract terms but embedded in the variables that capture the interaction between the performer and the environment. In this chapter, we have presented ways in which such analysis could be performed. First, we described how time series could be analyzed in the time domain and in the frequency domain. Moreover, we argued that the analysis of spatial patterns formed by a group of individuals could give insights about individual and collective behaviours. For this type of analysis, we presented a technique called the Voronoi diagrams, a two-dimensional spatial decomposition of geometrical space. The techniques described focus on the individual behaviour of the player and team and on the intra- and interteam interaction behaviour. These are possibilities that open new ways to understand the complexity of sport behaviour.

Questions for students

1. What are the major differences between time domain and frequency domain analysis and which are some relevant functions in each of these methodologies?
2. What does the stochastic memory of a process indicate about the dependence structure of that process over time?
3. Why may it be important for the statistical analysis of the underlying process to have time series that are relatively long?
4. In the sports context, what do the areas defined by the Voronoi diagrams represent?

5. What characteristics, besides spatial location and field area, could be considered to weight the Voronoi cell of each player?
6. What are, in principle, the spatial characteristics of the interaction behaviour between players in team sports that could be tested using any of the models presented?

References

Araújo, D. (2006) *Tomada de Decisão no Desporto*. [Decision-making in Sport]. Cruz Quebrada: Edições FMH.

Barris, S. and Button, C. (2008) A review of vision-based motion analysis in sport. *Sports Medicine*, 38 (12): 1025–43.

Brockwell. P. J. and Davis, R. A. (1991) *Time Series: Theory and Methods*, 2nd edn. New York: Springer.

Davids, K., Glazier, P., Araújo, D. and Bartlett, R. (2003) Movement systems as dynamical systems: the functional role of variability and its implications for sports medicine. *Sports Medicine*, 33 (4): 245–60.

Diniz, A., Barreiros, J. and Crato, N. (2010) Parameterized estimation of long-range correlation and variance components in human serial interval production. *Motor Control*, 14: 26–43.

Diniz, A., Wijnants, M. L., Torre, K., Barreiros, J., Crato, N., Bosman, A. M. T., Hasselman, F., Cox, R. F. A., Van Orden, G. C. and Delignières, D. (2011) Contemporary theories of 1/f noise in motor control. *Human Movement Science*, 30: 889–905.

Fonseca, S., Milho, J., Travassos, B. and Araujo, D. (2011) Modeling intra- and inter-team spatial interaction in team sports, Symposium on A Complex Systems Approach to Studying Behaviour in Sport. Organizer: Keith Davids. 13th FEPSAC European Congress of Sport Psychology, Madeira, Portugal.

Fonseca, S., Milho, M., Passos, P., Araújo, D. and Davids, K. (2012a) Approximate entropy normalized measures for analyzing social neurobiological systems. *Journal of Motor Behavior*, 44 (3): 179–83.

Fonseca, S., Milho, M., Travassos, B. and Araújo, D. (2012b) Spatial dynamics of team sports using Voronoi diagrams. *Human Movement Science*, 31 (6): 1652–9.

Fujimura, A. and Sugihara, K. (2005) Geometric analysis and quantitative evaluation of sport teamwork. *Systems and Computers in Japan*, 36 (6): 49–58.

Kim, S. (2004) Voronoi analysis of a soccer game. *Nonlinear Analysis: Modelling and Control*, 9(3): 233–40.

Law, J. (2005) Analysis of Multi-Robot Cooperation using Voronoi Diagrams. Proceedings of the 3rd International Kemurdjian Workshop 'Planetary rovers, space robotics and Earth-based robots-2005', St Petersburg, Russia, October 2005.

McGarry, T., Anderson, D. I., Wallace, S. A., Hughes, M. D. and Franks, I. M. (2002) Sport competition as a dynamical self-organizing system. *Journal of Sports Sciences*, 20 (10): 771–81.

Okabe, A., Boots, B., Sugihara, K., Chiu, S. N. and Kendall, D. G. (2008) *Spatial Tessellations: Concepts and Applications of Voronoi Diagrams*, 2nd edn. Hoboken, NJ: John Wiley.

Palma, W. (2007) *Long-Memory Time Series: Theory and Methods*. New Jersey: Wiley.

Passos, P., Araújo, D., Davids, K., Gouveia, L., Milho, J. and Serpa, S. (2008) Information-governing dynamics of attacker-defender interactions in youth rugby union. *Journal of Sports Sciences*, 26 (13): 1421–9.

Taki, T., Hasegawa, J. and Fukumura, T. (1996) Development of motion analysis system for quantitative evaluation of teamwork in soccer games, in *Proceedings of the International Conference on Image Processing, 16 September 1996, Lausanne*. IEEE, Vol. 3, pp. 815–18.

8 Self-organizing maps and cluster analysis in elite and sub-elite athletic performance

Wolfgang Schöllhorn, Jia Yi Chow, Paul Glazier and Chris Button

This chapter examines ways in which movement patterns can be analyzed as performance contexts change or as a function of learning and development. The methods described can be used to study the effects of important factors such as fatigue, injury, learning, development or training in motor performance.

Classifying objects can be considered as one of the major tasks in science (Slife 1995). Classifying usually occurs at the beginning of the research process and involves categorizing objects by criteria specified by the investigator. Most often, these criteria are associated with implicit assumptions and rely on a certain philosophical background. In the scientific literature, two general types of classification study can be identified; those adopting a confirmatory approach or an exploratory approach, with the former being more common (Tukey 1980; Jaeger and Halliday 1998). In confirmatory approaches, the classes are given in advance and are tested for statistical significance. In exploratory approaches, by contrast, only the criteria for the classification of the objects are provided. Once certain classes are identified, the explorative approach can be followed by the confirmatory approach so as to test the identified classes for significance.

For methodological and historical reasons, the quantitative investigation of movement has typically been focused on the classification of simple movements on the basis of time-discrete amplitudes of selected variables. In biomechanical studies, these time-discrete variables (also known as performance parameters) have typically been specified by deterministic or hierarchical models and have some relationship with performance outcome. Time-series data typically have to be reduced or collapsed to single data points (maximum, minimum, average, value at specific event, etc.) and pooled so that (confirmatory) statistical analyses can be performed. In parallel, the analysis of movements has been mainly limited to the statistical comparison of single variables. In cases where multiple variables have been analyzed, potentially more useful practical knowledge can be derived.

When movement patterns are classified by means of multiple time-continuous variables, a more holistic approach is pursued. The difference between a time-discrete and time-continuous movement description can be illustrated with an analogy. If we see a known person far away standing still, it is often difficult to identify that person. Once he/she starts to walk, our visual system receives additional information that increases the likelihood of recognizing that person.

Similarly, if only the left elbow of the person walking can be viewed, the probability of correctly identifying that person is rather low. However, if the motion of other joints and segments are presented simultaneously, the probability of recognizing the person improves. Indeed, Johansson (1973) showed that perception of biological motion relies more heavily on relative motion, rather than absolute motion characteristics of limb and torso segments.

While time-discrete variables focus on instantaneous characteristics of single joint or segment motion, time-continuous variables provide the opportunity to categorize movement qualities such as types of movement (jumping, running, etc.), modes of movement (springy, tentative, rushed, etc.) and individual styles (individual expressions of types and modes) of movements. According to pattern analysis, the quantification of coordination is initiated by means of the determination of a reference pattern to which all other patterns have to be compared with. Alternatively, the similarity of all patterns to each other can also be determined.

Numerous questions can be addressed through the quantitative description of movement patterns in sport on the basis of time-continuous variables. For example, how similar are the average patterns of movement within a class of movement? How are gait patterns similar within an individual across different performance context or between different individuals? Even in the study of plants or animals and their subordination into certain classes in biology, a first step for time-continuous movement patterns is their classification on the basis of certain criteria. Because the general classification of movements already has been performed successfully by numerous scientists (e.g. Hay 1993), mathematical algorithms are first required that are relevant to everyday experience and observations. Thus, plausible criteria for the classification of objects seem to be their relative similarity or proximity in a most abstract understanding. The quantitative sorting of objects by means of linear distances led to the development of different forms of cluster analysis (Everitt *et al.* 2001), while the mathematical simulation of neuronal assemblies was associated with artificial neural nets that meanwhile provided plausible nonlinear groupings.

Without delving too deeply into the problem of interpreting similarity or proximity (Everitt *et al.* 2001), the simplest procedure is to quantify a certain quality of all objects and to determine the relative distance of these quantities (e.g. three people walking should be clustered on the basis of their minimum knee flexion during single stance phase in gait). The first step in such a procedure would be to assign a quality or variable to 'knee flexion', such as 'knee angle'. This quality is typically represented by a unit such as radians or degrees. Hence, qualities can be compared by means of their relative size or a vector distance. A commonly used measure for mathematical comparisons is the Euclidean distance, which represents the distance between two objects on a straight line. If the distance between two knee angles of two participants is smaller than the distance relative to a third participant, the first two participants would be assigned to the first cluster and the third participant to another. Applying the same procedure to movement patterns that are described by means of multiple time course variables, some vector and matrix algebra is necessary that includes similarity and proximity measures analogously. In contrast to cluster analysis, which exclusively sorts objects, self-organizing maps (SOMS; as a specific form of artificial neural network [ANN]) have the additional ability to reduce high-dimensional data to low-dimensional data. Therefore, SOMs are often used as a preparatory tool for cluster analysis.

In the following sections, we examine the application of cluster analysis and SOMs to movement analysis in sport and human movement science.

Cluster analysis

As discussed earlier, the application of cluster analysis in sport can be divided into exploratory and confirmatory approaches. In the exploratory approach, hierarchical cluster analyses are typically applied to holistic descriptions of movements. Starting with a single object, all other objects are clustered successively by means of a chosen metric until all objects are included. The exploration of the number and size of the clusters along the relative metric provides either previously expected groups of movements or leads to a new categorization that has to be interpreted creatively. In summary, here the least information about the structure of the objects is included in the classification process. In the second case of plausible interpretations, the confirmatory approach, can be followed. Here, the classes or at least the number of classes are given in advance and the cluster analysis procedure classifies all objects accordingly on the basis of the chosen metric. Subsequently, the identified clusters have to be validated and any cluster differences has to be tested for significance. However, irrespective of the approach, a dominant influence on the results is given by the chosen variables as well as by their pre-processing. Thus, the selection of variables is directly connected with the specificity of the hypothesis and the expectation of the investigator while the pre-processing of the data has an indirect but strong influence on the relative weighting of the variables with respect to the resulting clusters (for further details, see Everitt *et al.* 2001; Rein *et al.* 2010a).

Owing to the increased processing capacity of computers by the end of the last century, cluster analysis has since been applied increasingly to large sets of time course oriented movement data without data reduction.

Exploratory approaches

One of the first exploratory applications of cluster analysis in the context of movement pattern analysis in sports was provided by Müller (1986). Several kinematic variable time courses and muscular activities were measured during the demonstration of different skiing techniques for downhill skiers. Discrete biomechanical parameters were extracted and classified by means of a cluster analysis. It was found that irrespective of the snow and slope conditions, the techniques could be classified as similar.

An explorative cluster analysis on the basis of time-continuous variables in discus-throwing movements during practice of a single high-performance athlete provided evidence for a successful learning process that led to enduring/lasting qualitative changes of the throwing technique (Schöllhorn 1993). Eight discus-throwing trials before and after a biomechanical feedback intervention were described by means of the time courses of 40 joint angles and angular velocities during the final throwing phase. Three trials were performed within one competition before the intervention and five trials during different competitions following the intervention. For data reduction, these high-dimensional data were factor analyzed. The resulting factor-loading matrices were compared by means of a structure comparison algorithm, which led to a distance matrix. The subsequent cluster analysis (Figure 8.1) clearly separated three trials (T791–T793) before a specific training intervention from five trials (T84–T88) performed after the biomechanical feedback. Figure 8.1 displays exemplarily the history of a hierarchical cluster analysis applied to eight discus throws during a learning process. The cluster analysis begins with determining the distances between all trials and is followed by determining the two most similar (smallest distance) trials (T791 and T793). The clustered trials are then considered as a single new trial. Subsequently, the next two trials with the smallest distance are clustered together and so on until all trials are clustered together. Similar results revealed the cluster analysis of the same data when data reduction was performed by means orthogonal reference functions (Schöllhorn 1995).

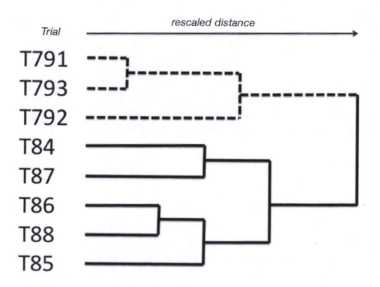

Figure 8.1 Clustering dendrogram resulting from an average linkage algorithm; horizontal lines indicate the level of the rescaled distance at which the respective movements are grouped into one cluster

Explorative cluster analysis of biomechanical data during several double steps in running provided a separation of left and right contact phase as well as of flight phase. Just by examining the ground contact phase of a single leg, 95% of the runners could be identified individually (Schöllhorn 1999). A similar application of cluster analysis to kinematic and muscular variables in long jumping allowed the identification of the athletes during take off (Jaitner *et al.* 2001a,b). Muscular variables pertaining to either the envelope of the rectified electromyography signals or their frequency spectra can be taken as input variables for the classification process for the cluster analysis. Different levels of expertise in handball players were also identified inter- and intra-individually on the basis of time-continuous, three-dimensional kinematic data of the hip, shoulder, elbow and wrist joint by Schorer *et al.* (2007). Cluster analysis yielded an assignment rate of 92% for the level of expertise.

A new direction in terms of cluster analysis applications in the field of elite sports was taken by Jäger *et al.* (2003) by analyzing tactical behaviour of teams in the form of player's coordinates during volleyball matches from the 2002 World Championships. Over 250 similar situations during a tournament where six participating teams competed against each other, were video recorded at 50 Hz. Positions (x and y coordinates) of the defending teams during a defensive move in time-discrete and time-continuous form were inputted to a cluster analysis that subsequently revealed team specific behaviours. Contrary to the opinions of a coach, who believed that all teams played with the same system, the specific behaviours of each team could be identified by means of the movement of all six players during the defence movement independent of the opponent. This individuality of team dynamics has a number of potential implications for tactical training.

Confirmatory approaches

A confirmatory approach of cluster analysis with a single discrete duration parameter was examined by Lames (1992). Using ideas from dynamical systems theory and with a focus on investigating the hysteresis effects (see Kelso 1995), the duration of the driving and pitching movement of several golfers was measured for different distances. In order to initiate a hysteresis effect, the golfers performed shots from 100 metres first, then decreasing down to ten metres in five-metre steps and then increasing back to 100 metres. The subsequent cluster analysis of the movement durations led to two, three, four or five clusters from which only the three-cluster solution could be interpreted plausibly in accordance with the assumed hysteresis phenomenon.

In a more recent study by Chow *et al.* (2008), which examined coordination changes of novice participants in a football (soccer)-kicking task, cluster analysis was also effectively used to determine intra-individual differences in kicking patterns. Key kinematic data of various joint motions were captured over a four-week intervention period (40 trials per session over 12 sessions) and the kinematic data were used as input for a cluster analysis procedure. Differences in coordination patterns within individual for each session were effectively determined and the information provided valuable insights about movement pattern variability, as well as the presence of preferred kicking patterns. Such information is extremely critical in helping researchers to understand the learning processes and to investigate nonlinearity in learning evidenced by sudden transitions from one movement pattern to another, as well as the emergence of pattern variability prior to a transition.

Another confirmatory application of cluster analysis was performed by Ball and Best (2007) to determine the presence of weight transfer for two styles of golf swing. Sixty-two golfers, from professionals to high-handicap players, performed simulated drives, hitting a golfball into a net. While standing on two force plates, the centre of pressure position relative to the feet was quantified at eight swing events identified from a 200-Hz video. Cluster analysis on the basis of these time-discrete parameters revealed two major styles of golf swing: a front-foot style and a reverse style. Nevertheless, validation procedures were required.

Validation of clusters

As cluster techniques will always identify groups of data depending on the identification parameters, it is important to consider additional procedures to validate them. For supporting and providing the statistical proof of the resulting clusters, different approaches have been suggested. According to Handl *et al.* (2005), cluster validation measures can be distinguished into internal and external measures:

> External validation measures comprise all those methods that evaluate a clustering result based on the knowledge of the correct class labels…Internal validation techniques do not use additional knowledge in the form of class labels, but base their quality estimate on the information intrinsic to the data alone.
>
> (Handl *et al.* 2005: 3203)

With further extension to the work by Lames (1992), Rein *et al.* (2010b) applied an internal validation approach to their cluster analysis of basketball shooting. The phenomenon of phase transition in basketball hook shots with decreasing and increasing distances from nine metres to two metres and back to nine metres, with one-metres increments was investigated. The input variables for the cluster analysis were 12 angle variables derived from a 13-segment, rigid, three-dimensional body model. The clusters were interpreted in the terminology of systems dynamics as attractors with certain criteria. Only two of eight participants showed a clear expected phase transition behaviour. Importantly, in this preliminary study, it was possible to identify three distinctive shooting patterns with varying frequencies at different shooting distances.

As three different shooting patterns had been previously established, the external validation procedures were adopted by Rein *et al.* (2010a). Two studies in basketball served for testing the sensitivity of cluster analysis to pre-processing and for testing the phenomenon of phase transitioning in hook-shot technique. For the first experiment, four professional basketball players had to throw from three different distances with three different techniques. Owing to the impact of data normalization, the same analysis was performed with z-transformed (average = 0, standard deviation = 1) and raw data. Both sets were validated by means of bootstrapping and Hubert-Gamma method. Overall, in the first experiment, the cluster analyses led to 'entirely feasible' results and were able to reproduce a priori known differences between diverse movement patterns. In the second validation study, two basketball players were instructed to shoot baskets by means of a hook-shot technique from distances between two to nine metres. In contrast to Rein *et al.* (2010b), the task was limited by a lowered ceiling to force flight curves of the ball that are dominated by the velocity of release than by the angle of release, with the aim of causing a phase transition in the movement pattern with increasing or decreasing distance. Only one participant showed strong indications of the use of two distinct patterns whereas another participant displayed 'distinctively fewer differences' as shooting distance was manipulated. Bootstrapping and Hubert-Gamma values showed that a validation procedure is necessary for the confirmatory approach of cluster analysis.

The external validation approach pursues the probability of ending up with certain clusters relative to arbitrary or accidental data. The internal approach compares the variation within a cluster relative to the variation between clusters (Bauer and Schöllhorn 1997). Both approaches demonstrate the problem and importance of variable selection and preparation that is known in the context of analyzing complex self-organizing systems (Haken *et al.* 1995). According to Haken *et al.* (1995), the selection of collective variables or order parameters is highly dependent on the investigator's intuition. The problem seems to become even bigger with increasing complexity of the movement task and the possibilities of compensations. Yet there are no general rules for the choice and selection of variables as well as for the preparation of the data before cluster analysis.

In summary, cluster analysis provides a powerful dimension reduction tool which can serve different purposes depending on the nature (i.e. explorative or confirmatory) of the research undertaken. In contrast to cluster analysis, ANNs have the ability to separate two classes nonlinearly (Figure 8.2) and therefore lead to higher recognition rates and potentially more flexibility in their use (Haykin 1994; Schöllhorn and Jäger 2006). As we discuss in the next section, ANNs can be administered independently or in combination with cluster analysis.

Self-organizing maps

SOMs, also known as Kohonen maps, are a specific type of ANN that can be used to mathematically model specific characteristics of neuronal cell assemblies. In contrast to supervised learning ANNs such as multi-layer-perceptrons (MLPs), SOMs are trained using unsupervised learning to typically produce a two-dimensional discrete representation of the input space of the training samples, called a map. A big advantage of SOMs is the way in which it captures

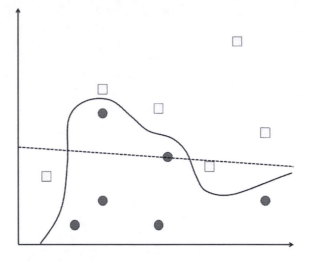

Figure 8.2 Linear versus nonlinear separation

low-dimensional views of high-dimensional data, akin to multidimensional scaling. SOMs are different from other ANNs because of their usage of a neighbourhood function that preserves the topological properties of the input space. Similar to most ANNs, SOMs operate in two phases. In the first phase, the map is trained using input examples. The second phase, called mapping, automatically classifies a new input vector. The competitive working process is also called vector quantization. Components of a SOM are called nodes or neurons that are associated with a weight vector of the same dimension as the input data vectors and a position in the map space. The usual arrangement of nodes is a hexagonal of rectangular grid. The procedure for placing a vector from input data space on to the map is to first find the node with the closest weight vector to the vector taken from input data space. Once the closest neuron is located, it is assigned the values from the vectors taken from the input data space. Mathematically, SOMs are sometimes associated with nonlinear forms of principal component analysis.

Owing to their capacity to map high-dimensional data to a low-dimensional map whilst preserving the topological characteristics of the original complex movement data, in principle, four different modes of application in the analysis of complex movement patterns can be distinguished (Figure 8.3A–D). In all approaches, an explorative strategy is pursued.

(A) In relation to describing a single movement by means of multiple time-discrete data, each movement is represented by a single vector that is mapped to a single node in the map space. By mapping several movements to the map space, SOMs function as classifiers that group similar movements to each other, owing to the characteristics of neighbourhood preservation.

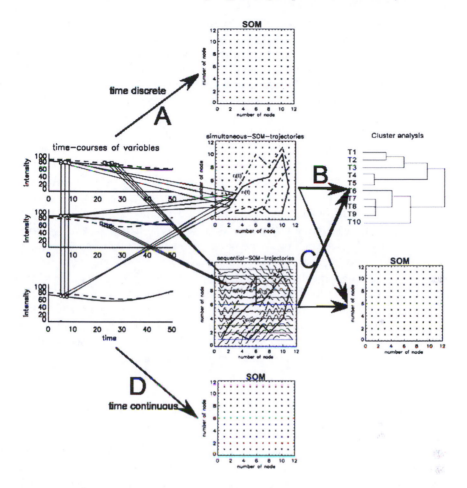

Figure 8.3 Variations of data processing by means of self-organizing maps

When the complex sport movement is described by means of time course data, three different approaches can be adopted. In all approaches, a single movement is described by means of several variable time courses.

(B) In the first time course oriented approach, the input vectors are constructed from all variable intensities at single instants. The number of vectors of a single movement is given by the number of instants the movement was measured with. Here, each feature vector is mapped to a single node in the map space and the whole movement is characterized by a two-dimensional trajectory in the map space (Figure 8.3).

(C) The second time course oriented approach considers each variable time-course as a single vector. Consequently, the number of input vectors per movement is given by the number of variables the movement was described with. The SOM maps each variable time course characteristics to a single node. Each resulting two-dimensional trajectory in the map space links the different time course characteristics of a single movement (Figure 8.3).

Once the movements are mapped to the node space (Figure 8.3B,C), the coordinates of the trajectories form new vectors, which can be either fed into another SOM or given into a cluster analysis to classify all movements by their relative similarity. When the trajectories are put into another SOM, the trajectories are mapped to different single nodes. The distribution of the nodes over the whole grid then displays the relative similarity of the movements in a two-dimensional space. However, these two-dimensional coordinates can be mapped with a cluster analysis to a linear grouping. When the coordinate vectors of the trajectories are directly put into a cluster analysis, the movements are grouped according to their one-dimensional similarity. In both cases (Figure 8.3B,C) when the SOMs are applied in a first-order form to the map, the movements on a trajectory in the low-dimensional node space the SOMs are taken for nonlinear data reduction comparable to linear analogies such as principal component analysis or Karhunen–Loève transformation. When SOMs are applied in the second-order form for the mapping of the trajectories, we can consider them as nonlinear classification procedures comparable to linear analogies such as cluster analysis.

(D) Instead of modelling the movement qualities by means of two SOMs or one SOM and a cluster analysis, a fourth approach is suggested. Here, all variable time courses of a single movement are put in a single, rather long, vector, which forms the input vector for the SOM. In this case, the SOM directly provides the two-dimensional map where each node corresponds to the model of a movement and the whole node grid provides the relative similarities of several movements.

In the following, the SOM research that is related to the area of movement execution in particular will be followed by the sport game related applications of SOMs.

To date, most applications of SOMs in elite sports can be found in the form of (B) or (C). An explorative combination of SOM and cluster analysis in form of (B) was applied by Bauer and Schöllhorn (1997). Two high-performance discus throwers were analyzed during different competition and training events over one year. The athletes' movement during the final throwing phase were described using a 14-segment, rigid body model by means of 13 joint angles and 13 angular velocities plus the trunk orientation angle and angular velocity, to achieve a physically complete description. Feature vectors of the variable time courses were mapped on a 10 × 10-node SOM. The resulting trajectories were subsequently placed into a cluster analysis. The results revealed, firstly, a clear differentiation of the two athletes. Secondly, they identified a successful intervention that resulted in a distinct separation of three trials before and five trials after the intervention period and, thirdly, sessions of training could be clearly separated from each other and provided evidence for day-dependent throwing strategies. However, the identification of signature movements for each discus thrower as well as continuous variations called traditional model- and repetition-oriented approaches into question.

Further evidence for the individuality of movement patterns in running patterns was found by Schöllhorn and Bauer (1997). By analyzing three to five double steps of 20 runners during a 2000-metre run by means of a SOM and cluster analysis, on the basis of the same variables as in Bauer and Schöllhorn (1997, it was possible to separate automatically contact phases of the right/left foot and the flight phase, as well as to identify the athletes by means of their kinematic data during a single ground contact phase. Identification was based on a 91 per cent recognition rate for the left foot and 96 per cent for the right foot but only 75 per cent for the flight phase.

The same approach with SOM and cluster analysis was pursued by Schöllhorn and Bauer (1998) in an investigation of world-class javelin throwers from different nations over several years in the search for individuality in elite sports. The same variables and data processing approach as in Bauer and Schöllhorn (1997) were used for describing and mapping the movements over a SOM towards a dendrogram. Most intriguingly, the results revealed the recognition of individual movement patterns of two female javelin throwers over several years. Obviously, the fingerprint-like throwing patterns were identifiable over several years. Furthermore, evidence was provided for a clear distinction of male and female throwing patterns as well as for nation-typical throwing patterns.

Two consecutive SOMs were applied to establish whether the order of movement executions affected variability over repeated trials (Janssen *et al.* 2010). Five participants performed ten first and ten second tennis serves in blocked and alternating (serial) series. The first serves were mainly accomplished with higher serving speed but less accuracy, whereas the second serves were mainly characterized by higher precision, lower serving speed. As the input dimension of the kinematic data (15 angles) was high, a self-implemented network called 2-SOM (because of its structure, which consisted of two series-connected SOMs) was chosen for analysis purposes. Within the 2-SOM, the first SOM was used to reduce data dimension, whereas the second SOM was used to classify the serve patterns. The 2-SOM revealed a person recognition rate of 100 per cent using all serves of all participants for only the blocked or serial condition. Within the 'person clusters', a network that was trained either with all individuals' data from the blocked or serial condition was able to distinguish between an individual's first and second serve with an accuracy of 99 per cent (in the blocked condition) and 90 per cent (in the serial condition), respectively. In general, movement variability was greater for the serial condition compared with the blocked condition over all participants.

Lees *et al.* (2003) reported the results of a study that applied SOMs with 12 × 8 neurons to analyze instep kicks by two soccer players for distance or accuracy.

The output patterns were repeatable for the same task for one player. The authors claimed that the trajectories in the output map were related to characteristics of the movement technique, although these characteristics were not determined. In a subsequent study, Lees and Barton (2005) used a similar approach to model several kicks by six soccer players. Fourteen joint angles were obtained from three-dimensional coordinates for 80 equispaced time instants from take off for the last stride to the end of the follow through of the kick. The output maps distinguished between right and left-footed groups. Intra-player differences were small.

The analysis of 60 golf chip shots of four low-handicap male golfers over distances of 4–24 metres in four-metre intervals, randomly assigned, was the objective of the investigation of Lamb *et al.* (2011). From a 16-segment model, a 24-dimensional input dataset consisting of joint angle time courses was derived. Because of high heterogeneity in the training data between the golfers, separate SOMs were trained on each player's respective kinematic data. Subsequently, a second SOM was trained using the best-matching nodes from the previous SOM for each respective player. The first SOMs varied between 24 × 16 and 25 × 15 nodes, the second SOMs had in general 32 × 1 nodes. A U-matrix representation for each player allowed a phase specific comparison within each player. The attractor layout diagrams were presented as evidence of nonlinear phase transitions for three of the four shot distances.

A confirmatory approach was pursued as well when data were reanalyzed from Bartlett *et al.* (2006) with respect to differences in treadmill running with marker and no-marker conditions (Lamb *et al.* 2008). Kinematic time course data were analyzed using a 29 × 23 hexagonal lattice. In general, the findings of Bartlett *et al.* (2006) could be replicated. However, SOMs do require more work to be applied properly. The ability to represent high-dimensional coordination patterns on visualizable low-dimensional map hold great potential (Bartlett *et al.* 2006).

In another study by this group, Lamb *et al.* (2010) showed how SOMs could be used to objectively distinguish between three types of basketball shots. Two SOMs were used in this investigation. Kinematic data from right and left ankles, knees, hips and shoulder were processed and input to the first SOM. Each variable was range normalized to maximum and minimum values of +1 and −1. The map size of the first SOM was 42 × 13 nodes and was used to analyze different phases of the movements, while the second SOM had 9 × 6 nodes and was used for the classification of the complete trials. There remains some debate over the best way to represent data (i.e. complete or broken down into key phases). In particular, the trial SOM was considered more relevant in providing a macro representation (see Lamb *et al.* 2010).

In contrast to this confirmatory approach, Beckmann *et al.* (2012) employed a more exploratory approach for the possibility of identifying individual-specific movement characteristics in different athletic events. Specifically, five decathletes were recorded using two high-speed video cameras and three-dimensionally reconstructed during the final throwing phases of shot put, discus and javelin movements while competing in the same decathlon. On the basis of a rigid 14-segment body model, time-normalized angle and angular velocity time courses formed the input vectors for the SOM and was compared with support vector machines. By inclusion of all variables, the disciplines could be distinguished at a 100 per cent level. When the throwing or shot put arm was excluded, no individual could be identified by means of the SOM but an individual recognition rate over all throwing disciplines by means of the support vector machines achieved at 98.5 per cent.

By coding the rallies as a series of zones, from where the players were hitting the volleyball, an intriguing approach was suggested by Perl and Lames (2000) that transferred the modelling by means of dynamic SOMs to game sports. Approximately 5000 rallies of men and women's volleyball matches of first and second German division formed the training set for the 20 × 20 node grid. However, the only plausible rallies that could be identified were those in which single nodes corresponded to characteristic events in a single rally; e.g. serve or offence smash. A similar approach has also been applied to squash (Perl 2002) and table tennis (Perl and Baca 2003).

Summary

Overall, cluster analysis and SOMs enjoy increasing popularity among movement scientists, owing to their capacity to explore and validate different qualities in movement science and match analysis. Both methods of analysis offer a fruitful basis for characterizing and interpreting high-dimensional datasets. The need to balance exploratory and confirmatory approaches in combination with time-continuous and time-discrete approaches is one of the biggest challenges for the coming years. The willingness to apply most recent methodological developments from related disciplines is growing and offers a promising wide new field of research.

References

Ball, K. A. and Best, R. J. (2007) Different centre of pressure patterns within the golf stroke I: Cluster analysis. *Journal of Sports Science*, 25: 757–70.

Bartlett, R., Bussey, M. and Flyger, N. (2006) Movement variability cannot be determined reliably from no-marker conditions. *Journal of Biomechanics*, 39: 3076–9.

Bauer, H. U. and Schöllhorn, W. (1997) Self-organizing maps for the analysis of complex movement patterns. *Neural Processing Letters*, 5: 193–9.

Beckmann, H., Janssen, D. and Schöllhorn, W. I. (2012) *Identifikation individueller disziplinübergreifender Bewegungsstile* [Identification of individual and discipline independent movement styles], in Bundesinstitut für Sportwissenschaft (ed.) *BISp-Jahrbuch Forschungsförderung* [Federal Institute of Sport Science (ed.) *Annual Report of Governmental Funded Research Projects*]. Bonn, Germany.

Chow, J. Y., Davids, K., Button, C. and Rein, R. (2008) Dynamics of movement patterning in learning a discrete multiarticular action. *Motor Control*, 12: 219–40.

Everitt, B. S., Landau, S. and Leese, M. (2001) *Cluster Analysis*, 4th edn. New York: Arnold.

Haken, H., Wunderlin, A. and Yigitbasi. A (1995) An introduction to synergetics. *Open Systems and Information Dynamics*, 3 (1): 97–130.

Handl, J., Knowles, J. and Kell, D. B. (2005) Computational cluster validation in post-genomic data analysis. *Bioinformatics*, 21 (15): 3201–12.

Hay, J. G. (1993) *The Biomechanics of Sports Technique*, 4th edn. Englewood Cliffs, NJ: Prentice Hall.

Haykin, S. (1994) *Neural Networks: A Comprehensive Foundation*. New York: Macmillan.

Jaeger, R. G. and Halliday, T. R. (1998) On confirmatory versus exploratory research. *Herpetologica*, 54: S64–6.

Jäger, J., Schöllhorn, W. I. and Schwerdfeger, B. (2003) A pattern recognition approach for an opponent specific classification of tactical moves in team sports, in E. Müller, H. Schwameder, G. Zallinger and V. Fastenbauer (eds) *Proceedings of the 8th Annual congress of the European College of Sport Science*. Salzburg: Institute of Sport Science, pp. 370.

Jaitner, T., Mendoza, L. and Schöllhorn, W. I. (2001a) Analysis of the long jump technique in the transition from approach to takeoff based on time-continuous kinematic data. *European Journal of Sport Science*, 1: 1–12.

Jaitner, T., Ernst, H., Mendoza, L., Schöllhorn, W. I. (2001b) Changes of EMG patterns during motor learning of ballistic movements, in: H. Gerber and R. Müller, R. (eds) Proceedings of the XVIIIth Congress of the International Society of Biomechanics (ISB). Zürich: ETH.

Janssen, D., Gebkenjans, F., Beckmann, H. and Schöllhorn, W. I. (2010) Analyzing learning approaches by means of complex movement pattern analysis. *International Journal of Sport Psychology*, 41 (Special Issue): 18–21.

Johansson, G. (1973) Visual perception of biological motion and a model for its analysis. *Perception and Psychophysics*, 14: 201–11.

Kelso, J. A. S. (1995) *Dynamic Patterns: The Self-Organization of Brain and Behavior*. Cambridge, MA: MIT Press.

Lamb, P., Bartlett, R. M., Robins, A. and Kennedy, G. (2008) Self-organizing maps as a tool to analyze movement variability. *International Journal of Computer Science in Sport*, 7: 28–39.

Lamb, P., Bartlett, R. and Robins, A. (2010) Self-organising maps: an objective method for clustering complex human movement. *International Journal of Computer Science in Sport*, 9: 20–9.

Lamb, P. F., Bartlett, R. M. and Robins, A. (2011) Artificial neural networks for analyzing inter-limb coordination: the golf chip shot. *Human Movement Science*, 30: 1129–43.

Lames, M. (1992) Synergetik als Konzept in der Sportmotorik. [Synergetics as a concept for sport movements]. *Sportpsychologie*, 6 (3): 12–18.

Lees, A., Barton, G. and Kershaw, L. (2003) The use of Kohonen neural network analysis to qualitatively characterize technique in soccer kicking. *Journal of Sports Sciences*, 21: 243–4.

Lees, A. and Barton, G. (2005) A characterisation of technique in the soccer kick using Kohonen neural network analysis, in T. Reilly, J. Cabri and D. Araújo (eds) *Science and Football V: The Proceedings of the Fifth World Congress on Science and Football*. London: Routledge, pp. 83–8.

Müller, E. (1986) *Biomechanische Analyse alpine Schilauftechniken*. [Biomechanical analysis of skiing techniques.] Innsbruck: Inn-Verlag.

Perl, J. (2002) Game analysis and control by means of continuously learning networks. *International Journal of Performance Analysis of Sport*, 2: 21–35.

Perl, J. and Baca, A. (2003) Application of neural networks to analyze performance in sports, in E. Müller, H. Schwameder, G. Zallinger, V. Fastenbauer (eds) *Book of*

Abstracts of the 8th Annual Congress of the European College of Sport Science in Salzburg, Austria, 9–12 July 2003. Available online at www.informatik.uni-mainz.de/dycon/ABS_2003__Perl_Baca_Appl_NN.pdf (accessed 7 June 2013).

Perl, J. and Lames, M. (2000) Identifikation von Ballwechselverlaufstypen mit Neuronalen Netzen am Beispiel Volleyball. [Identification of rallies in Volleyball by means of SOMs], in W. Schmidt and A. Knollenberg (eds) *Sport – Spiel – Forschung: Gestern. Heute. Morgen*. Hamburg: Czwalina, pp. 211–16.

Rein, R., Button C., Davids, K. and Summer, J. (2010a) Cluster analysis of movement patterns in multiarticular actions: a tutorial. *Motor Control*, 14: 211–39.

Rein, R., Davids, K. and Button, C. (2010b) Adaptive and phase transition behavior in performance of discrete multi-articular actions by degenerate neurobiological systems. *Experimental Brain Research*, 201: 307–22.

Schöllhorn, W. I. (1993) *Biomechanische Einzelfallanalyse im Diskuswurf.* [Biomechanical single case study of discus throwing]. Frankfurt: Harri Deutsch.

Schöllhorn, W. I. (1995) Time course oriented analysis of biomechanical movement patterns by means of orthogonal reference functions. Paper presented at the XVth Congress of the International Society of Biomechanics (ISB) 2–6 July, Jyväskylä.

Schöllhorn, W. I. (1999) Complex individual movement styles identified by means of a simple pattern recognition method, in P. Parisi, F. Pigozzi and G. Prinzi (eds) *Book of Abstracts of the 4th Annual Congress of the European College of Sport Science, Rome, Italy, 14–17 July 1999*. Cologne: European College of Sport Science.

Schöllhorn, W. I. and Bauer, H. U. (1997) Linear–nonlinear classification of complex time course patterns, in J. Bangsbo, B. Saltin, H. Bonde, Y. Hellsten, B. Ibsen, M. Kjaer and G. Sjogaard (eds) *Conference Proceedings of the 2nd European College of Sport Science*. Copenhagen: University of Copenhagen, pp. 308–9.

Schöllhorn, W. I. and Bauer, H. U. (1998) Identifying individual movement styles in high performance sports by means of self-organizing Kohonen maps, in H. Riehle, and M. Vieten (eds) *XVI International Symposium on Biomechanics in Sports*. Konstanz: Universitätsverlag, pp. 574–77.

Schöllhorn, W.I. and Jäger, J. M. (2006) A survey on various applications of artificial neural networks in selected fields of healthcare, in R. Begg, J. Kamruzzaman and R. A. Sarker (eds) *Neural Networks in Healthcare: Potentials and Challenges*. Hershey, PA: Idea Group Inc., pp. 20–58.

Schorer, J. Baker, J. Fath, F. and Jaitner, T. (2007) Identification of interindividual and intraindividual movement patterns in handball players of varying expertise levels. *Journal of Motor Behavior*, 39: 409–21.

Slife, B. D. and Williams, R. N. (1995) *What's Behind the Research? Discovering Hidden Assumptions in the Behavioral Sciences*. Thousand Oaks, CA: Sage Publications.

Tukey, J. W. (1980) We need both exploratory and confirmatory. *American Statistician*, 34 (1): 23–5.

9 Single camera analyses in studying pattern-forming dynamics of player interactions in team sports

Ricardo Duarte, Orlando Fernandes,
Hugo Folgado and Duarte Araújo

A network of patterned interactions between players characterizes performance in team ball sports. Thus, interpersonal coordination patterns are an important topic in the study of performance in such sports. A very useful method has been the study of inter-individual interactions captured by a single camera filming an extended performance area. The appropriate collection of positional data allows investigating the pattern forming dynamics emerging in different performance sub-phases of team ball sports. This chapter outlines: (i) a simple and flexible motion analysis procedure to capture the movement displacement trajectories of performers using a single camera; and (ii) exemplar data illustrating the analysis methods employed in the identification of pattern forming dynamics in a three-versus-three sub-phase of association football near the scoring areas.

This chapter focuses on the methodological procedures for capturing the relative positions of team players on the field using a single camera, as well as appropriate analysis methods to analyze the pattern-forming dynamics of player interactions. Team sport competitions can be characterized as complex systems in which players continuously interact to contest ball possession and positional advantage (Correia *et al.* 2012). This complex system regulates and is regulated by players' individual and collective interactions, which destabilize or stabilize the system accordingly (Davids *et al.* 2005). The inspirational background to the study of pattern forming dynamics in team sports comes from coordination dynamics frameworks (Kelso 2009). The ecological dynamics approach adopted some of those concepts and tools to investigate emergent pattern-forming dynamics in decision making (Araújo *et al.* 2006), adaptive behaviour (Davids *et al.* 2006) and social movement coordination (Duarte *et al.* 2012a) at the individual environment scale in representative sports settings. An important concept in these approaches is the 'order parameter'. Order parameters are collective variables synthesizing the complementary relations of cooperation and competition among the individual parts of a system, which may be used to capture and describe the self-organizing patterns emerging in a complex, dynamical system (Kelso 2009). Given its dynamical nature and sensitivity to environmental changes, when a system is displaced from equilibrium a phase transition in the 'order parameter' occurs, switching from one coordinated pattern to another (McGarry *et al.* 1999).

Compound kinematic variables integrating relevant ecological constraints are commonly used as order parameters, such as the distance between the basket and attacking/defending players (Araújo *et al.* 2006) or angles formed between vectors linking players and an imaginary line parallel to the try line in rugby union (Passos *et al.* 2009). To identify the existence of an order parameter, changes in the state of a system must be identified as consequences of variations in the 'control parameter' (Kelso 2009). Control parameters are variables that 'move' a complex system (i.e. the order parameter) through different states, inducing nonlinear qualitative behavioural changes (Kelso 2009). They can help explain why the interactions of opposing players remain stable (despite the inherent variability) or, in contrast, why attackers gain spatial and temporal advantage over defenders, creating a phase transition in the system (Passos *et al.* 2008). Interpersonal distance and relative velocity were often demonstrated to act as control parameters in one-on-one performance sub-phases of invasion team sports (Araújo *et al.* 2006; Passos *et al.* 2008; Duarte *et al.* 2010a).

To accurately determine and measure these order and control parameters specific methodologies are needed for collecting the relative positions of players in the pitch. One of the main methods for time–motion analysis of player positions that has been widely used is the video-based system (Dobson and Keogh 2007). These video-based systems are often used to analyze the physical conditioning of players (e.g. Di Salvo *et al.* 2007) or capturing player coordination dynamics (e.g. Travassos *et al.* 2012) and can be divided into manual and automated video-tracking systems (Barris and Button 2008). Despite providing a more time-efficient collection, automated video-based systems are frequently expensive and rely on several pieces of fixed apparatus (Barris and Button 2008), making it difficult to implement in some research scenarios and on a large scale. Manual tracking video-based systems, on the other hand, are often a more time-dependent method, which leads frequently to a focus on a smaller number of players, with reliability (i.e. intra or inter-observer reliability) frequently described as a potential limitation of these methods (Dobson and Keogh 2007).

This chapter presents a tutorial on how to implement a straightforward and low-cost method to capture the relative players' positions on the pitch, with a high degree of flexibility and reliability. The application of this method is illustrated with the identification of pattern-forming dynamics in three-versus-three sub-phases of association football near the scoring areas. The emphasis is on the description of motion-analysis procedures and data-analysis methods.

Motion analysis procedures applied to a three-versus-three small-sided game

To illustrate the motion analysis procedures, a representative experimental task was developed stimulating the creation of shooting opportunities near the scoring area in a seven-a-side association football competition of youth football players (age 11.8 ± 0.4 years). The task consisted of a goalkeeper plus three-versus-three plus goalkeeper small-sided game, where, to create shooting opportunities, the attacking team needed to make penetrating passes into the space behind the defending team (Figure 9.1). The central performance space was 20 × 20 metres and the scoring areas measured 14.5 metres in length, to simulate the goal-keeper's area according to International Federation of Association Football (FIFA) rules. Thus, the off-side rule was associated as a task constraint only inside the scoring areas. Six outfield players were divided in two teams by their coaches. The small-sided game lasted for six minutes.

Single-camera recordings

An important methodological issue of the present method is that camera position-ing does not need to be perpendicular with the field of performance; i.e. the camera lens does not need to be perpendicular in relation to the pitch plane of motion. Particularly in this experimental task, participants' on-field movement displace-ments were recorded using a regular digital video camera statically positioned at approximately 30 metres from the pitch, to capture the whole playing area. Owing to the facilities available in the stadium, the camera was placed five metres above the ground, perpendicular to the longitudinal component of the pitch and with an angle of depression of approximately ten degrees. However, this method can be used with other camera placements and specifications without losing accuracy (e.g. Duarte *et al.* 2010b; Correia *et al.* 2012; Travassos *et al.* 2012). Before the beginning of the experiment, several non-collinear control points corresponding to specific landmarks visible in the video camera were measured for later calibrations (see the camera calibration and object-plane reconstruction section below). Previous studies showed that seven control points were sufficient to obtain adequate accuracy levels in movement data (Fernandes *et al.* 2007).

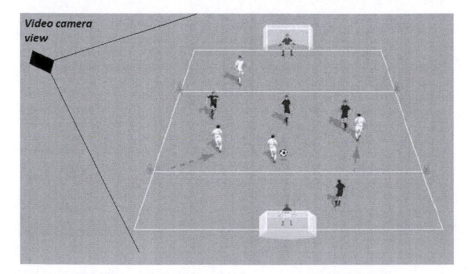

Figure 9.1 Schematic representation of single-camera video motion capture

Image treatment

Video-recorded images of the small-sided game were transferred to digital support, coded and saved as '.avi' format and goal-scoring opportunities identified throughout the game. From the 21 goal-scoring opportunities occurred during the game, only ten plays were analyzed further, in which: (i) the ball was not projected into an aerial trajectory; and (ii) there were no changes in ball possession between teams. The video recordings of these situations were split into unique video files, with minimum file size to increase the computational performance during extraction of positional variables and analysis.

The software package TACTO 8.0 (Figure 9.2; Fernandes *et al.* 2010) was used to extract the virtual positional coordinates (measured in pixels units) from participants' movement displacement trajectories. The procedure consisted of following with a computer mouse cursor the middle point located between the feet of each participant (chosen as working point). This working point was used because it represents an estimate of the projection of the player's centre of gravity on the pitch (Duarte *et al.* 2010a). Data were obtained at 25 Hz as recommended by Fernandes and Caixinha (2004). The TACTO package was also used to assess the virtual coordinates of the seven control points previously selected that afterwards were used for calibration. During these procedures, the computer resolution was set at 1280 × 800 pixels and the TACTO 8.0 window was fixed on a permanent position on screen. It is necessary to keep this procedures unchanged during the digitization of all trials to avoid improper data transformation owing to changes in the image plane reference frame.

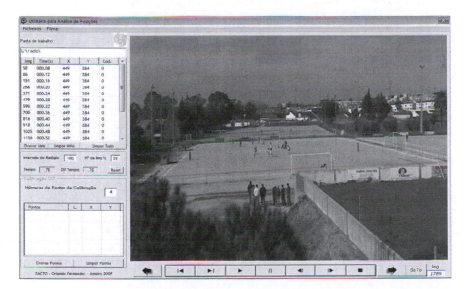

Figure 9.2 The TACTO 8.0 device window; manual tracking of a selected working point with a computer mouse allows virtual coordinates of the tracked player/object to be obtained

Camera calibration and object-plane reconstruction

Camera calibration and object-plane reconstruction were made using bi-dimensional (2-D) direct linear transformation (2D-DLT) method (Abdel-Aziz and Karara 1971). This planar analysis used algorithms adapted by Reinschmidt (1996) from the original DLT method formulated for tri-dimensional analysis (Woltring and Huiskes 1990). The MATLAB® (MathWorks Inc.) files used in these steps can be found at the website of the International Society of Biomechanics (Reinschmidt 1996). The DLT method is thought to deal reliably with some measurement errors such as optical distortion and decentring distortion reported by other methods (Marzan and Karara 1975; Kwon 2008). This method directly relates an object point located in the object-space/plane and the corresponding image point on the image-plane of the camera/digitizer unit. Two reference frames are defined: the object-space/plane reference frame (the *XYZ*-system) and the image-plane reference frame (the *UV*-system; Figure 9.3). The [*x*, *y*, *z*] is the object-space coordinates of point *O* (i.e. the pitch coordinates attributed to the working point of each digitized player in which *z* coordinates were always equal to zero), while [*u*, *v*] is the image-plane coordinates of the image point *I* (i.e. the virtual coordinates obtained with the TACTO package). The mathematical description of the 2D-DLT method can be found online (Kwon 2003). In the current study, owing to the use of 2-D analysis, eight DLT coefficients were automatically determined to reflect the relationships between the object-plane reference frame (i.e. the pitch coordinates) and the image-plane reference frame (i.e. the digitized virtual coordinates). This procedure was used twice for camera calibration and 2-D reconstruction of the players' pitch coordinates in each time instant (Figure 9.4).

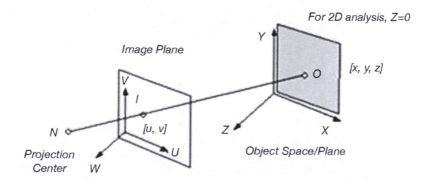

Figure 9.3 The direct linear transformation (2D-DLT) method for camera calibration and bi-dimensional reconstruction

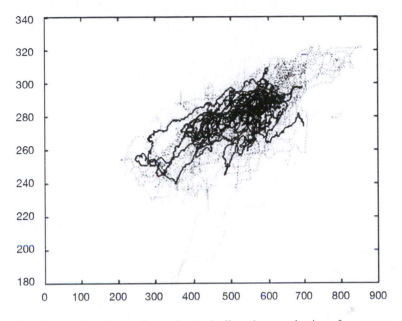

Figure 9.4 Converted pitch coordinates (metres) allow the reproduction of movement displacement trajectories of players in the space of action

Quality control procedures

An important methodological issue when dealing with signal processing in behavioural studies is to ensure that variations in the time-series data (e.g. Cartesian coordinates of players' movement displacement trajectories) are only due to the natural and inherent variability in performance. As mentioned by Goto and Mascie-Taylor (2007), variability in continuous quantitative data may be due to the inherent variance but also human measurement error (e.g. lack of consistence in digitizing) and/or instrumentation error (e.g. lack of accuracy in the calibration process). Failure to treat these errors properly results in amplified noisy velocity and acceleration data (Kwon 2008). To guarantee the fidelity of the obtained positional data earlier described, three steps were fulfilled: (1) using appropriate data *filtering*; (2) testing the *accuracy* of the instrument; (3) training and testing the *consistency/reliability* of the digitations.

Filtering

A widely accepted recommendation when working with kinematic data is the use of appropriate data filtering to remove some data fluctuations due to human or instrumentation error (Winter 2005). Signals with predominant lower frequencies such as the ones used in our experimental task are more suitable to possess higher frequencies of noise (Giakas 2004). Taking these recommendations, we used a Butterworth low-pass filter to maintain the original lower frequencies and remove the higher ones above a specific cut-off frequency. The original (unfiltered) dataset was compared with different cut-off frequencies. The similarity between unfiltered and the various filtered datasets was taken as a criterion to select the cut-off frequency of 6 Hz for all the analyzed trials based on residual analysis technique (Winter 2005).

Accuracy

To test the accuracy and validity of the instrument for the specific task under analysis, we used the procedures suggested by Fernandes and Caixinha (2004). We compared the distances obtained from digitization with a fine path of a player from which we knew the real distances (i.e. a circuit on the pitch with changing directions). The mean absolute percentage error showed values less than five per cent for all the measurements, which were taken as indicative of high accuracy (Fernandes and Caixinha 2004).

Consistence and reliability

To decrease the human measurement error and increase the internal consistence of the tracking operator, a digitizing training programme of seven consecutive days was completed. The protocol consisted of digitizing one random trial/play per day (i.e. six outfield players involved in each play). On the seventh day, the tracking operator completed the same protocol performed in the pretest as post-test measures, digitizing the same players twice interspersed by a break of five hours (see protocol details in Duarte *et al.* 2010a). To assess the internal consistence and reliability between the digitized trials, we used the coefficient of reliability (R) derived from the intra-technical error of measurement (intra-TEM) as suggested by Goto and Mascie-Taylor (2007). This accuracy index is based on the standard deviation between repeated measures. In this illustrative case, results showed an improvement from the pretest to post-test measurements. In the pretest, values of R between the two measurements were higher than 94% for longitudinal (goal-to-goal) component of motion and 84% for the lateral (side-to-side) component. In post-test measurements, R values were higher than 95% for both components of motion in all digitized players, which ensures internal consistence of the tracking operator (Ulijaszek and Kerr 1999). High values of reliability between different tracking operators (i.e. inter-operator reliability) are also available in the literature (Serrano and Fernandes 2011).

Variables computation

For the study of team sports as multi-agent dynamical systems, there are some compound-motion variables that might capture the complex dynamics of players' interpersonal interactions during competitive performance (see Chapter 6). With the individual kinematic data of each player obtained by the aforementioned procedures it is possible to obtain specific compound motion variables. A previous study identified a high coupling tendency between the movements of attacking and defending players in the three-versus-three sub-phase of association football (Duarte *et al.* 2012b). Thus, based on players' positional data, a single centroid value (i.e. the geometrical centre) for the six outfield players was calculated. The centroid or group 'centre of mass' was calculated as the mean position of the six outfield players over time (Frencken *et al.* 2011). Next, using the longitudinal component of motion, we calculated for each time instant the smallest distance of this centroid to the defensive line (i.e. the boundary line between the central performance space and the scoring area, see Figure 9.1) as a potential order parameter.

The inter-centroid distance (i.e. distance between the centroid of the attacking and defending players; Folgado *et al.* 2012) and the relative stretch index (i.e. the mean vectorial distances of players to their team centroid; adapted from Bourbousson *et al.* 2010) were tested as control parameter candidate variables. As suggested by Frencken *et al.* (2011) the inter-centroid distances tend to decrease immediately before the creation of a shooting opportunity, suggesting that the closeness of the two sub-groups of players can influence the stability of the competing team relations. Our purpose was also to assess whether differences in the relative stretch index of teams influenced the stability of the relative positioning in reference to the goals. Specifically conceived MATLAB files were used to compute these time-series data.

Illustrative data on pattern-forming dynamics in association football

The exploratory analyses of the centroid distances to the defensive line suggested the existence of two behavioural states, before and after the instant of an assisting pass (i.e. the last pass before a shot occurred; see top panel of Figure 9.5).

Using normalization procedures that did not alter the structure of the time-series data, we subtracted each value of the order parameter from the own mean (Rosenblum *et al.* 2001). This procedure allowed us to find a mean point between the two states corresponding to values of zero (see bottom panel of Figure 9.5). Thus, the first state displayed positive values of the order parameter corresponding to the initial stable relations between teams (i.e. where the defending sub-group successfully interacted together to prevent shooting opportunities). The second state displayed negative values of the order parameter that emerged from an arrangement of interpersonal relationships that led to defensive system instabilities and goal-scoring opportunities. The qualitative changes between the two identified states observed in the bottom panel of Figure 9.5 by the shift from positive to negative values suggested that the emergence of instabilities within these small-groups (i.e. changes in their relative positioning leading to penetrations in the scoring areas) may be characterized by some nonlinear properties such as order–order transition (Kugler and Turvey 1987).

Analysis of first derivative values of the order parameter also revealed a high

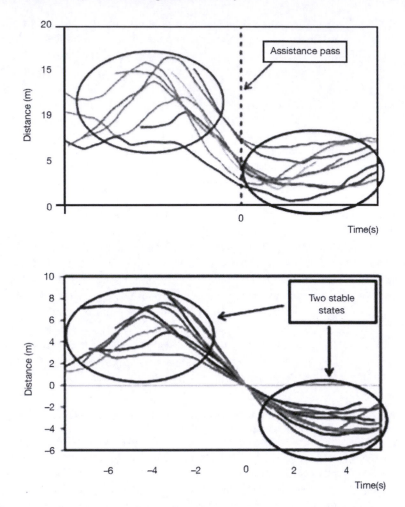

Figure 9.5 The two behavioural states of the order parameter; top panel shows the
distance of the single centroid to the defensive boundary line of all the
analyzed trials, synchronized by the assistance pass instant; bottom panel
shows the order parameter subtracted by the own mean to highlight the
qualitative changes associated with perturbations of the initial stability of
teams (see text for details)

rate of change at the moment prior to the appearance of system instabilities
(Figure 9.6). These results reinforced the idea that transitions between the two
identified states occurred suddenly from one state to another, and not by a cumulative linear process.

To better understand how the stability of the competing teams was perturbed
in the studied sub-phases of play, we tested whether the two control parameters

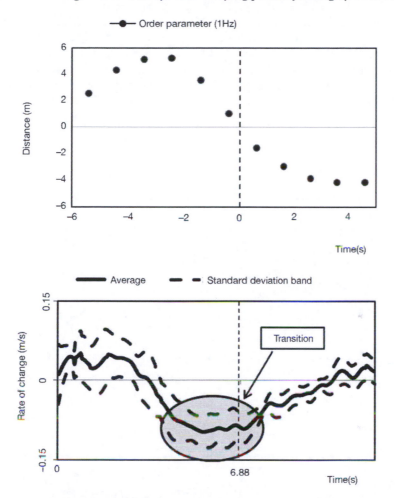

Figure 9.6 Identification of the nonlinear qualitative changes between the two
behavioural states; top panel displays an exemplar play with increased slope
in the transition between the two system states (down-sampled to 1 Hz);
bottom panel shows the average and standard deviation bands of the first
derivative of the order parameter in all plays, highlighting with an ellipse the
high rate of change of the order parameter; the slope or high rate of change
indicates the order–order transition

influenced the stability of the order parameter. Inter-centroid distances revealed a
trend for consistently present lower values (minimum of 1.89 ± 1.0 metres) at the
instants immediately before the loss of stability in teams (see top panel of Figure
9.7). Standard deviations also showed a convergence towards low values at these
instants. As these values were observed only at these instants of play, it suggests
that a decrease in the distance between teams seemed to influence the emergence
of instabilities in the three-versus-three sub-phases near goal scoring areas.

Relative stretch index measures demonstrated a trend for increasing positive values (2.56 ± 1.4 metres), with increased stability (low standard deviation) before the perturbation of system stability (see bottom panel of Figure 9.7). Positive values meant that attacking teams were more stretched than defending teams. This finding implies that the instabilities characterizing the movement of these small groups into the goal-scoring areas were associated with a high dispersion of the attackers compared to the spatial arrangement of the defending players.

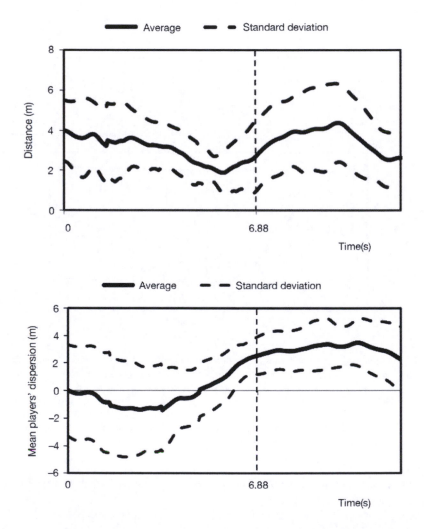

Figure 9.7 Moving average and standard deviation values of the inter-centroid distances (left panel) and relative stretch index (right panel); vertical dashed lines highlight the instant of the instabilities corresponding to the zero crossing of the order parameter previously identified in Figure 9.5

Concluding remarks and future implications

This chapter outlined a low-cost and straightforward method to reconstruct the players' movement displacement trajectories in the performance context using a single camera. The high values of accuracy and reliability, as well as its flexibility, suggest the possibility of using this method in a wide range of training and competitive performance settings. Special care is recommended with signal processing in which appropriate data filtering and short-term digitization training programmes should be undertaken to remove high-frequency content noise (i.e. human and instrumentation error) from the inherent performance variability.

Obtaining positional data from players' on-field performance allowed us to identify the pattern forming dynamics emerging from players' interactions during a three-versus-three sub-phase of association football near the scoring areas. A functional relevant order parameter was proposed based on previous qualitative examinations of collective movement data. Sudden transitions associated to qualitative behavioural changes were identified in this order parameter (i.e. distance from a single centroid to the defensive boundary line) by the influence of two intertwined control parameters (i.e. the inter-centroid distance and relative stretch index).

More specifically, low values of inter-centroid distance and increasing positive values of relative stretch index were shown to influence the emergence of instabilities in the small-sided game that led to goal-scoring opportunities. The complementary relations between these two control parameters suggested that goal-scoring opportunities created at this level of interpersonal interactions resulted from a combined influence of the attacking and defending sub-groups. This influence was characterized by an approaching of the two sub-groups to each other and an increase in the difference between the dispersion values of the attacking and defending players. Folgado *et al.* (2012) demonstrated that more skilled footballers achieved higher inter-centroid distances during three-versus-three small-sided games compared to less-skilled players. In the illustrative experiment presented in this chapter, it was observed that inter-centroid distance values tended to decrease to the lowest values only in the moments before the loss of stability between the small groups of attacking and defending players. These findings are in agreement with the results of Frencken *et al.* (2011) on four-versus-four small-sided games, reporting a trend towards a decrease in this variable when teams scored goals. Concerning the relative stretch index data, Bourbousson *et al.* (2010) observed that basketball teams followed a counter-phase relation as a function of changes in ball possession. However, in the plays presented here, no changes in ball possession between teams occurred. The presented analyses revealed that the stability of the game was perturbed only when the relative dispersion of the players showed a consistent pattern, indicated by the low standard deviation towards increasing positive values.

Analysis of group motion dynamics of attacking and defending sub-phases of performance can allow to identify pattern forming dynamics of players' interactions related to the emergence of instabilities in sub-groups relations, such as goal-scoring opportunities. Coaches and practitioners can enhance their training programmes by using these data to constrain small-sided games for training inter-personal interactions during attacking and defending sub-phases of team sport. On the other hand, researchers can use this approach from nonlinear dynamical systems to investigate how key relational system variables evolve over time and influence the interactional behaviour of team players during performance.

References

Abdel-Aziz, Y. I. and Karara, H. M. (1971) Direct linear transformation from comparator coordinates into object space coordinates in close-range photogrammetry, in *Proceedings of the Symposium on Close-Range Photogrammetry*. Falls Church, VA: American Society of Photogrammetry, pp. 1–18.

Araújo, D., Davids, K. and Hristovski, R. (2006) The ecological dynamics of decision making in sport. *Psychology of Sport and Exercise*, 7 (6): 653–76.

Barris, S. and Button, C. (2008) A review of vision-based motion analysis in sport. *Sports Medicine*, 38 (12): 1025–43.

Bourbousson, G., Sève, C. and McGarry, T. (2010) Space-time coordination dynamics in basketball: Part 2. The interaction between the two teams. *Journal of Sports Sciences*, 28: 349–58.

Correia, V., Araújo, D., Duarte, R., Travassos, B., Passos, P. and Davids, K. (2012) Changes in practice task constraints shape decision-making behaviours of team games players. *Journal of Science and Medicine in Sport*, 15 (3): 244–9.

Davids, K., Araújo, D. and Shuttleworth, R. (2005) Applications of dynamical systems theory to football, in T. Reilly, J. Cabri and D. Araújo (eds) *Science and Football V*. Abingdon: Routledge, pp. 547–50.

Davids, K., Button, C., Araujo, D., Renshaw, I. and Hristovski, R. (2006) Movement models from sports provide representative task constraints for studying adaptive behavior in human movement systems. *Adaptive Behavior*, 14: 73–94.

Di Salvo, V., Baron, R., Tschan, H., Calderon Montero, F., Bachl, N. and Pigozzi, F. (2007) Performance characteristics according to playing position in elite soccer. *International Journal of Sports Medicine*, 28: 222–7.

Dobson, B. P. and Keogh, J. W. L. (2007) Methodological issues for the application of time-motion analysis research. *Strength and Conditioning Journal*, 29 (2): 48–55.

Duarte, R., Araújo, D., Fernandes, O., Fonseca, C., Correia, V., Travassos, B., Esteves, P., Vilar, L. and Lopes, J. (2010a) Capturing complex human behaviors in representative sports contexts with a single camera. *Medicina-Lithuania*, 46: 408–14.

Duarte, R., Araújo, D., Gazimba, V. and Fernandes, O. (2010b) A time-motion analysis method to study people interactions in human movement science, in *Conference Proceedings of the 3rd Mathematical Methods in Engineering International Symposium*. Coimbra: Polytechnic Institute of Coimbra, pp. 408–15.

Duarte, R., Araújo, D., Correia, V. and Davids, K. (2012a) Sport teams as superorganisms: implications of sociobiological models of behaviour for research and practice in team sports performance analysis. *Sports Medicine*, 42 (8): 633–42.

Duarte, R., Araújo, D., Freire, L., Folgado, H., Fernandes, O. and Davids, K. (2012b) Intra- and inter-group coordination patterns reveal collective behaviours of football players near the scoring zone. *Human Movement Science*, 31 (6): 1639–51.

Fernandes, O. and Caixinha, P. (2004) A new method of time–motion analysis for soccer training and competition. Part II: Game activity and analysis. *Journal of Sports Sciences*, 22 (6): 505.

Fernandes, O., Caixinha, P. and Malta, P. (2007) Techno-tactics and running distance analysis by camera. *Journal of Sports Science and Medicine*, 6 (Suppl.10): 204–5.

Fernandes, O., Folgado, H., Duarte, R. and Malta, P. (2010) Validation of the tool for applied and contextual time-series observation. *International Journal of Sport Psychology*, 41: 63–4.

Folgado, H., Lemmink, K., Frencken, W. and Sampaio, J. (2012) Length, width and centroid distance as measures of teams tactical performance in youth football. *European Journal of Sport Science*, 1–6, iFirst article; doi: 10.1080/17461391.2012.730060

Frencken, W., Lemmink, K., Delleman, N., Visscher, C. (2011) Oscillations of centroid position and surface area of soccer teams in small-sided games. *European Journal of Sport Science*, 4: 215–23.

Giakas, G. (2004) Power spectrum analysis and filtering, in N. Stergiou (ed.) *Innovative Analyses of Human Movement*. Champaign, IL: Human Kinetics, pp. 223–58.

Goto, R. and Mascie-Taylor, C. (2007) Precision of measurement as a component of human variation. *Journal of Physiological Anthropology*, 26: 253–6.

Kelso, J. A. S. (2009) Coordination dynamics, in R. A. Meyers (ed.) *Encyclopedia of Complexity and System Science*. Berlin: Springer, pp.1537–64.

Kwon, Y. H. (2003) DLT method. Available online at www.kwon3d.com/theory/dlt/dlt.html (accessed 7 June 2013).

Kwon, Y. H. (2008) Measurement for deriving kinematic parameters: numerical methods, in Y. Hong and R. Bartlett (eds) *Handbook of Biomechanics and Human Movement Science*. Abingdon: Routledge, pp. 156–81.

McGarry, T., Khan, M. and Franks, I. (1999) On the presence and absence of behavioural traits in sport: an example from championship squash match-play. *Journal of Sports Sciences*, 17: 297–311.

Marzan, G. T. and Karara, H. M. (1975) A computer program for direct linear transformation solution of the collinearity condition, and some applications of it, in *Proceedings of the Symposium on Close-Range Photogrammetric Systems*. Falls Church, VA: American Society of Photogrammetry, pp. 420–76.

Passos, P., Araújo, D., Davids, K., Gouveia, L., Milho, J. and Serpa, S. (2008) Information-governing dynamics of attacker–defender interactions in youth rugby union. *Journal of Sports Sciences*, 26 (13): 1421–9.

Passos, P., Araújo, D., Davids, K., Gouveia, L., Serpa, S., Milho, J. and Fonseca, S. (2009) Interpersonal pattern dynamics and adaptive behavior in multiagent neurobiological systems: conceptual model and data. *Journal of Motor Behavior*, 41: 445–9.

Reinschmidt, C. (1996) Movement Analysis Software (2D-DLT) [Matlab code]. International Society of Biomechanics. Available online at http://isbweb.org/software/movanal.html (accessed 7 June 2013).

Rosenblum, M., Pikovsky, A., Kurths, J., Schafer, C. and Tass, P.A. (2001) Phase synchronization: from theory to data analysis, in R. Lipowsky, E. Sackmann and A. J. Hoff (eds) *Handbook of Biological Physics*. Leiden: Elsevier, pp. 279–321.

Serrano, J. and Fernandes, O. (2011) Reliability of a new method to analyse and to quantify athletes' displacement. *Portuguese Journal of Sport Sciences*, 11, (Suppl 2): 935–6.

Travassos, B., Araújo, D., Duarte, R. and McGarry, T. (2012) Spatiotemporal coordination patterns in futsal (indoor football) are guided by informational game constraints. *Human Movement Science*, 31 (4): 932–45.

Ulijaszek, S. A. and Kerr, D. A. (1999) Anthropometric measurement error and the assessment of nutritional status. *British Journal of Nutrition*, 82: 165–77.

Winter, D. A. (2005) *Biomechanics and Motor Control of Human Movement*, 3rd edn. New York: John Wiley and Sons.

Woltring, H. J. and Huiskes, R. (1990) Stereophotogrammetry, in N, Berme and A, Capozzo (eds) *Biomechanics of Human Movement*. Worthington, OH: Bertec Corporation, pp. 108–27.

10 Using virtual environments to study interactions in sport performance

Vanda Correia, Duarte Araújo, Gareth Watson and Cathy Craig

This chapter highlights the potential of immersive, interactive virtual reality technology to study dynamical interactions in sport performance. In view of the continuous advances in this technology, the dilemma between maintaining task representative design and guaranteeing experimental control has ceased to exist. The advantages and disadvantages of this methodological tool for the design of both practice and research-based experimental tasks that intend to improve and investigate the dynamics of environment–agent systems and information–action coupling in sports, are reviewed and discussed. Virtual reality technology is highlighted, as it allows us to capture the complexity of actions yet to control the presentation of information (mainly visual and auditory but also haptic/tactile) that guides action.

Although the use of virtual reality environments has been extensively used to investigate social interactions in many different fields of research (e.g. neuroscience, journalism, therapy in treatment of psychological disorders) only a few researchers have addressed its potential application to sport (e.g. Bideau *et al.* 2010; Watson *et al.* 2011). In this chapter, we review and discuss the advantages and disadvantages of this methodological tool for improving and investigating the dynamics of environment–agent systems in sports. That is to say, how this technology could be used to enhance sports performance from a complex sciences perspective, by allowing for the examination of individual athletes and sports teams' behaviours as they emerge as a result of the informational constraints imposed by and controlled in the virtual environment. In other words, how the perceptually based information guides decisions about how and when to act.

We will outline the importance of examining interpersonal goal-directed interactions under simulated dynamic task constraints that warrant the active exploration of information. This exploration is important to continuously guide on-going action. We emphasize also how crucial it is to simultaneously guarantee that relevant action information present in the 'real'[1] context of performance is also available in virtual contexts to support functional behaviour. In view of that, we provide illustrative empirical evidence of recent applications of virtual environments for sports research, addressing the implications for the design of both practice and research related tasks.

Dynamic interactions in sport performance

Players in teams are constantly interacting, co-adapting towards shared (i.e. between teammates) and opposing (i.e. between opponents) performance goals (e.g. Marsh, Richardson, Baron, and Schmidt 2006; Passos *et al*. 2011; McGarry, Anderson, Wallace, Hughes, and Franks, 2002). Multiple constraints are responsible for multiple effects in both interpersonal interaction processes and outcomes (e.g. Passos 2010). That is to say, that different dynamic interactions and consequent performance outcomes may emerge as a function of many interacting individual, task and environment constraints. Namely, in team ball games, players display functional coordination tendencies, based on local interaction rules acting during performance (Passos *et al*. 2011). These local interaction rules are context dependent, expressing the performance task constraints influencing players' behaviours (Passos *et al*. 2011).

The emerging interpersonal coordination patterns are functional spatiotemporal adjustments or adaptations to changing circumstances (Araújo *et al*. 2006; Kelso 1995; Kelso 2002; Warren 2006). In view of this fact, a growing body of research on sport performance has been concerned with interpersonal interactions phenomena (e.g. Araújo *et al*. 2004; Correia *et al*. 2012a; Esteves *et al*. 2011; Passos *et al*. 2008). Interpersonal coordination emerges from interactions during performance, shaped by contextual, individual and task constraints (Araújo *et al*. 2004; McGarry and Franks 2007; Passos *et al*. 2008). It is important to note that behaviour emergent from the interaction of a subject with the context can be expressed by the action and transitions in the course of the action (Araújo *et al*. 2006). It is thus important to formalize this dynamic behaviour in 'real contexts' and to identify potential informational constraints in these 'less controlled' *in situ* situations, which can be then used as manipulated parameters or variables in 'virtual environments' to help not only to describe but also to explain how emergent behaviour emerges under (manipulated) informational task constraints.

Virtual environment technology

Virtual environment technology has been used for the simulation of domain-specific environments of human behaviour in research, training and education. A virtual environment consists of an artificial (i.e. synthesized) environment generated using software and is mostly experienced via vision and sound. This approach has been successfully applied to the study of human behaviour in varying domains, such as neuroscience (e.g. Bohil *et al*. 2011; Tarr and Warren 2002); journalism (e.g. de la Peña *et al*. 2010); therapy in the treatment of anxiety disorders (e.g. Gerardi *et al*. 2008; Villani *et al*. 2007). The key element of a virtual environment system is the visual display. This display can either be an enclosed head-mounted display (HMD; Figure 10.1) or an open display such as a computer monitor or projection screen. A higher level of immersion is possible with the HMD. Owing to the diversity of HMDs, virtual environment systems vary with respect to their field of view, resolution and weight, amongst other characteristics

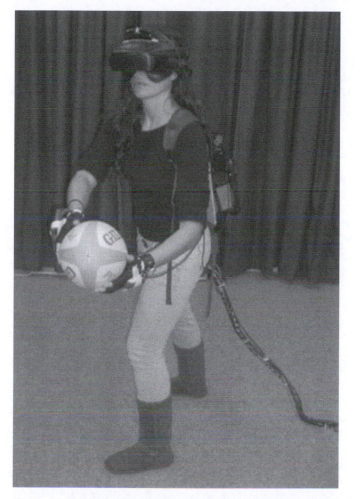

Figure 10.1 Illustrative immersive interactive virtual reality apparatus in the Movement
Innovation Laboratory at Queen's University, Belfast. It shows a participant
wearing a pair of gloves with attached hand trackers, a head-mounted
display with attached head tracker and a back-pack housing the control unit

(see, e.g. Stanney *et al.* 1998). Alongside, and sometimes integrated within the
same visual display device (e.g. as part of the HMD), auditory stimulation is often
used in the form of three-dimensional spatial surround sound (Bohil *et al.* 2011).
The use of devices providing haptic or tactile feedback is also increasing.

Although participants' performance in the virtual environment simulated task
may be captured by means of a keyboard, mouse, joystick or other device, the use
of immersive and interactive virtual environments is growing. Immersive interactive virtual environments must thus incorporate highly sensitive tracking

systems with head or body tracking devices (fixed to the head or body segments, such as the hands, see Figure 10.1). These systems are used to update in real time an egocentric viewpoint, besides allowing for the capture of the action being performed. That is, these tracking systems monitor in 'real' time (i.e. online) behavioural responses (e.g. biomechanical data). Any movement in the real world is therefore updated in the virtual context (i.e. data from the tracking system updates the participant's or user's viewpoint of the unfolding action in the virtual context). Online updating using a tracking system and HMD means that the participant is fully immersed (i.e. they never leave the virtual world, even by averting their gaze). Of note here is that the participants are allowed to choose where they look in the virtual context. These features of recent virtual environment technology help to enhance levels of immersion. A number and assortment of sensory and motor channels linked to the virtual environment, which simultaneously allows for the matching of motor inputs (such as unrestricted body movements), amplifies feelings of *immersion* (Bohil *et al*. 2011).

The discussion of assumptions, concepts and underlying paradigms or ontological positions is beyond the scope of this chapter but we briefly mention some issues related to virtual environment use. A notion commonly related with virtual environment simulations is that of *presence*, otherwise known as *subjective experience* or *experiential fidelity* (Riccio 1995; Stoffregen *et al*. 2003). It may be said that 'the psychological product of technological immersion' (Bohil *et al*. 2011, p. 754) and its influence on performance is regularly argued (e.g. Bideau *et al*. 2010; Craig and Watson 2011; Krijn *et al*. 2004; Villani *et al*. 2007). Presence is generally evaluated by the use of subjective measurements (i.e. dependent on the expertise of the researcher in using such instruments) such as self-reports, questionnaires and interviews, and is based on attribute category rating scales (e.g. Sheridan 1992, 1996; Wagner *et al*. 2009) but also uses objective measurements such as physiological indicators (Bohil *et al*. 2011; Wagner *et al*. 2009).

Another important issue is the notion of *action* (or *functional*) *fidelity* (e.g. Moroney and Moroney 1998; Stoffregen *et al*. 2003). Action fidelity is the relationship between behaviour in the simulator and behaviour in the simulated system and it is essentially measured in terms of task performance (Stoffregen *et al*. 2003). That is, it can be assessed by measures such as time to perform the task, emergent action similar to that observed in the situation being simulated. The simulation should primarily simulate the functions (i.e. it should demand the same type of interaction and the same goals) of the simulated context rather than prioritizing the 'fidelity of the stimuli' (Araújo *et al*. 2005; Stoffregen *et al*. 2003). The subjective feeling of being there (i.e. presence or experiential fidelity) can be seen as more concerned with enhancing stimulus fidelity (of the virtual environment) (Stoffregen *et al*. 2003). Conversely, action fidelity puts emphasis on simulation adequacy in terms of research, training and learning purposes (Stoffregen *et al*. 2003). Therefore, it must be guaranteed that the functions or action demanded by the simulation are similar to those of the simulated (natural) context of performance.

The virtual environment has many advantages over video presentation or natural practice or game performance situations for improving our understanding of the complexity of action in sport (see, e.g. Vignais *et al.* 2009). The virtual environment is about simplifying the complexity of sport by computer generating performance contexts and thus reducing the multitude of variables that may be influencing the emergent behaviour. In spite of this, it can be seen as shedding light on the complexity of action by exerting control over some variables and observing their effect on the dynamics of behaviour that emerges likewise in the complex natural context. One of the advantages is based on the ability to precisely control the presentation of sensory information (mainly visual and auditory but also haptic/tactile) that is involved in the guidance of action. It also makes it possible to couple and decouple perception and action (Craig *et al.* 2011; Craig and Watson 2011). As Bohil *et al.* (2011) have stated in a recent review, 'Virtual reality provides a middle ground, supporting naturalistic and contextually rich scenarios along with an exacting degree of control over key variables' (p. 752). This technology makes it possible to simulate a varying number of performance situations using immersive, interactive virtual environments. That is, visual information made available (manipulated) can be displayed to both stationary and moving participants by means of combined use of the HMD and motion-tracking systems.

Advantages of virtual environments over screen displays or video playback have also been pointed out (Bideau *et al.* 2010). Some attempts have been made to improve the recorded viewpoint of the match (e.g. in tennis: Farrow and Abernethy 2003; Williams *et al.* 2002; in soccer: Savelsbergh *et al.* 2002; Petit and Ripoll 2008). That is, this research attempts to provide participants with the perspective of the game nearest to what they would experience if they were performing in the game. However, the viewpoint is still not controlled by the observer (i.e. an egocentric viewpoint). An egocentric viewpoint refers to the naturalistic interaction between the head movements of the observer and the updating in real time of the optical information presented to the eyes of the observer. In other words the observer can 'move to perceive and perceive to move' (Gibson 1979). In addition to the automatic updating of viewpoint, the virtual environment allows for a binocular field of vision or stereopsis (i.e. visual field calculated for each eye). In addition, it allows for complete control of the information presented to performers and the movement trackers or controllers allow for diverse types of behavioural data to be captured (e.g. Craig and Watson 2011; Bideau *et al.* 2010; Brault *et al.* 2012).

A potential limitation of these studies is the lack of tactile/force feedback that may reduce performance on the virtual environment simulated task. When a cable is used to connect the visual display device to the central computer, a limitation that may be pointed out is the eventual restricted movement (McMenemy and Ferguson 2007). Another potential limitation is that the HMD may affect distance and depth perception (e.g. Willemsen *et al.* 2009) and the limited field of view restricts the level of peripheral vision that is available to the observer (e.g. Knapp and Loomis 2004). Finally, accessibility, costs and the required specialized technical assistance may also limit the use of this technology (e.g. Rizzo and Kim 2005).

Research on expertise in sport, namely on visual perception in sport, has focused on what discrete 'cues' may be used by individuals for effective perform-ance. The information sources under study are commonly hidden by means of temporal and/or spatial occlusion paradigms and motor responses are combined with eye movement registration techniques (e.g. Müller and Abernethy 2006; Vaeyens *et al.* 2007; for a review see, e.g. Williams and Ericsson 2005). To inves-tigate information sources used for perceptual judgments and actions, researchers have also made use of virtual environments to manipulate information in a contin-uous rather than a discrete fashion (e.g. Vignais *et al.* 2009; Bideau *et al.* 2003, 2004). Investigations in sport carried out using a virtual environment have demonstrated the influence of spatiotemporal optical invariants as information that shapes actions (e.g. restricted movements, e.g. Dessing and Craig 2010) and judgments on actions to be performed (e.g. by button pressing; e.g. Watson *et al.* 2011; Craig *et al.* 2006, 2009). However, more work is needed to understand how performers interact and create goal-directed adaptive behaviour, coupled with the many dynamic information sources in performance contexts (Correia *et al.* 2012).

This remits to the importance of guaranteeing representative design for sport psychology, practice and experimental design (Araújo *et al.* 2005; Pinder *et al.* 2011). Representative design (put forward by Brunswik 1956; see also Hammond and Stewart 2001) means that experimental task constraints, representative from the context for which the findings are intended to be generalized are essential in investigating performance in sports but also for the design of training and evalu-ation tasks meant to improve players' and teams' performance (Araújo *et al.* 2006; Davids *et al.* 2007; Pinder *et al.* 2011). An indicator that a task situation might not be representative of a specific domain is that expert performance can drop to the level of novices (Allard *et al.* 1980; Araújo *et al.* 2005). As virtual environment technology progresses, it has progressively become more financially accessible to research laboratories and, as a result, the potential dilemma of task representative design versus experimental control grows fainter and more outdated.

We next depict the potential contribution of immersive and interactive virtual reality setups to investigate behaviour in various sport performance tasks and contexts. To accomplish this, we consider illustrative empirical studies that have applied this technology to sports.

Designing virtual contexts of representative interpersonal interactions

Coupling perception and action

Gibson (1979) advocated that behaviour is grounded on perception–action couplings. That is, information is picked up from the surrounding environment and optic flow (i.e. the pattern of light generated by a particular animal–environment interaction). Optic flow is generated by action so that visual perception guides the action and, in turn, the action changes perception. It has been suggested that virtual environments are good tools for studying the perception–action loop in athletes (e.g. Bideau *et al*. 2010; Craig and Watson 2011) by simulating the perceptual information and measuring the resulting actions. Simulations of performance contexts and situations must allow participants to explore the task constraints so that they can pick up relevant information to guide goal-directed behaviour. In immersive, interactive virtual environment setups, movement through the optic array is simulated. This means that by moving, participants bring about transformations in the optic array to create an optic flow. It is this detection of the transformation in the optic array (i.e. picking up relevant information) that guides movement. This is accomplished by means of the aforementioned tracking systems that track the head and body so that the visual display changes accordingly. This advanced virtual environment setup guarantees 'forces resulting in flows and flows resulting in forces – of perception entailing action and of action entailing perception' (Richardson *et al*. 2008, p. 174). Hence, the specific perception–action couplings are maintained (Araújo *et al*. 2005). Representative functional interactions arise when participants continuously act to perceive information from the visual context of performance and this information in turn shapes action. Experimental designs, including using virtual contexts, should maintain specific and functional perception–action couplings and allow and potentiate interpersonal coordination.

A study by Watson *et al*. (2011) used an immersive interactive environment with a button-pressing response task to investigate 'pass-through-ability' in rugby union. Though decoupling action responses from perception by relying on judgments alone (button-press responses), this was an important study in highlighting how virtual environment technology can be used to understand affordances that emerge in dynamic rugby situations and how they may be defined in terms of the spatiotemporal dynamics of the optics of the unfolding events.

Importantly, existing technological advances are keeping with the ecological psychology hallmark of perception–action coupling, given that participants are able to act instead of 'perceive only'; i.e. they can move and, for this forward movement, optic flow information is provided. For instance, in the study by Dessing and Craig (2010) on how goalkeepers save curved free kicks, hand movements in the direction of the approaching ball were considered to be measures of task performance. In a recent study by Correia *et al*. (2013), the influence of emerging gaps between defenders on a ball-carrier's choice of action was investigated. In this experiment, participants acted freely (owing to the task characteristics, they could essentially run or pass the ball to one of two attacking teammates). Note, though, that it is important to avoid a discrete look at actors performing discrete actions when faced with virtual simulations of natural performance tasks; i.e. not only considering the actions performed but their dynamics and how they are related to the unfolding information dynamics. There is a lack of systematic research about how performers are continuously using information throughout the dynamic course of goal-directed action (Correia *et al*. 2013). Although the action informs about perception, thus far, continuous action or, better, the dynamics of that action has not been considered in sport research.

Dynamics of the athlete–environment system

It is important to consider that goal-directed action in interpersonal interactions is dependent on initial conditions, emerging from perception–action couplings under the influence of the local constraints and that understanding the resultant variability is a key feature of behaviour (e.g. Davids 2009; Newell 1986). This means that more individualized analyses may be needed and the virtual environment may be a fine tool to accomplish this. For instance, this could be investigated on different timescales of sport performance, learning and development. Besides, the emphasis on constraints in understanding individual differences must consider not only the perception–action coupling but also the degeneracy property. Degeneracy essentially concerns the capacity to make use of structurally different components to achieve the same functional outcomes (Edelman and Gally 2001; Hong and Newell 2006; Davids *et al.* 2006). This property expresses the flexibility and adaptability to fit task constraints for performance goal-achievement (Edelman and Gally 2001; Davids *et al.* 2006) and may be investigated by means of the manipulation of virtual environment task constraints. That is, it is possible, by having full control over the manipulation of task features, such as the kinematics of teammates and opposing players' behaviours, to assess the same individuals exploitation of structurally different components to achieve the same functional outcomes.

The perception of what action is possible in a given task is also said to be body and action scaled (e.g. Warren 1984; Warren and Whang, 1987; Oudejans *et al.* 1996; Turvey *et al.* 1999; Marik 1987). Dimensionless body ratios and individual action capabilities (i.e. intrinsic functional properties of the individual) have been shown to relate directly to the environmental properties. This individual scaling may also be considered in the build-up of sports interaction research by means of virtual environment technology.

Online updated interaction between the participant's actions and the virtual performance context are still scarce. Although there is a functional relationship between the participants and the virtual context, the virtual environment does not allow for true reciprocity as in the simulated athlete–environment system. The influence of the environment on the participant is present in most immersive interactive virtual environment designs. However, the influence of the participant on the environment, such as on the behaviour of other players involved in the virtual environment task (avatars), is not. This should not be a problem, given that the great advantage of these systems over the natural performance context is actually to have control over the visual context and information made available (e.g. avatar movements).

One foremost characteristic is that this kind of setup overcomes some difficulties that are found *in situ*, such as the impracticality of examining sport-specific decision making of non-players (e.g. studying non-rugby players in a rugby task where significant physical contact is allowed by the game rules; Araújo *et al.* 2005).

Empirical evidence has also been provided supporting the role of visual and

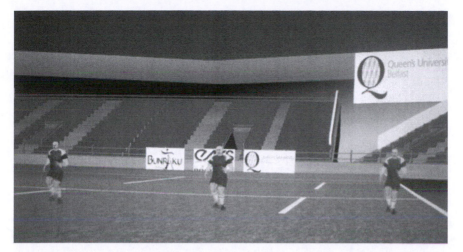

Figure 10.2 A schematic representation of what the ball-carrying participant could see in front of him/her (i.e. the defensive line) in a virtual environment simulated three-versus-three rugby task

nonvisual sensory information in the perception and realization of the possibilities of action (e.g. Stoffregen and Riccio 1988). Emergent behaviour expressed in interpersonal sport interactions depends also on multiple sensory modalities, including information from both vestibular and kinaesthetic modalities. Technological possibilities of a multimodal interface combining three-dimensional visual and sound displays, together with other sensory modalities would be helpful for better investigating interpersonal interactions in complex systems such as sport.

Implications of virtual environments for sport performance research and practice organization

There is still a need to bridge the natural–virtual context gap. For instance, descriptive or experimental investigations undertaken in the field of performance may provide evidence of how the key constraints in natural contexts influence behaviour. By way of virtual contexts (use of immersive and interactive virtual reality technology), a coach, a psychologist or player/athlete, may reproduce and experience those performance challenges and thus potentiate not only the diagnostic of performance but also the subsequent intervention (Craig *et al*. 2011; Watson *et al*. 2011). Virtual environments could be helpful in off-field training in cases of injury, to increase training load without significant increases in fatigue or even when there are no facilities available for training because of weather conditions.

Key constraints on performers' behavioural events and outcome found in natural contexts of performance, such as interpersonal distance and relative velocity

(Duarte *et al.* 2010; Passos *et al.* 2008), initial interpersonal distance (Correia *et al.* 2012a) could be reproduced and manipulated in virtual contexts. This potentially facilitates practising off field some aspects of performance, which, owing to various aspects (e.g. excessive opportunities to be tackled in the natural context may restrict the number of trials suitable to avoid injury and excessive fatigue), cannot be performed with such a high frequency on the field.

In tasks designed for both research and practice, the possibility of actually intercepting or running through spaces, for example, must be provided to the participants. Designed tasks must also contain objects in the virtual environment context with properties that are relevant to an individual's purpose within the task (i.e. that afford desired skills and adaptive and functional behaviours).

As mentioned before, the types of cross-modal interactions that take place during direct perception in the natural context should also be exploited. Moreover, to our knowledge, immersive and interactive virtual environment tasks applied to sports research has focused on the study of one participant interacting with an entirely controlled a priori virtual simulated performance context (including the behaviour of other players). Taking advantage of the advance in technology, such as tracking systems and vision display devices, further research could use more elaborated virtual worlds and could investigate also the interpersonal coordination between players and teams, by immersing more than one participant in the virtual environment simulated sport task; i.e. to investigate interactions between teammates or opposing players when facing pre-established movements of the other virtual players involved. Although this might be not possible at the moment, it is certainly being worked on (e.g. a simple Kinect4® or a Nintendo Wii®, has interaction between players/participants) and this is of great interest for furthering this area of research.

Considering the dynamics in the individual–environment relationship and scaled to the individual (Marik 1987; Oudejans *et al.* 1996; Warren 1984; Warren and Whang 1987; Turvey 1999), we may incorporate these characteristics within virtual environments. For instance, when catching a ball in a virtual context, the participant could see a longer arm or a faster arm movement, and participants' height or jumping reach could be changed. This would not be possible except through virtual means.

Conclusion

The potential for studying behaviour in sport through virtual environment technology has been outlined. One of the main advantages it offers is to experimentally control the information available and examine how this information guides action in sport. Although such technologies are not yet widely accessible, large displays and body-based interactive devices are becoming increasingly advanced and accessible (e.g. Kinect4, Nintendo Wii®), and immersive and interactive sport situations will be easier to simulate while maintaining their functional fidelity.

Questions for students

1. How is perception–action reciprocity assumed to be sustained in a virtual environment?
2. What role do tracking systems and displays play in providing a realistic representation of a sporting context? How does the level of immersion differ between an HMD-based display and a desktop/screen-based projection?
3. What are the advantages and disadvantages of using immersive, interactive virtual environment over more traditional methods (e.g. video or eye tracking) when trying to understand performance?
4. How can you recreate a representative sports experimental setup in a virtual environment?
5. How do you think virtual environment technology should be used to improve performance in sport?

Note

1 We avoid using the term real context or real behaviour because interacting with virtual contexts does not imply unreal behaviour or that the virtual context is unreal.

References

Allard, F., Graham, S. and Paarsalu, M. (1980) Perception in sport: basketball. *Journal of Sport Psychology*, 2: 14–21.

Araújo, D., Davids, K., Bennett, S., Button, C. and Chapman, G. (2004) Emergence of sport skills under constraints, in A. M. Williams and N. J. Hodges (eds) *Skill Acquisition in Sport: Research, Theory and Practice*. Abingdon: Routledge, pp. 409–34.

Araújo, D., Davids, K. and Serpa, S. (2005) An ecological approach to expertise effects in decision-making in a simulated sailing regatta. *Psychology of Sport and Exercise*, 6 (6): 671–92.

Araújo, D., Davids, K. and Hristovski, R. (2006) The ecological dynamics of decision making in sport. *Psychology of Sport and Exercise*, 7 (6): 653–76.

Bideau B., Kulpa, R., Menardais, S., Fradet, L., Multon, F., Delamarche, P. and Arnaldi, B. (2003) Real handball goalkeeper vs. virtual handball thrower. *Presence: Teleoperators and Virtual Environments*, 12 (4): 411–21.

Bideau, B., Multon, F., Kulpa, R., Fradet, L., Arnaldi, B. and Delamarche, P. (2004) Using virtual reality to analyse links between handball thrower kinematics and goalkeeper's reactions. *Neuroscience Letters*, 372: 119–22.

Bideau, B., Kulpa, R., Vignais, N., Brault, S., Multon, F. and Craig, C. (2010) Using virtual reality to analyze sports performance. *IEEE Computer Graphics and Applications*, 30 (2): 14–21.

Bohil, C. J., Alicea, B., and Biocca, F. A. (2011) Virtual reality in neuroscience research and therapy. *Nature Reviews*, 12: 752–62.

Brault, S., Bideau, B., Kupla, R. and Craig, C. M. (2012) Detecting deception in movement: the case of the side step in rugby. *PLoS ONE*, 7 (6): e37494; doi:

10.1371/journal.pone.0037494 (accessed 7 June 2013).

Brunswik, E. (1956) *Perception and the Representative Design of Psychological Experiments*, 2nd edn. Berkeley: University of California Press.

Correia, V., Araújo, D., Cummins, A. and Craig, C. (2012) Perceiving and acting upon spaces in a VR rugby task: expertise effects in affordance detection and task achievement. *Journal of Sport and Exercise Psychology*, 34: 305–21.

Correia, V., Araújo, D., Vilar, L. and Davids, K. (2013) From recording discrete actions to studying continuous goal-directed behaviours in team sports. *Journal of Sports Sciences*, 31 (5): 546–53.

Craig, C. and Watson, G. (2011) An affordance based approach to decision making in sport: discussing a novel methodological framework. *Revista Psicologia del Deporte*, 20 (2): 689–708.

Craig, C., Berton, E., Rao, G., Fernandez, L. and Bootsma, R. (2006) Judging where a ball will go: the case of curved free kicks in football. *Naturwissenschaften*, 93 (2): 97–101.

Craig, C., Goulon, C., Berton, E., Rao, G., Fernandez, L. and Bootsma, R. J. (2009) Optic variables used to judge future ball arrival position in expert and novice soccer players. *Attention, Perception, and Psychophysics*, 71 (3): 515–22.

Craig, C. M., Bastin, J. and Montagne, G. (2011) How information guides movement: intercepting curved free kicks in soccer. *Human Movement Science*, 30 (5): 931–41.

Davids, K. (2009) The organization of action in complex neurobiological systems, in D. Araújo, H. Ripoll and M. Raab (eds) *Perspectives on Cognition and Action in Sport*. New York: Nova Science Publishers, pp. 3–13.

Davids, K., Bennett, S. J. and Newell, K. (2006) *Movement System Variability*. Champaign, IL: Human Kinetics.

Davids, K., Araújo, D., Button, C. and Renshaw, I. (2007) Degenerate brains, indeterminate behavior and representative tasks: implications for experimental design in sport psychology research, in G. Tenenbaum and R. Eklund (eds) *Handbook of Sport Psychology*, 3rd edn. New York: John Wiley, pp. 224–44.

de la Peña, N., Weil, P., Llobera, J., Giannopoulos, E., Pomés, A., Spanlang, B., Friedman, D., Sanchez-Vives, M. V. and Slater, M. (2010) Immersive journalism: immersive virtual reality for the first-person experience of news. *Presence*, 19 (4): 291–301.

Dessing, J. C. and Craig, C. M. (2010) Bending it like Beckham: how to visually fool the goalkeeper. *Plos ONE*, 5 (10): e13161; doi:10.1371/journal.pone.0013161 (accessed 7 June 2013).

Duarte, R., Araújo, D., Gazimba, V., Fernandes, O., Fologado, H., Marmeleira, J. and Davids, K. (2010) The ecological dynamics of 1v1 sub-phases in association football. *Open Sport Science Journal*, 3: 16–18.

Edelman, G. M. and Gally, J. (2001) Degeneracy and complexity in biological systems. *Proceedings of the National Academy of Sciences of the USA*, 98: 13763–8.

Esteves, P. T., de Oliveira, R. F. and Araújo, D. (2011) Posture-related affordances guide attacks in basketball. *Psychology of Sport and Exercise*, 12: 639–44.

Farrow, D. and Abernethy, B., (2003) Do expertise and the degree of perception–action coupling affect natural anticipatory performance? *Perception*, 32 (9): 1127–39.

Gerardi, M., Rothbaum, B. O., Ressler, K., Heekin, M. and Rizzo, A. (2008) Virtual reality exposure therapy using a virtual Iraq: case report. *Journal of Traumatic Stress*, 21: 209–13.

Gibson, J. J. (1979) *The Ecological Approach to Visual Perception*. Hillsdale, NJ: Lawrence Erlbaum Associates.

Hammond, K. R. and Stewart, T. R. (eds) (2001) *The Essential Brunswik: Beginnings, Explications, Applications*. New York: Oxford University Press.

Hong, S. L. and Newell, K. M. (2006) Practice effects on local and global dynamics of the ski-simulator task. *Experimental Brain Research*, 169: 350–60.

Knapp, J. M. and Loomis, J. M. (2004) Limited field of view of head-mounted displays is not the cause of distance underestimation in virtual environments. *Presence: Teleoperators and Virtual Environments*, 13 (5): 572–7.

Kelso, J. A. S. (1995) *Dynamic Patterns. The Self-Organization of Brain and Behavior.* Cambridge, MA: MIT Press.

Kelso, J. A. S. (2002) The complementary nature of coordination dynamics: selforganization and agency. *Nonlinear Phenomena in Complex Systems*, 5 (4): 364–71.

Krijn, M., Emmelkamp, P. M. G., Biemond, R., de Wilde de Ligny, C., Schuemie, M. and van der Mast, C. A. P. G. (2004) Treatment of acrophobia in virtual reality: the role of immersion and presence. *Behavior Research and Therapy*, 42: 229–39.

Marik, L. S. (1987) Eye height-scaled information about affordances: a study of sitting and stair climbing. *Journal of Experimental Psychology: Human Perception and Performance*, 13 (3): 361–70.

Marsh, K. L., Richardson, M. J., Baron, R. M. and Schmidt, R. C. (2006) Contrasting approaches to perceiving and acting with others. *Ecological Psychology*, 18, 1–38.

McGarry, T. and Franks, I. (2007) System approach to games and competitive playing: reply to Lebed (2006) *European Journal of Sport Science*, 7: 47–53.

McGarry, T., Anderson, D. I., Wallace, S. A., Hughes, M. D. and Franks, I. M. (2002) Sport competition as a dynamical self-organizing system. *Journal of Sports Sciences*, 20, 771–81.

McMenemy, K. and Ferguson, S. (2007) *A Hitchhiker's Guide to Virtual Reality.* Wellesley, MA: A. K. Peters.

Moroney, W. F. and Moroney, B. W. (1998) Simulation, in D. J. Garland, J. A. Wise, V. D. Hopkins (eds) *Human Factors in Aviation Systems.* Hillsdale, MI: Lawrence Erlbaum Associates, pp. 358–88.

Müller, S. and Abernethy, B. (2006) Batting with occluded vision: an in situ examination of the information pick-up and interceptive skills of high- and low-skilled cricket batsmen. *Journal of Science and Medicine in Sport*, 9: 446–58.

Newell, K. M. (1986) Constraints on the development of coordination, in M. G. Wade and H. T. A. Whiting (eds) Motor Development in Children: Aspects of Coordination and Control. Dordrecht, Netherlands: Martinus Nijhoff, pp. 341–60.

Oudejans, R. R. D., Michaels, C. F., Bakker, F. C. and Dolne, M. A. (1996) The relevance of action in perceiving affordances: perception of catchableness of fly balls. *Journal of Experimental Psychology: Human Perception and Performance*, 22 (4): 879–92.

Passos, P. (2010) *Rugby.* Cruz Quebrada: Faculdade de Motricidade Humana.

Passos, P., Araújo, D., Davids, K., Gouveia, L. F., Milho, J. and Serpa, S. (2008) Information-governing dynamics of attacker-defender interactions in youth rugby union. *Journal of Sport Sciences*, 26 (13): 1421–9.

Passos, P., Milho, J., Fonseca, S., Borges, J., Araújo, D. and Davids, K. (2011) Interpersonal distance regulates functional grouping tendencies of agents in team sports. *Journal of Motor Behavior*, 43 (2): 155–63.

Petit, J. P. and Ripoll, H. (2008) Scene perception and decision making in sport simulation: a masked priming investigation. *International Journal of Sport Psychology*, 39 (1): 1–19.

Pinder, R., Davids, K., Renshaw, I. and Araújo, D. (2011) Manipulating informational constraints shapes movement re-organisation in interceptive actions. *Attention, Perception, and Psychophysics*, 73: 1242–54.

Riccio, G. E. (1995) Coordination of postural control and vehicular control: implications for multimodal perception and simulation of self-motion, in P. Hancock, J. Flach, J. Caird and K. Vicente (eds) *Local Applications of the Ecological Approach to Human-Machine Systems*, Hillsdale, NJ: Lawrence Erlbaum Associates, pp. 122–81.

Richardson, M. J., Shockley, K., Fajen, B. R., Riley, M. A. and Turvey, M. T. (2008) Ecological psychology: six principles for an embodied–embedded approach to behaviour, in P. Calvo and A. Gomila (eds) *Handbook of Cognitive Science: An Embodied Approach*. San Diego, CA: Elsevier, pp. 161–87.

Rizzo, A. and Kim, G. J. (2005) A SWOT analysis of the field of virtual reality rehabilitation and therapy. *Presence: Teleoperators and Virtual Environments*, 14 (2): 119–46.

Runeson, S. and Frykholm, G. (1981) Visual perception of lifted weight. *Journal of Experimental Psychology*, 7 (4): 733–40.

Savelsbergh G. J. P., Williams A. M., van der Kamp J. and Ward P. (2002) Visual search, anticipation and expertise in soccer goalkeepers. *Journal of Sports Sciences*, 20: 279–87.

Sheridan, T. B. (1992) Musings on telepresence and virtual presence. *Presence: Teleoperators and Virtual Environments*, 1 (1): 120–6.

Sheridan, T. B. (1996) Further musings on the psychophysics of presence. *Presence: Teleoperators and Virtual Environments*, 5: 241–5.

Stanney, K. M., Mourant, R. R. and Kennedy, R. S. (1998) Human factors issues in virtual environments: a review of the literature. *Presence: Teleoperators and Virtual Environments*, 7 (4): 327–51.

Stoffregen, T. A. and Riccio, G. E. (1988) An ecological theory of orientation and the vestibular system. *Psychological Review*, 95: 3–14.

Stoffregen, T. A., Bardy, B. G. Smart, L. J. and Pagulayan, R. J. (2003) On the nature and evaluation of fidelity in virtual environments, in L. J. Hettinger and M. W. Haas (eds) *Virtual and Adaptive Environments: Applications, Implications, and Human Performance Issues*. Mahwah, NJ: Lawrence Erlbaum, pp. 111–28.

Tarr, M. J. and Warren, W. H. (2002) Virtual reality in behavioural neuroscience and beyond. *Nature Neuroscience*, 5: 1089–92.

Turvey, M. T., Shocklet, K. and Carello, C. (1999) Affordance, proper function, and the physical basis of heaviness. *Cognition*, 73: B17–26.

Vaeyens, R., Lenoir, M., Williams, A. M., Mazyn, L. and Philippaerts, R. M. (2007) The effects of task constraints on visual search behavior and decision-making skill in youth soccer players. *Journal of Sport Exercise Psychology*, 29: 147–69.

Vignais, N., Bideau, B., Craig, C., Brault, S., Multon, F., Delamarche, P. and Kulpa, R. (2009) Does the level of graphical detail of a virtual handball thrower influence a goalkeeper's motor response? *Journal of Sports Science and Medicine*, 8: 501–50.

Villani, D., Riva, F. and Riva, G. (2007) New technologies for relaxation: the role of presence. *International Journal of Stress Management*, 14: 260–74.

Wagner, I., Broll, W., Jacucci, G., Kuutii, K., McCall, R., Morrison, A., Schmalstieg, D. and Terrin, J.-J. (2009) On the role of presence in mixed reality. *Presence: Teleoperators and Virtual Environments*, 18 (4): 249–76.

Warren W. (2006) The dynamics of perception and action, *Psychological Review*, 113: 358–89.

Warren, W. H., Jr. (1984) Perceiving affordances: visual guidance of stair climbing. *Journal of Experimental Psychology: Human Perception and Performance*, 10 (5): 683–703.

Warren, W. H., Jr. and Whang, S. (1987) Visual guidance of walking through apertures:

body-scaled information for affordances. *Journal of Experimental Psychology: Human Perception and Performance*, 13 (3): 371–83.

Watson, G., Brault, S., Kulpa, R., Bideau, B., Butterfield, J. and Craig, C. (2011) Judging the 'passability' of dynamic gaps in a virtual rugby environment. *Human Movement Science*, 30 (5): 942–56.

Willemsen, P., Colton, M. B., Creem-Regehr S. H. and Thompson, W. B. (2009) The effects of head-mounted display mechanical properties and field-of-view on distance judgments in virtual environments. *ACM Transactions on Applied Perception*, 6 (2): article no. 8; doi: 10.1145/1498700.1498702

Williams, A. M. and Ericsson, K. A. (2005) Perceptual–cognitive expertise in sport: some considerations when applying the expert performance approach. *Human Movement Science*, 24: 287–307.

Williams, A. M., Ward, P., Knowles, J. M. and Smeeton, N. J. (2002) Anticipation skill in a real-world measurement, and transfer in tennis. *Journal of Experimental Psychology: Applied*, 8 (4): 259–70.

11 Methods of measurement in studying team sports as dynamical systems

Daniel Memmert and Jürgen Perl

The theoretical roots of the approach of an artificial simulation by means of neural networks lie back in the 1940s. Meanwhile, the claim of modelling biological dynamics has been reduced to a more pragmatic application of the great abilities of net-based concepts and tools. Today, two approaches are mainly in use. They can complement each other, in particular in decision making processes that occur in team sports. Unsupervised or self-organizing maps or networks (SOM) can learn and recognize the patterns of match situations on their own (Figure 11.1, left graphic), whereas supervised or feed forward networks (FFN) can learn by supervision what are the best solutions for a situation, once recognized (Figure 11.1, right graphic; see also Kohonen 1995; Hopfield 1982).

An FFN consists of a number of layers, each of which contains a number of neurons. The layers are arranged in a sequential order. The neurons of each layer can change the states of the neurons of the following layer by means of specific functions ('feed forward'), which, as a whole, model the network behaviour. During the learning phase, every step from input to output layer is completed by

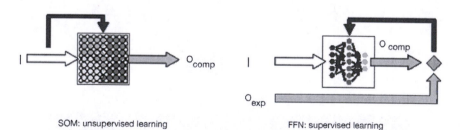

SOM: unsupervised learning   FFN: supervised learning

white: input; gray: output; black: data depending (re)organization of neurons

Figure 11.1 (left) Self-organizing map (SOM: neurons are grouped to clusters which form the output; (right) feed-forward network (FFN): comparison of expected output O_{exp} and computed output O_{comp} is feedback and so changes the neuron connections to minimize the difference between expected and computed output

a comparison of calculated and expected results, the difference of which is then used for feedback (e.g. back propagation): the feedback is combined with a deviation-depending reinforcement and so adjusting the parameters of the functions that calculate the changes of the neuron states. After the learning phase; i.e. as soon as the calculated results are satisfyingly accurate, the network can calculate output value-like actions to given input value-like situations.

A self-organizing network also consists of neurons which are not organized in layers but are regularly arranged in a matrix. As opposed to FFNs, the connections between neurons do not define possible signal pathways but describe a topological neighbourhood relation. During the learning phase, an input affects a particular neuron, to which it is closest or most similar, by moving it towards the input. The neurons of a number of neighbour shells are moved in the same direction, with decreasing intensity at increasing distance. Owing to the similarity of controlled neuron movements, the input values eventually cause a distribution of the neurons that is topologically similar to the distribution of the input values. In particular, classes of input values are mapped to clusters of neurons. After the learning phase, input values can be classified as belonging to specific clusters. This way, the high variety of datasets can be reduced to a small set of characteristic types.

In this chapter, the focus is on pattern recognition and SOMs. Supporting games by means of decision-optimizing FFNs has been done with simulated games, e.g. in the field of robot soccer, but currently is still too complicated for original games played by humans.

Developments and derivations of the basic SOM approach

Static and dynamic pattern analyses

There are two ways of net-based pattern analysis in sport. The first and comparably simple one is that of analyzing time- or space-oriented distributions, as for example player positions on the pitch. During a game, every player distributes their positions over the pitch in a characteristic way, depending on their tactical tasks and their technical and conditional skills. The net can then find the typical clusters; i.e. specific areas with the most frequented positions. In every moment, a group of players – defence or offence – form patterns of positions on the pitch, depending on their tactical task and the actions of the respective opponent group. The net can again find typical clusters; i.e. the most frequent formations.

Different to this static pattern analysis – and significantly more difficult – is a dynamic pattern analysis of complex game processes. For this purpose, trajectories are very helpful. They connect situation-representing neurons to a process-representing sequence of neurons. The advantage of trajectories is that they reduce the sequence of high-dimensional process datasets to a simple two-dimensional sequence of neuron coordinates, which is much easier to handle (see detailed explanations below). Moreover, they can be taken as input to a second net in order to analyze trajectories as dynamic process patterns. On the other hand, we are then confronted with two basic disadvantages of SOMs: the number of available trajectories is much smaller than that of the contained data sets and therefore it is normally not sufficient for SOM training. They are also unable to learn continuously and follow development of team behaviour over time. The approach of the dynamically controlled network 'DyCoN', which has been developed by one of the authors (Perl 2002a), is able to solve the problem.

DyCoN-approach

Owing to the fact that SOM training is controlled by an external algorithm using parameters that run down to final values and so eventually cause the end of the training process, a SOM that has been trained once cannot be reactivated for further training. Therefore, continuing training would require a complete rearrangement of the net and all controlling parameters, a practice that cannot be done in a satisfying way.

The DyCoN concept, however, is different: each neuron contains an internal memory and a self-controlling algorithm. The effect of the individual neural self-control is that a DyCoN has no final state but it can always adjust its internal memory to new input and can therefore learn continuously as well as in separate phases (see Perl 2002a; Perl and Dauscher 2006).

Trajectories and two-level pattern analysis

Figure 11.2 shows how trajectory analysis works; the matrix represents the trained network in which the small, grey shaded squares represent situations of a game – as for instance are formations (i.e. sets of x–y coordinates) of selected groups of players. Each grey shade stands for a specific type of such situation (e.g. the rhombic formation of the back four in soccer), while areas of the same grey shade represent variants of the same type (e.g. different geometric forms of that rhombus). The situation datasets of the game activate corresponding neurons of the network: starting with the light grey square that is marked by an dark frame, the process runs through some light grey neurons followed by some grey and dark, and so on. The resulting trajectory – i.e. the embedded sequence of black arrows – is a two-dimensional mapping of the process; i.e. the time series of recorded situations.

To analyze such trajectories, they are taken as training data for a second network, which is then able to cluster the set of trajectories and find out the characteristic types of processes. An example would be to assume that the colour sequence 'light grey, medium grey, dark grey, light grey' from Figure 11.2 means a sequence of formations 'rhombus, line, square, rhombus' of the back four, which might be corresponding to a particular defence strategy of a soccer team. The second network learns those sequences, compresses them to clusters or types and therefore represents the defence patterns of that team.

However, the combinatorial variety of such trajectories through some hundreds of neurons is so large that it makes sense to reduce the original neuron-oriented

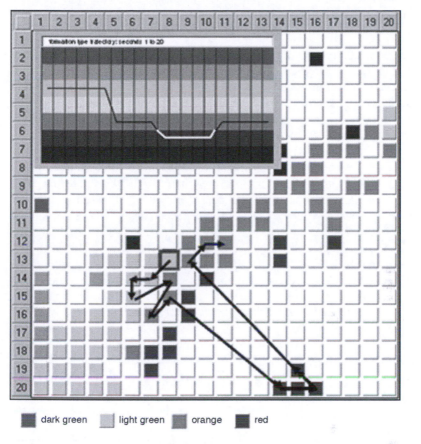

Figure 11.2 Network with a process trajectory and the corresponding type profile

trajectories to type-oriented trajectories, as is shown in the small embedded diagram of Figure 11.2: the trajectory has been replaced by the sequence of corresponding colours/type numbers, resulting in the sequence (5,5,5,5,5,5,3,3,3,3,2,2,2,2,2,3,3,3,3,3), which can be taken as an input vector for the second network, as described above. One serious problem remains: normally, a set of about 5400 input data (one per second) is available from a soccer game to train a net. The procedure of dividing the stream of input data into trajectories reduces the number of available data objects dramatically to some hundreds, often missing the necessary amount for a successful training by a long way. The advantage of DyCoN, however, can compensate for the lack of data by two steps:

- Monte Carlo simulation multiplies the original trajectories by varying the values of their components without changing the trajectory types;
- repeated training phases (as described above) help to acquire more information from the available data.

Overview on the development of game analysis: concepts, devices and tools

There are three main tracks of technical development that can be observed since the early 1990s (see also Figure 11.3). Data have normally been acquired manually by extraction from the video recording. Since around 2010, position recording has been supported by automatic devices, whereas ball recording using automatic video analysis and action recording using net-based pattern recognition have just started very recently (Perl *et al.* 2012). Methods of analysis have mainly been reduced to event analysis, using statistical approaches and mapping the complex game to simple numbers and/or distribution. First approaches to process-oriented analyses started in the second half of the 1990s in tennis, table tennis and handball (working group of Mainz; Perl 2001), followed by net-based approaches in squash, volleyball, soccer and general game analysis (working groups of Mainz and Heidelberg; Memmert and Perl 2005) starting around the year 2000. Early data processing tools mainly used video recorders and databases, while neural networks increased their influence in game analysis around the late 2000s (Perl 2002b). Again, the working groups of Mainz, Heidelberg and, more recently, Cologne, have been the leading centres of that development (e.g. Memmert and Perl 2009a,b). Currently, the research focus is on creativity and game simulation in particular.

Meanwhile, neuronal networks have become a frequently studied and commonly recognized possibility for data analysis and data simulation in sport. By means of neuronal networks, different kinds of human movements and several

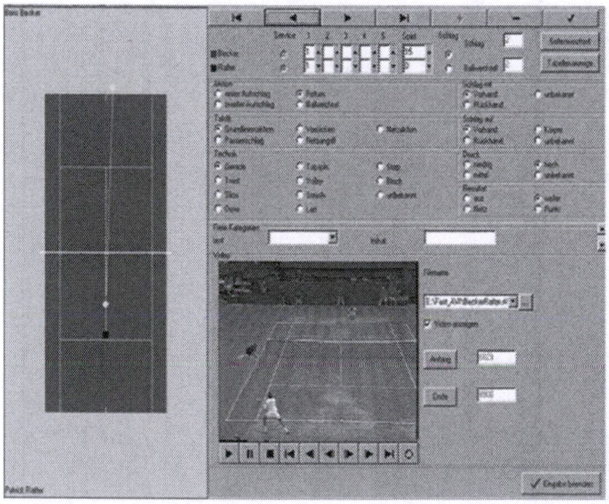

frequency	BL	BR	FL	FR	Σ
BL	0.3	0.5	0.1	0.1	1.0
BR	0.4	0.4	0.2	0.0	1.0
FL	0.1	0.1	0.4	0.4	1.0
FR	0.1	0.2	0.4	0.3	1.0

success	BL	BR	FL	FR	Σ
BL	0.8	0.9	0.4	0.5	2.6
BR	0.9	0.7	0.3	0.2	2.1
FL	0.3	0.5	0.7	0.8	2.3
FR	0.3	0.2	0.7	0.6	1.8

BL:back-left	FL:front-left
BR:back-right	FR:front-right

Figure 11.3 (left): TeSSy input interface with video control (bottom), animation interface (left), attribute selection and input panel (top); (right): examples of a stroke frequency matrix and a stroke success matrix representing tactical concepts and technical skills, respectively

skills in sport can be analyzed. For example, handball (Memmert and Perl 2009a), soccer (Memmert and Perl 2009b), squash (McGarry and Perl 2004), field hockey (Memmert and Perl 2005), arm movements (Draye *et al.* 1995; Cheron *et al.* 1996), arm and stand-up movements (Draye *et al.* 2002), as well as walking (Aminian *et al.* 1993; Köhle and Merkl 1998; Schöllhorn *et al.* 2002; Tucker and White 1999; Schöllhorn 2004) were modelled by means of neural nets. These studies demonstrate that additional research questions linked with pattern learning, gate analysis, game analysis, motor analysis and simulation processes can profit from using neuronal networks. All in all, the role and development of neuronal networks is a topic of current discussions in computer sport science and a new method of analysis in studying team sports as dynamical systems.

Game complexity: from simple to complex game dynamics

The first approaches to video-based game data recording and analysis date back to the late 1970s. While many modern concepts and methods of game analysis have already been developed, the weakness was – and still is – the data extraction process, which normally had to be done manually. Thus, the first case studies were restricted to structurally simple two-person games such as tennis or squash, later followed by games like volleyball, in which the teams are separated, acting like (abstract) super-players.

During the past five years or so, the combination of automatic position data extraction and net-based process pattern analyses has made great progress, with analyses of complex game processes such as those from handball, basketball or even soccer (Perl and Memmert 2011).

Tennis

The first computer-based tennis analyses were restricted simply to strokes, which were simply be described by the 'from' position and the 'to' position. Figure 11.3 shows the interface of TESSY® (Razorcat Development GmbH, Berlin), a video- and computer-based tennis analysis tool which was developed during the 1990s, offering a collection of complex game-process analysis features (Mussel *et al.* 2001).

TESSY enabled statistical evaluations of game situations and stroke sequences, including stroke combinations within single rallies. Moreover, tactical patterns, e.g. position clouds or stroke bundles, could be presented graphically. Finally, simulations of games and their tactical concepts were possible, as is shown in Figure 11.3. A player's technical skills (against a fixed opponent or as mean values) can be characterized by a matrix of success values of those 'from–to' strokes, while tactical concepts are represented by a similar matrix containing the frequencies of strokes. Obviously, as was in fact done in practice, such matrices can be used to simulate the effects of tactical concepts and technical skills by just changing the corresponding matrix values and analysing the changing game dynamics.

Squash

A player-specific process in squash can be defined as sequence of stroke positions (cf. tennis) of a player (see McGarry *et al.* 1999). Figure 11.4 shows an example of two strokes (left) and a net trained with the positions of four-stroke sequences, taken from games of an international tournament in 1988.

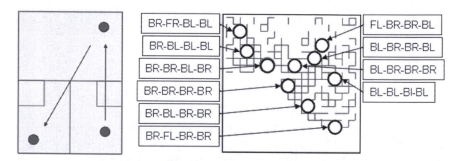

Figure 11.4 Squash court with game process BR–FR–BL (left); trained net representing the most frequent 4-position-sequences (right); BL = backhand left side, BR = backhand right side, FR = forehand right side

The tactical pattern of a player in a game is the collection of all action sequences in which he has been involved. In the case of stroke positions as actions, however, it has to be considered that the stroke position of a player is the target position of his opponent's stroke and therefore reflects the tactical pattern of the opponent and not of the actual player.

In Figure 11.5, it can be seen that, in the semi-final, the tactical patterns of both players mainly consisted of the same two sequences BR–BL–BL–BL and BL–BL–BL–BL (see Figure 11.3); i.e. both players trying to keep their opponent

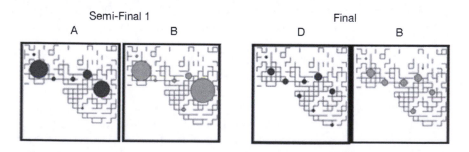

Figure 11.5 Tactical patterns of players depending on their opponents; A, B and D are the players. The squares represent the corresponding networks, where the circles represent the players' tactical concepts. Each circle corresponds to a stroke sequence, the frequency of which is encoded by the diameter of the circle

on the backhand side. In the final, the winner of semi-final 1, player B, showed a quite different tactical behaviour (i.e. varying much more between long line and cross playing). Again, both players showed nearly identical patterns. It seems that even top players are not able to play tactical patterns independently of their opponents but find a common rhythm, which is not specific for a player but for the pair of players.

Of course, analyses dealing with complex game dynamics based on tactical patterns can also be done without neural networks. However, the main advantage of self-organizing neural networks is that they are able to select the most important 10–20 types of sequences themselves, instead of having to manually select from 256 different possibilities – or even millions as is the case in football. In the example of squash, the sequences are of length four, where each component of the sequence can have the four entries BL, BR, FL, FR, therefore summing up to $4^4 = 256$. The same calculation with soccer sequences of length 10 (meaning a duration of only 10 seconds) and only six different formation types already sums up to $10^6 = 1.000.000$ different sequence types.

Volleyball

The first net-based approach to volleyball from 1999 (Perl and Lames 2000) was similar to the squash approach above, resulting in a characterization of the most important sequences and their frequencies as is presented in Figure 11.6.

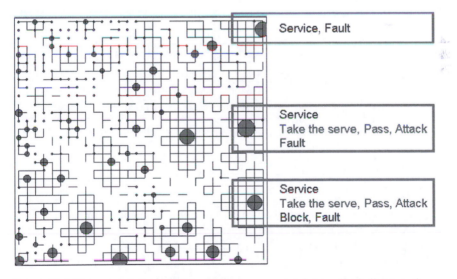

Figure 11.6 The network was trained with game processes from volleyball, presenting the most important sequences as circles, whose diameters represent the frequencies of the corresponding sequences, three of them being explained in more detail

Different to squash, however, this network could not give information about the individual technical or tactical behaviour and therefore its use was restricted to statistical analyses of frequencies and distributions of typical game processes only. The simple reason is that the net was unable to give information about the actions of single players, owing to its conceptual design.

In a second approach, the focus was on the formation of the players of a team on the playground (Figure 11.7, right-hand graphic), resulting in a much better insight into the tactical behaviour of the teams. After training, the two-dimensional neuron grid of the artificial neural network is organized into clusters of similar configurations. Figure 11.7 shows a trained net with such separated clusters (left). One cluster, which could, for example, correspond to the presented formation type – is highlighted by a thick black frame.

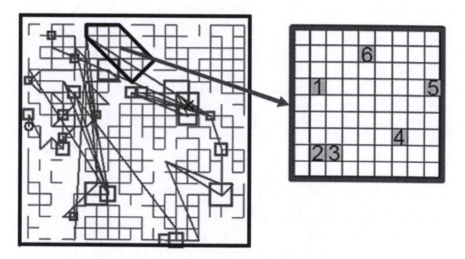

Figure 11.7 (left): Trained net with a trajectory representing a sequence of player formations starting at the 'O' and ending at the 'X'; (right): scheme of a configuration prototype of a team formation, which could, for example, correspond to the marked cluster

Testing original game data on the trained net again (as in squash) results in activations of neurons, representing the types and frequencies of the activated formations. Moreover, the order of appearance of the configurations can also be transferred onto the net and results in a trajectory (grey line).

By way of example, Figure 11.8 shows the differences between two top teams in the game of an international women's tournament: both nets show the defence's preparation for the expected service of the opponent team. It can easily be seen that Germany and Italy prefer quite different formations when it comes to taking the service. Moreover, there is another remarkable difference: while the

Germany   Italy

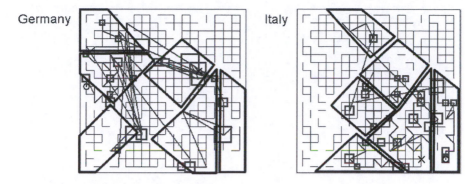

Figure 11.8 Trajectories showing the preparation of the defence against the opponent's
service

Italian team obviously finds the optimal formation comparably fast, only adjusting the formation itself (most of the moves are inside the marked clusters), the German team prepares by changing the whole formation (most of the moves are between the marked clusters), which means much more movement and a certain restlessness that later affects their actions negatively.

Football (soccer)

Neural networks can already be used for the computer-supported analysis of several more complex tactical performance factors in soccer. Based on position data (Figure 11.9), soccer-specific situations can be objectivized by using analysis software for the assessment of match situations (see Grunz *et al.* 2009, 2012; Memmert and Perl 2006, 2009a,b; Memmert *et al.* 2011; Perl *et al.* 2011).

The basis for the generation of the data is the collection of the *x*–*y* coordinates of all 22 players and the ball for the entire match time of 90 minutes ('tracking'). Using a sampling rate of 25 frames per second, an amount of 135,000 *x*–*y* data per player is generated which equals a total amount of 3,105,000 *x*–*y* data per game, including the ball. The basic idea is that the developed neural networks make it possible to compare match scenes from one or more games, to discover which sequences have led to which results. As described for volleyball, the neurons activated by the single datasets are being connected to trajectories that represent the two-dimensional patterns of the match sequence.

Similar patterns of such match sequences are then assigned to a common neuron or a cluster of adjacent neurons on a neural net of the second level and form a characteristic type. The aim is to group sequences, e.g. a 'quick build-up' on to the net in according clusters during the training, to automatically detect the respective realizations during the game analysis. In this way, it is possible to analyze extensive amounts of data online and to classify them with regard to differences and similarities.

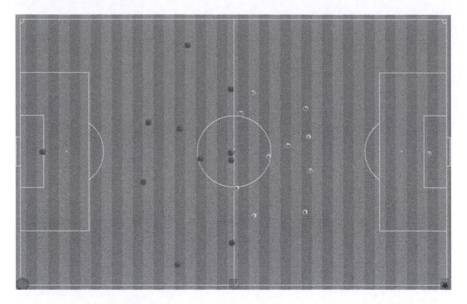

Figure 11.9 A two-dimensional replication of a match situation by means of position data

Another crucial aspect of the evaluation of a team's tactical behaviour is the interaction of specific tactical groups, such as offence and defence. The problem is that, despite the availability of the position data, an analysis of, for example, tactical movements of a team formation is hardly operable with conventional methods, owing to above-mentioned amount of data. Here, the ability of neural networks to recognize patterns offers new possibilities (as indicated in Figure 11.10). Specific match situations can be isolated from the rest of the game and,

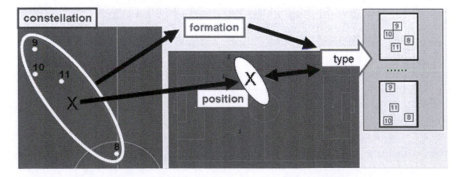

Figure 11.10 Net-based recognition of formation types and the recombination with position and time information (Perl and Memmert 2011)

thus, specific player positions can be learned by the net as characteristic formations. In this way, it is possible to identify frequency distributions of typical group formations as well as tactical interaction processes. At the same time, the degree of the implementation of tactical patterns can be identified, together with the ability of a team, to situationally generate new patterns.

First validation studies show that approximately 90% of the match events that are collected by means of traditional game analysis can also be detected by neural networks (Grunz *et al*. 2012). These events include various group tactics such as build-ups and set pieces (further differentiated into throw-ins, free kicks and corner kicks) as well as goal scoring.

From quantitative to qualitative analysis – and back

Analyses of complex behavioural processes – such as team sports – are intended to map the time-oriented flow of situations and actions to a time series of data packages, which then have to be transferred and condensed into a sequence of the characteristic and/or relevant pieces of information. Obviously, statistical numbers like mean values or even distributions of types of activities are neither sufficient nor adequate to characterize or analyze such complex behaviour. In 1971, Günter Hagedorn formulated the problem of the high time- and space-related meaning of qualitative game situations (Hagedorn 1971), also called the context orientation of activities (e.g. see Perl 1999). It turns out that patterns are, for instance, useful for the necessary quantitative–qualitative transfer (see Pattern recognition, below) and, as described above, that self-organizing neural networks can be used to find, characterize and analyze those patterns (e.g. Perl and Dauscher 2006).

Owing to the massive lack of game data, these first steps were normally case studies, demonstrating ways and dealing with aspects as well as basic phenomena. Of course, a well-based research requires information not only about one game but about a collection of games, to recognize standards, invariants, opponent-dependent behaviour and so on. By now, automatic position recording is one very important step towards developing standard routines for analyzing games and collecting information about them, which opens the way to a high-level empirical analysis. Not only is this the necessary step from data-based qualitative analysis to information-based quantitative statistics; the approaches that have been developed in the meantime allow much more: the combination of behavioural patterns and statistical distributions of frequencies and success can be used for simulation of training effects as well as tactical innovations (see Simulation, below). Moreover, the combination of advanced network skills and statistical analyses can help to recognize tactical creativity – and to improve it by means of net-based simulation. Two examples are given in the next chapter.

Pattern recognition

Based on the approach depicted in Figure 11.10, Figure 11.11 exemplarily shows some of the possibilities of the formation-based quantitative and qualitative

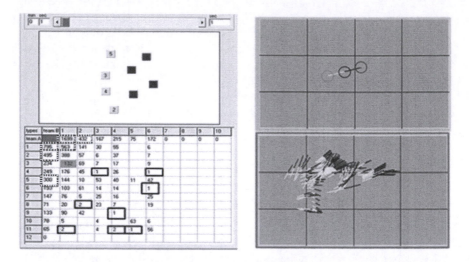

Figure 11.11 Example of the user interface of a tool for the combined quantitative and qualitative analysis of formations in football (see explanation in the text)

pattern analysis of game processes in soccer. On the left of Figure 11.11, the inter-action analysis with the selection tool for the data of both teams (here, the back-four of Team A (in light grey) and four offensive players of Team B (in dark grey), the scrollbar for a review of the entire match, the window to display the respective formation and the synoptic table which lists the number of formations as well as the coincidence frequencies for the entire match. Very frequently occurring formations are framed in a dotted line, very rarely occurring ones in solid black. On the top right, the window of a simplified formation, the group's field of attention and of the combined formation of the offence and defence group. On the bottom right, the window with the interaction process of the observed offence/defence formation for a certain period of the match (Perl and Memmert 2011).

Another example from team sport research illustrates the pattern-recognition phenomenon by means of neural networks with regard to tactical creativity. In team sports, tactical creativity at a behavioural level is defined as unusualness, innovativeness, statistical rareness or even uniqueness of solutions to a related sport situation (Memmert and Roth 2007; Memmert 2011). Using the example of tactical creativity, different types of creative learning behaviour can be differen-tiated by means of neural networks. Such a process-oriented analysis can help to find reasons for specific distinctive features. In this specific case, the different learning patterns could be explained by the fact that the training process was char-acterized by various types of learning behaviour in the different training groups (Memmert and Perl 2009b).

Figure 11.12 exemplarily shows an array of trajectories representing the

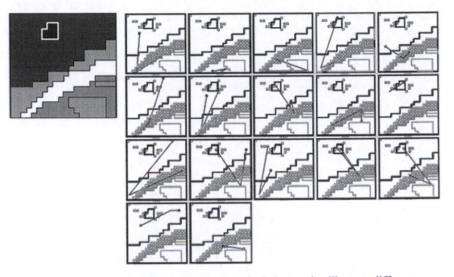

Figure 11.12 Trained neural network with grey shaded areas that illustrate different quality levels (top left) and a representation of the trajectories of hockey training. The learning process begins in the dark grey square and ends in the light grey square (Memmert and Perl 2009b); the colours of the neurons correspond to those in the large net graphic (top left)

individual training process of the athletes; beginning with the dark grey and ending with the light grey square, the individual sub-steps of the respective process are displayed as red lines on the net. In the three steps of the process, the trajectory runs through the grey shaded areas that depict the different quality levels of the net (from light grey = very good to black = extremely bad). After the entry on the net, the mean values of the qualitative analysis between the groups were compared by means of c^2 tests for the nominal-scaled variable.

The development of hockey-specific tactical creativity of the 20 hockey players represented in Table 11.1 shows very varied results over the 15 months of training: in 5 of 20 cases (25%), the performance increases at the beginning but turns out to be worse in the end than in the middle of the training process (up–down fluctuation process). The contrary behaviour was observed for 30% of the subjects (down–up fluctuations). In 25% of the cases, the performance increased monotonically, whereas it decreased monotonically in 10% of the cases. In 10% of the cases, the performance remained almost entirely the same.

Table 11.1 represents the collected results of the hockey, the soccer and the control group regarding the development of tactical creativity. Interestingly, the hockey group shows different result patterns than the soccer group. Only a comparison of the c^2 statistics of both fluctuation processes showed a significant effect between the hockey and the soccer group. The subjects of the hockey group showed stronger up–down fluctuations than those from the soccer group and vice

Table 11.1 Summary of the results of all trajectories of all three groups (hockey, soccer, control); the five different types of learning behaviour are outlined in the second column

Type of learning behaviour	Trajectory	Number of developments		
		Hockey	Soccer	Control
$a = b = c$	———————	3	5	4
$a \leq b \leq c$		10	11	11
$a \geq b \geq c$		12	8	17
$a < b > c$		24	11	11
$a > b < c$		1	17	6

Source: Memmert and Perl 2009b

versa. Compared with the control group, there were no significant differences regarding the fluctuations between the soccer and the hockey group. Concerning the other three types of learning processes, no crucial differences between the groups were found.

Such a process-oriented comparison of the results can help to detect problems and to find reasons for specific distinctive features. In this specific example, the different learning patterns could, for example, be explained by the fact that the training process was characterized by various types of learning behaviour in the different training groups.

Simulation

An advanced application of neural networks is the simulation of tactical behaviour, creative actions and dynamic learning in games. The current step of the game process is tested on the network, activating the corresponding neuron, which then returns information in different semantic categories such as type of activity, degree of creativity, probability of success or probability of transition to other activities. The idea is to replace the current activity by a simulated one, which could be more creative or successful, and to further simulate the resulting process by means of transition and success matrices (see Figure 11.3) and then to analyze the resulting simulated process with the intention of improving the team's tactical behaviour. Mapped to a network, this means that neurons should have the ability to represent not only frequent but also – and in particular – rare actions. If such a net is calibrated with respect to success or adequacy, the time series of a process is mapped to a trajectory, where the neurons can be recognized to correspond to creative actions (Grunz *et al.* 2009).

Questions for students

1. Characterize the differences between SOMs and FFNs.
2. Depict the differences between static and dynamic pattern analyses.
3. How does the DyCoN approach work?
4. Which are the three crucial technical developments for the analysis of sport games by means of neural networks during the last couple of years?
5. Describe the possibilities of the net-based game analysis in different team sport games.
6. What are the differences between racket and team sports with regard to the analysis by means of neural networks?
7. Which new results can be found by means of analysis of the tactical creativity when using neural networks for pattern recognition?

References

Aminian, K., Robert, P., Jéquier, E. and Schutz, Y. (1993) Level, downhill and uphill walking identification using neural networks. *Electronics Letters*, 29 (17): 1563–5.

Cheron, G., Draye, J. P., Bourgeois, M. and Libert, G. (1996) A dynamic neural network identification of electromyography and arm trajectory relationship during complex movements. *IEEE Transactions on Biomedical Engineering*, 43 (5): 552–8.

Draye, J. P., Cheron, G., Bourgeois, M., Pavisic, D. and Libert, G. (1995) *Identification of the Human Arm Kinetics using Dynamic Recurrent Neural Networks*. Neuro-COLT Technical Report Series NC-TR-95-017. ESANN'1995 Proceedings, European Symposium on Artificial Neural Networks, Brussels (Belgium), 19–21 April 1995. Egham: Royal Holloway University of London, Department of Computer Science, pp. 33–8.

Draye, J. P., Winters, J. M. and Cheron, G. (2002) Self-selected modular recurrent neural networks with postural and inertial subnetworks applied to complex movements. *Biological Cybernetics*, 87: 27–39.

Grunz, A., Memmert, D. and Perl, J. (2009) Analysis and simulation of actions in games by means of special self-organizing maps. *International Journal of Computer Science in Sport*, 8: 22–36.

Grunz, A., Memmert, D. and Perl, J. (2012) Tactical pattern recognition in soccer games by means of special self-organizing maps. *Human Movement Science*, 31: 334–43.

Hagedorn, G. (1971) Beobachtung und Leistungsmessung im Sportspiel [Observation and performance measures in team sports]. *Leistungssport*, 1: 17–22 [German].

Hopfield, J. J. (1982) Neural networks and physical systems with emergent collective computational abilities. *Proceedings of the National Academy of Sciences of the USA*, 79: 2554–8.

Köhle, M. and Merkl, D. (1998) Experiments in gait pattern classification with neural networks of adaptive architecture, in *Proceedings of the 8th International Conference on Artificial Neural Networks, Skövde, Sweden*. Perspectives in Neural Computing. New York: Springer.

Kohonen, T. (1995) *Self-Organizing Maps*. New-York: Springer.

McGarry, T. and Perl, J. (2004) Models of sports contests: Markov processes, dynamical systems and neural networks, in M. Hughes and I. M. Franks (eds) *Notational Analysis of Sport*. London and New York: Routledge, pp. 227–42.

McGarry, T., Khan, M. A. and Franks, I. M. (1999) On the presence and absence of behavioural traits in sport: an example from championship squash match play. *Journal of Sports Science*, 17: 297–311.

Memmert D. (2011) Sports and Creativity, in M. A. Runco and S. R. Pritzker (eds) *Encyclopedia of Creativity*, 2nd edn. San Diego: Academic Press, 2: 373–8.

Memmert, D. and Perl, J. (2005) Game intelligence analysis by means of a combination of variance-analysis and neural networks. *International Journal of Computer Science in Sport*, 4 (1): 29–38.

Memmert, D. and Perl, J. (2006) Analysis of game creativity development by means of continuously learning neural networks, in E. F. Moritz and S. Haake (eds) *The Engineering of Sport 6*. New York: Springer, 3: 261–6.

Memmert, D. and Perl, J. (2009a) Analysis and simulation of creativity learning by means of artificial neural networks. *Human Movement Science*, 28: 263–82.

Memmert, D. and Perl, J. (2009b) game creativity analysis by means of neural networks. *Journal of Sport Science*, 27: 139–49.

Memmert, D. and Roth, K. (2007) The effects of non-specific and specific concepts on tactical creativity in team ball sports. *Journal of Sport Science*, 25: 1423–32.

Memmert, D., Bischof, J., Endler, S., Grunz, A., Schmid, M., Schmidt, A. and Perl, J., (2011) World-level analysis in top level football. Analysis and simulation of football specific group tactics by means of adaptive neural networks, in C. L. P. Hui (ed.) *Artificial Neural Networks: Application*. Rijeka, Croatia: InTech, pp. 3–12. Available from: www.intechopen.com/articles/show/title/world-level-analysis-in-top-level-football-analysis-and-simulation-of-football-specific-group-tactic (accessed 10 June 2013).

Mussel, D., Perl, J. and Schröder, H.-J. (2001) TeSSy 2000: Erfassungs- und Analysesystem für Tennis. [TeSSy 2000: system for collecting and analysing tennis], in J. Perl (ed.) *Sport and Informatik VIII*. Köln: Strauß, pp. 111–21.

Perl, J. (1999) Aspects and potentiality of unconventional modeling of processes in sporting events, in B. Scholz-Reiter, H.-D. Stahlmann and A. Nethe (eds) *Process Modelling*. Berlin-Heidelberg: Springer, pp. 74–85.

Perl, J. (2001) DyCoN: Ein dynamisch gesteuertes Neuronales Netz zur Modellierung und Analyse von Prozessen im Sport, in J. Perl (ed.) *Sport and Informatik VIII*. Köln: Strauß, pp. 85–98.

Perl, J. (2002a) Adaptation, antagonism, and system dynamics, in G. Ghent, D. Kluka and D. Jones (eds) *Perspectives – The Multidisciplinary Series of Physical Education and Sport Science, 4*. Oxford: Meyer and Meyer Sport, pp. 105–25.

Perl, J. (2002b) Game analysis and control by means of continuously learning networks. *International Journal of Performance Analysis of Sport*, 2: 21–35.

Perl, J. and Dauscher, P. (2006) Dynamic pattern recognition in sport by means of artificial neural networks, in R. Begg and M. Palaniswami (eds) *Computational Intelligence for Movement Science*. Hershey, ID: Idea Group Publishing: pp. 299–318.

Perl, J. and Lames, M. (2000) Identifikation von Ballwechselverlaufstypen mit Neuronalen Netzen am Beispiel Volleyball. [Identification of rallies in Volleyball by means of SOMs], in W. Schmidt and A. Knollenberg (eds) *Sport – Spiel – Forschung: Gestern. Heute. Morgen*. Hamburg: Czwalina, pp. 211–15.

Perl, J. and Memmert, D. (2011) Net-based game analysis by means of the software tool SOCCER. *International Journal of Computer Science in Sport*, 10: 77–84.

Perl, J., Memmert, D., Bischof, J. and Gerharz, Ch. (2006) On a first attempt to modelling creativity learning by means of artificial neural networks. *International Journal of Computer Science in Sport*, 5 (2): 33–8.

Perl, J., Memmert, D., Baca, A., Endler, S., Grunz, A., Rebel, M., and Schmidt, A. (2011) Sensors, monitoring, and model-based data analysis in sports, exercise and rehabilitation, in D. T. H. Lai, R. K. Begg and M. Palaniswami (eds). *Healthcare Sensor Networks: Challenges Toward Practical Application*. Boca Raton, FL: CRC Press, pp. 375–405.

Schöllhorn, W. (2004) Applications of artificial neural nets in clinical biomechanics. *Clinical Biomechanics*, 19 (9): 876–98.

Schöllhorn, W. I., Schaper, H., Kimmeskamp, S. and Milani, T. L. (2002) Inter- and intra-individual differentiation of dynamic foot pressure patterns by means of artificial neural nets. *Gait and Posture*, 16: 159.

Tucker, C. A. and White, S. C. (1999) Neurocomputational approaches to pattern recognition and time series analysis, in W. Herzog and A. Jinha (eds) *International Society for Biomechanics Congress XVIII*, p. 2.

12 Team sports as dynamical systems

Tim McGarry, Jürgen Perl and Martin Lames

The challenge for understanding coordination was introduced by Meijer (2001) as 'Charles' problem' (Charles V, 1500–1558) in reference of the longstanding difficulty in comprehending how coordination might be explained using mechanical (machine) metaphor. In short, Charles was reportedly preoccupied with getting mechanical clocks (or pendulums) to strike together in unison but was unsuccessful in doing so. Unfortunate for Charles, an answer to the coordination problem was not discovered until much later when Huygens, in 1664, reportedly sympathetic, behaviour between pendulums when swung separately but suspended from a common frame. Thus, two pendulums swinging from a common frame, given sufficient time, self-coordinate into one of two possible rhythmic patterns, that of in-phase or anti-phase (Meijer 2001). In-phase and anti-phase coordination therefore constitute separate attractors for the coupled pendulums with both pendulums drawn to one or the other attractor. Importantly then, coordinated behaviours between coupled pendulums emerges not from prescriptive control design by some outside agency (like Charles) but, instead, from within by virtue of common information (energy) flows. In short, coupled pendulums produce self-organized behaviours by means of shared information exchange.

Relative phase

Relative phase is a metric that indicates the relative position of two points in their given cycles at any instant. In-phase (zero or unity) represents the same positions in the given cycles at any instant whereas half-phase (or anti-phase) represents opposite positions, with other phase relations expressed within the limits of zero through unity (or 360 degrees). For example, in-phase represents two pendulums at the same points in their respective cycles with both pendulums reaching the same zeniths at the same time whereas anti-phase represents the anti-symmetric relation with the two pendulums reaching opposing zeniths at the same time.

Human rhythmic coordination

Relative phase was used to describe the coordination features of simple rhythmic coordinated actions expressed in the well-known 'finger waggling' experiments of Kelso and colleagues (Kelso *et al.* 1981; Kelso 1984; Haken *et al.* 1985). The task was to flex and extend the index fingers of both hands in the transverse plane paced at different oscillating frequencies. Increasing coordination instabilities leading to spontaneous transition from anti-phase to in-phase were reported as a result of increasing the cycling frequencies beyond some critical value. Haken *et al.* (1985) modelled these dynamics results using two coupled oscillators (pendulums) representing the two index fingers, a theory of self-organizing behaviour subsequently applied to other rhythmical movements, including coordination between different limbs (Kelso and Jeka 1992), multi-limb movements (Kelso *et al.* 1991) and other coordination patterns (deGuzman and Kelso 1991), including coordination processes between the legs of different persons (Schmidt *et al.* 1990). The same system description predicated on coupled oscillator dynamics therefore describes coordination for many different complex rhythmic actions including coordinated actions produced between persons. This latter finding, in particular, prompted McGarry *et al.* (2002) to propose coupled oscillator dynamics between players and teams as the theoretical underpinning for the many and varied unique but nonetheless patterned game behaviours that typify different sports.

Game sports: self-organizing dynamics and behavioural perturbations

In consequence of results from investigating sports (squash) game behaviours as a probability-based (Markov) process, McGarry and Franks (1996) suggested that sports contest behaviours instead be considered as open (complex) self-organizing systems attracting to certain (stable) patterns of behaviour at the expense of other ones. In this context, the idea of 'perturbations' prompting temporary instabilities in otherwise coordinated game behaviours was introduced as a key concept for developing appropriate new descriptions for different sports. Perturbations in squash game behaviours were subsequently affirmed by McGarry *et al.* (1996), who reported good agreement among independent observers tasked with identifying them. Similar evidence on perturbation behaviours in squash games presented in the added context of dynamical self-organizing systems are reported in McGarry *et al.* (1999). Further evidence of perturbations identified from visual inspection has been reported for tennis (Jörg and Lames 2009) and football (Hughes *et al.* 1998). Thus, behavioural perturbations disrupt game equilibrium by producing system instability that is recognized by simple observation. Relative phase offers the prospect of identifying perturbations using a quantitative metric leading, possibly, to a new paradigm for investigating game sports behaviours in future research.

The underlying premise for considering sports behaviours as self-organizing dynamical systems is that, just as relative phase represents coordination for rhythmic movement behaviour, including between persons (Schmidt *et al.* 1990), so relative phase represents the spatiotemporal coupling of players and teams underpinning the behavioural rhythms that characterize the different game sports. In net games, anti-phase coordination is predicted on the basis of alternating strokes, such that, as one player leaves some neutral position to strike the shot, the other player waits for the pending stroke in the same or equivalent neutral position (see later comment on a common locus or separate loci of oscillations for the different racket sports). In invasion games, however, since both teams want to score against each other while preventing being scored against, in-phase behaviour between the two teams is expected as the opposing players locomote in tandem with each other. These are the basic hypotheses when considering relative phase in game sports.

Preliminary analysis of player movement data using radial distance from the T-position (approximate centre court location) provided good indication of anti-phase attraction in squash dyads, as hypothesized (McGarry *et al.* 1999). From these results, McGarry *et al.* (2002) proposed an accounting of sports game behaviours predicated on coupled oscillator dynamics. Put simply, the common descriptions of self-organizing behaviours resulting from the coupling dynamics of pendulums (Huygens), waggling fingers (Haken *et al.* 1985), different legs of different persons (Schmidt *et al.* 1990) and squash players (McGarry *et al.* 1999) was extended to include team sports as follows. Firstly, the reasoning of squash players oscillating about a common locus (the T) in coupled fashion by virtue of shared information exchanges was applied to the other racket sports, for example tennis and badminton, while acknowledging the separate and different loci of oscillation for the tennis players (e.g. the mid-point of the baseline) and badminton players (e.g. centre half-court). Secondly, this same reasoning was extended to include doubles play in these same sports, suggesting then that tennis players couple with their double (teammate) as well as with their opponents, thereby introducing the concept of multiple couplings as well as layered, or nested, couplings – a coupling of couplings, if you will. Thirdly, this same reasoning was further extended to speculate on other team sports, for example basketball and football. The next section reports subsequent research on these suggestions.

Attractors

Lames (1991) identified game sports as comprising 'two parties (teams, doubles or singles) that interact dynamically in order to score a goal/point and simultaneously to prevent the opponent from scoring' (p. 33), a definition that acknowledges unique performance structure for game sports with both parties sharing mutual competing objectives. Two main points should be emphasized here. Firstly, strong couplings between two interacting parties are typical of sports games. In most situations, the actions of one team cannot properly be understood without knowing the actions of the opponent. Secondly, these interactions are dynamic, acknowledging that intentions and behaviours change in time. If a certain game action is successful for a given player or team then the opponent has reason to change his (her) behaviour. If the action is unsuccessful however, then the player or team will look for something better to do. These interactions may further be understood in regards to the enslavement principle that is typical for complex systems (Haken 1993). The game state as order parameter enslaves the scope of actions possible for the players and teams. For example, the actions of a tennis player are constrained in part by the position and actions of the opponent and ball. Similarly, the actions of a football player are likewise constrained by game context, such as position of ball, teammates and opponents. Thus, lower-level behaviours of players and teams are influenced by higher-level game behaviours and, on the other hand, these higher-level game behaviours emerge from the lower-level behaviours produced by the interactions between players and teams.

At this point, we trust that striking analogies are apparent between features of game sports and properties owned by dynamical systems. As such, it may be useful to consider the ultimate objectives of both parties as attractor states in which a game exists in phase space containing all possible game states. Figure 12.1 offers an abstract model of football game behaviour with goal scoring considered as possible attractor states for both teams. Here, the game progresses from top to bottom with game behaviour observed as meandering in phase space between the two attractors. The state of attraction for one team necessarily constitutes a state of repulsion for the opposing team. In this accounting, the phase meandering between the two attractors is a product of the constant interactions of opposing players and teams as they pursue their competing objectives of attraction (repulsion) and repulsion (attraction). Beyond general abstraction however, the challenge is to identify appropriate variables that might adequately describe the spatial, temporal and/or situational state of a football match at any given point in time. Possible considerations for addressing this challenge using artificial neural networks are presented later in this chapter.

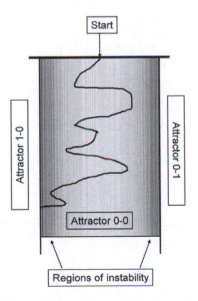

Figure 12.1 Illustration of football as a complex dynamical system (Lames and McGarry 2007)

Net games

Tennis

Palut and Zanone (2005) first presented relative phase analysis in tennis. Four tennis players of national level were instructed to play a rally from the baseline while not trying to win the point in the first seven strokes. Two-dimensional coordinate positions of the players on the tennis court were recorded at 25 Hz for 40 rallies, from which lateral distances from the centre line of the tennis court (i.e. the longitudinal line that divides the tennis court into two equal parts) were obtained. Relative phase of the two players in the lateral direction was then computed using the Hilbert transform procedure. The results reported a bimodal distribution demonstrating approximate anti-phase and in-phase behaviours corresponding with baseline exchanges between line and cross-court shots, respectively. For example, a player producing a line shot thereafter moves in the direction of the midline while the opponent retrieving the shot moves from the midline in the opposite direction to the player, thus yielding anti-phase. Alternatively, a player producing a cross-court shot once more travels towards the midline following the shot, whereas the opponent this time leaves the midline in the same direction as the player to retrieve the shot, thereby producing in-phase. As such, the rallies exhibited intermittent phase transitions between the generally stable properties of in-phase and anti-phase, indicating phase attractions within the tennis dyads as hypothesized by virtue of shared information exchange between the players.

Lames and Walter (2006) analyzed a single rally in a top women's tennis game with the aim of investigating relative phase in reference to game behaviour. Firstly, it was demonstrated that a rally in tennis produced cyclical behaviours as demonstrated in the circles observed in the phase plane results (Figure 12.2). Secondly, transitions between in-phase and anti-phase as reported by Palut and

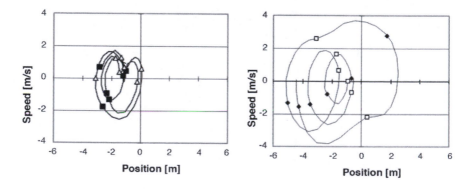

Figure 12.2 Phase space for two players in a tennis rally (Lames and Walter 2006); Serena Williams (left) Justine Henin (right); △, □ = strokes of Williams; ■, ◆ = strokes of Henin; going for the ball to strike and returning to a neutral position results in cyclical structures in a speed/position phase space

Zanone (2005) were once more observed (not shown). Since these phase transitions occurred by regular switching between cross play and line play, however, the more important challenge for game understanding is that of identifying the 'critical fluctuations' in relative phase (cf. perturbations), indicating the destabilizing of a phase relation before a possible phase transition. In addition, relative phase measures in both lateral and longitudinal directions are required for a more complete accounting of tennis behaviour, as information pertaining to important tactical aspects of game behaviour such as approaching the net cannot be obtained from lateral data.

Squash

McGarry *et al.* (1999) used radial distance from the T to investigate interaction among squash dyads and consequently reported single anti-phase coordination for all four squash rallies investigated. Radial distance was selected on the reasoning that it offers a single metric to express the two-dimensional movement kinematics of both players at any instant. As noted, however, when investigating baseline tennis behaviour as a dynamical self-organizing system, Palut and Zanone (2005) restricted analysis to the lateral direction only and, moreover, selected velocity instead of displacement as the kinematic metric of choice. To address these issues, McGarry and Walter (2012) applied Hilbert analysis to squash game behaviour for purposes of investigating the movement kinematics of squash dyads separately in lateral, longitudinal and radial directions using displacement and velocity metrics, with the aim of reporting on the similarities and dissimilarities that exist between these various selected measures. Speaking generally, the findings demonstrated strong phase attractions within squash dyads with varying combinations of direction and kinematic metrics producing varying results. More specifically, bimodal phase attractions were reported for both lateral and longitudinal directions for both displacement and velocity metrics, although the phase attraction values differed depending on the kinematic metric, whereas the radial direction produced only single anti-phase attraction for both metrics. As with the results from Palut and Zanone (2005), the bimodal phase relations of the squash dyad in the lateral directions are attributed to transitions between line and cross-court shots and, similarly, to transitions between short and long shots in the longitudinal direction. These results furthermore indicate that additional information for understanding game behaviour is derived from analyzing movement kinematics in both directions instead of a single direction which results necessarily in some loss of information.

The different results reported by McGarry and Walter (2012) were interpreted to indicate that selection of direction and kinematic metrics are important considerations when investigating coordination dynamics of game sports. Of more importance, however, was the observation that the varying outcomes from the varying initial conditions for analysis nonetheless conformed to common dynamical system descriptions, as expected given the universal underpinnings of self-organizing complex systems.

Invasive games

Basketball

Team sport behaviour in basketball resulting from dynamical interactions of dyads comprising players (Bourbousson *et al.* 2010a) and teams (Bourbousson *et al.* 2010b) was investigated. These authors recorded the kinematic trajectories of individual players and then undertook relative phase analysis of all possible player combinations, yielding dyads comprising players from the same team and from opposing teams. The results indicated in-phase coordination between dyads, with stronger attractions observed in the longitudinal direction (basket-to-basket) than the lateral (side-to-side) direction. Moreover, the phase attractions were influenced by the particular make up of the playing dyad, with dyads comprising direct opponents identified from playing position reporting stronger phase attractions than other permutations. This result is explained by the basketball teams using individual marking defensive strategy rather than zone defence. Other phase attractions reported were anti-phase in the lateral direction observed for the playing dyads comprising the wing players from the same teams, a result attributed to these players working in concert to increase width when attacking and decrease width when defending.

The kinematic data for each team were obtaining from the geometric means of the individual players data. These data were then subjected to relative phase analysis as before, thereby investigating game dynamical behaviour at the level of team instead of the level of players. As expected, similar results regarding in-phase attractions between teams was reported, with stronger phase locking in the longitudinal direction than the lateral direction. In-phase attraction between teams was furthermore stronger than between players as anticipated from statistical considerations.

Football

Frencken *et al.* (2011) also used team centroids (geometric means) as well as surface areas to analyze playing behaviours in small-sided (five versus five) football games. The distance between team centroids was taken as an indication of game pressure with lesser distances between teams indicating higher pressure exerted by one or both teams on the other. The surface area contained within the perimeter of a team configuration was interpreted as an index of player (or team) distribution with higher values indicating higher dispersion of players (Frencken and Lemmink 2008). Visual inspection indicated strong in-phase couplings between teams on both variables. A crossing of team centroids was also reported before some of the goals were scored possibly representing behavioural perturbation in these instances.

Lames *et al.* (2010) also reported dynamical analysis of a football game using relative phase (see also Cordes *et al.* 2011; Siegle and Lames 2013). Position data of all players from the 2006 FIFA (International Federation of Association Football) World Championship final were recorded at 25 Hz using automated image processing techniques (Beetz *et al.* 2005) and relative phase between teams was obtained from centroid data aggregated to 1 Hz using Hilbert transform. Figure 12.3 presents data for both team centroids from the first half and demonstrates strong in-phase coupling in the longitudinal (forward–backward) direction (Xrp = 0.002° ± 5.254°). Three main perturbations from in-phase are noted from data inspection, each of which is associated with significant breaks from open play. The first perturbation (minute 6) was associated with a penalty kick resulting in a goal to France, the second perturbation (minute 19) corresponded to the equalizing goal by Italy and may well be a result of the time taken to restart the game, and the third perturbation (minute 33) was attributed to game injury lasting more than a minute. These results highlight the strong in-phase couplings attributed to behavioural interactions between teams produced in open play, as contrasted against the weaker coupling behaviours observed during periods of inactive game behaviour, as expected. As before, strong in-phase couplings between teams is predicted on the basis of shared information exchanges between players and teams as they contest the game using common, if competing, objectives.

The coupling of teams in the lateral (side-to-side) direction was marginally stronger than the longitudinal direction as indicated in reduced phase variability (Xrp = 0.010° ± 3.844° versus Xrp = 0.002° ± 5.254°). In contrast to the results from the team centroids just noted, the coupling of the team ranges was weaker in both lateral (Xrp = 0.130° ± 18.250°) and longitudinal (Xrp = 0.128° ± 18.319°) directions as represented by increased phase variability. Since the lateral and longitudinal range values for a team are determined from the maximum and

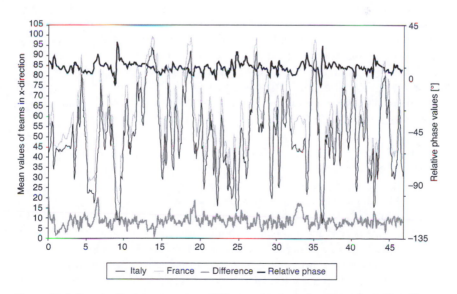

Figure 12.3 Longitudinal team centres, differences and relative phase for Italy and France during the first half of the 2006 World Cup final game

minimum player coordinates within a team configuration, this finding is expected, as the range is more sensitive than the centroid (mean) to changes in player movements. Regarding game behaviour, the result indicates that the teams are less coupled on measures of dispersion (cf. surface area) than on measures of central tendency.

Relative phase in the longitudinal direction for the midfield lines comprising four players per team ($Xrp = 0.000° \pm 5.398°$) returned similar values as the entire teams, although higher sensitivity to tactical behaviour was noted. For example, perturbation in relative phase in the corresponding midfield lines was observed in the ninth minute. This perturbation was due to a free kick awarded to France producing attacking play and leading to a goal-scoring opportunity. Similar observation of a scoring opportunity created by one of the French midfield players was noted in the 36th minute. Further analysis of a single playing dyad comprising a French attacker and Italian defender showed strong attraction to in-phase ($Xrp = 0.000° \pm 11.223°$), as expected, with three main perturbations from this phase relation. The first perturbation was associated with the scoring opportunity for France in the ninth minute noted above for the midfield line associations. The second perturbation in the playing dyad occurred in the 24th minute and was attributed to dribbling action by the French attacker ultimately leading to a scoring opportunity. The last perturbation was produced in the 43rd minute when the French attacker entered the penalty box without attention from the defender, who was preoccupied with assisting a teammate in tackling another opposing player. The coupling of a second playing dyad comprising an Italian attacker and French defender demonstrated stronger in-phase attraction than the first playing dyad ($Xrp = 0.000° \pm 6.551°$ versus $Xrp = 0.000° \pm 11.223°$) with two main perturbations identified from the data. The first perturbation was associated with the ninth-minute scoring opportunity for France mentioned already, with the French defender leaving defending duties temporarily to join the attack. The second perturbation was associated with a failed attack by France during which the French defender moved towards the halfway line while the Italian attacker remained in vicinity of the penalty box.

In short, these summary findings together with results from other investigations of football games revealed strong in-phase attractions in both longitudinal and lateral directions, from which it is suggested that coupling attraction may serve as an indicator of game quality. The more a team acts as a single unit with its behavioural organization coupled to the opposing team, then perhaps the better is the tactical performance. The coupling attractions should furthermore be considered in context of ball possession, however, with the defending players and team looking to establish in-phase associations with their opponents and the attacking players and team seeking simultaneously to break from it and free space, perhaps by way of perturbation. These assertions are consistent with the interpretation of results from futsal (indoor football) game behaviour (Travassos *et al.* 2011, 2012), although additional evidence is required to elucidate further on these possible important associations.

Artificial neural networks

In this section, we extend consideration of game sports behaviours as self-organizing dynamical systems by using artificial neural networks for identifying patterned behaviours in large data sets. Indeed, artificial neural networks themselves contain self-organizing features derived from rule-based approximations of nervous system function that, importantly, allow for automated learned recognition of structured patterns. For purposes of continuity, the following section relates only to uses of neural networks for analysis of football.

Football behaviour results from complex dynamic processes that make understanding difficult beyond the limits provided by simple comparisons such as action frequencies. For example, the vast amounts of data obtained by automated position recording methods are often reduced to providing general information on position distributions of players and their corresponding movement kinematics. In contrast, self-organizing neural networks such as dynamically controlled networks, DyCoN (Perl 2001), are useful for game analysis in their ability for recognizing dynamic behavioural patterns associated with playing strategies of tactical groups, such as offence and/or defence. One example for sports practice is identifying patterned behaviours in the changing time-dependent constellations of the playing configurations. For obvious reasons, automated position records are most useful for obtaining the required data, although in many instances the amount of data available is too large for detecting important information, even for artificial neural networks, which require large data sets. The data must therefore be reduced before analysis by neural networks, as detailed in Perl and Memmert (2011). For additional detail on research in football behaviour using neural networks, the reader is referred to Perl (2008), Grunz *et al.* (2009), Memmert and Perl (2009a, 2009b) and Grunz *et al.* (2011).

One way to reduce the amount of data is to separate the playing constellations from their positions on the playing surface denoted by geometrical centre, as demonstrated in Figure 12.4. This technique reduces the large number of

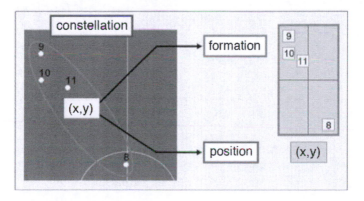

Figure 12.4 Separating a constellation of players on the playground into its formation and position

constellations to smaller numbers of formations, which can be learned by the network and reduced further to characteristic types by virtue of patterned features. Applying this protocol for each time point produces information regarding the playing formations, the formation types and their positions. These data, combined with other corresponding information added manually regarding activities and outcomes, enables wide ranging analyses, from the analysis of dynamic processes regarding tactical behaviours to statistical analysis.

Following training of the network, the formations and formation types contained in each dataset of the position data can be recognized and mapped as a trajectory (Figure 12.5). Figure 12.5 shows a net of neurons depicted in white and/or grey-shaded squares, where each shade represents a formation type, as exemplified in Figure 12.4. Neurons of equal shade represent variant formations of the same characteristic type; representing these variants by single type reduces the number of different formation types to approximately ten. This reduction of formation types has two important advantages. Firstly, it enables statistical analyses on reasonable distribution numbers and, secondly, the formation trajectories are smoothed, thus allowing easier comparisons.

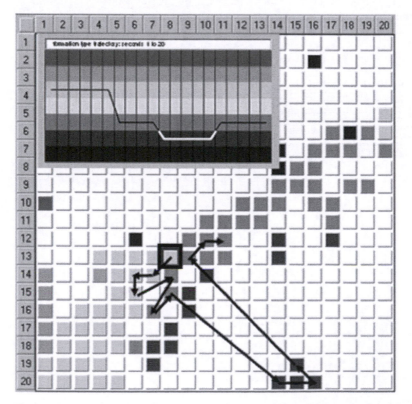

Figure 12.5 A trajectory of formations on the net and its reduction to a formation type
trajectory

Figure 12.5 demonstrates operation of the network. The position datasets of the game activate corresponding neurons within the network, starting with the one identified with the black mark (bordered square). The process then passes through some light-grey neurons, followed by some middle-grey and some dark-grey ones, and so on. Reduced to the most important formation types, which represent the specific behaviours of the corresponding tactical groupings (see embedded graphic at top left, Figure 12.5), the trajectories become much simpler to follow and comprehend. For example, the formation types could represent various defensive formations, with different formations indicated in the changing colours from light grey to medium grey to dark grey and back to medium grey. Thus, an advantage of net-based analysis is that the net is able to recognize different formation types and their dynamic transitions within a team automatically without need of additional information.

Net-based approaches for analyzing football behaviour: SOCCER

In this section, some net-based approaches of behavioural (tactical) and statistical analyses are introduced. This research uses the software application SOCCER developed by Perl in 2010. For more information on SOCCER and the spectrum of analyses it offers, see Perl and Memmert (2011). Figure 12.6 addresses the distribution of formations of tactical groupings and their interactions with opponent groupings. In Figure 12.6, the defence group of team A and the offence group of team B during the first half is represented, where the defence types 3 (890) and 5 (1,689) and the offense types 2 (1,428) and 4 (1,039) are most frequent. Note that frequency values denote time (in seconds) – for example, team B played formation 4 against different formations of team A for an aggregate of 1,039 seconds, that is for approximately 17 minutes of the first half. The formation of offence type 4 for team B is shown in the left-hand box, while the right-hand box demonstrates the formation of defence type 5 for team A. As can be seen from the matrix, the combination of both types appeared to be an aggregate of 624 seconds in the first half, comprising multiple separate instances of varying durations.

offense type 4	types	team B	1	2	3	4	5	6	7	defence type 5
	team A		0	1428	144	1039	118	2	9	
	1		35	13	1	21				
	2		110	82	1	27				
	3		890	451	60	367	3		9	
	4		0							
	5		1689	865	81	624	113	2		
	6		19	17			2			
	7		1		1					

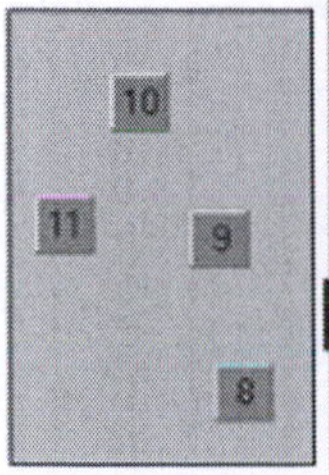

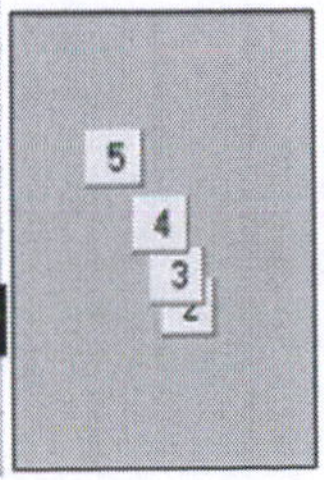

Figure 12.6 Frequencies of formations and their correlations

These data denote playing configurations representing the situational context of the game at the respective points in time. They should not necessarily be taken as indicating ball-related interactions between offensive and defending units, however, as the ball may or may not be possessed by players within these particular formations. This said, the most recent version of SOCCER distinguishes between team formations with ball-related and non-ball-related associations.

SOCCER offers many types of distribution analyses but little information by way of underlying game dynamics that produced these frequency counts. Regarding game dynamics, the phase trajectories of formation types of offence group B and defence group A are presented in Figure 12.7 (from the 21st to the 30th minute). Here, the meaning of phase is somewhat different from earlier usage reported in this article. Unlike before, phase does not represent position relations between the players or teams but, instead, it represents the formation relations between the tactical groupings being investigated. In the example presented, the time-depending distribution of the correspondences between type B4 and type A5 is highlighted for approximately 200 of the 640 seconds observed in the first half. These B4–A5 playing formation frequencies indicate this particular combination of playing configurations between the two teams as being a common phase of game behaviour.

Specific phase patterns may be of interest to sports practitioners for addressing questions regarding particular tactical concepts in the context of specific formation conditions, as well as for evaluating them by the success/failure outcomes of certain team activities (e.g. ball possession, goal scoring opportunities). In fact, such tactical phase patterns could be detected using neural networks on a second level of analysis. In the following, we offer an example of a feature analysis which demonstrates the usefulness of combining quantitative and qualitative aspects for advancing understanding of game behaviour.

Figure 12.8 presents the time section from Figure 12.7. First inspection of the formation phases shows that team B has frequent changes between 2 and 4 while team A has similar changes between 5 and 3, an expected finding, given that these are the most frequent formations of the respective teams. Second inspection shows correspondences between these changes, two of which are marked in Figure 12.8. The process starts in T21 with a phase of [B,A] = [4,5] and, ignoring spikes, is followed by change in B to [**B,A**] = [**2**,5], and then change in A to [**B,A**] = [2,**3**] before change in B to [**B,A**] = [**4**,3]. This sequential change in

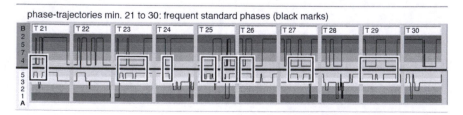

Figure 12.7 Distribution of a typical pair of formations between minutes 21 and 30

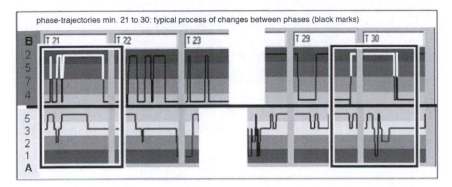

Figure 12.8 Example of a typical tactical pattern produced between the two teams

formation combinations between the two teams, which appears in similar fashion between T29 and T30, is represented in the preceding sentence by the use of bold-face type.

Initial impressions may suggest randomness in these patterns, the more so since the phase changes are not observed as idealized (error free) patterns but instead appear disturbed by secondary formation types (error). Restated, the patterned formations are not obvious and unambiguous but, instead, demonstrate variability typical of real-world data. Taking the respective success of the team actions into consideration offers additional information and perspective. In addition to the automated position data, there are corresponding success valuations of time-dependent team activities, such as flanking, tackling and shooting. Here, 'success' is not used in a game theoretical way where the aggregate of win and loss equals some fixed value (e.g. zero or unity). For example, a successful ball win by team A may be accompanied with successful tackling by team B without necessarily reducing the success awarded either team. In addition, success in the context of a formation does not necessarily mean success of the corresponding tactical group, simply that while the tactical group was in that formation the team was awarded a successful action.

Figure 12.9 demonstrates the results of combining quantitative and qualitative analysis. By way of example of combining SOCCER-based analysis formations with corresponding success values, we introduce the following nomenclature: SB([B,A] = [4,5]) = 0.89 which means that the tactical formation (type 4) of team B when competing against the tactical formation of team A (type 5) yielded an 89% success rate for Team B. Note that references to tactical formations of both teams represent specific playing configurations within these teams and not necessarily either or both teams in their entirety. Given the nomenclature explained above, the sequences that yielded most success were SB([B,A] = [4,5]) = 0.89, SB([B,A] = [2,5]) = 0.82, SB([B,A] = [2,3]) = 0.83, SB([B,A] = [4,3]) = 0.84, SA([A,B] = [5,4]) = 0.87, SA([A,B] = [5,2]) = 0.84, SA([A,B] = [3,2]) = 0.91 and SA([A,B] = [3,4]) = 0.94.

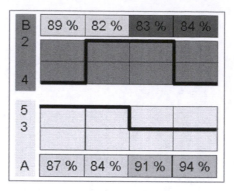

Figure 12.9 Prototype of the tactical pattern from Figure 12.5, together with success values

Figure 12.9 shows the simplified phase diagrams of teams A and B combined with the corresponding success values. The figure is reminiscent of the strategic trees of game theory, where the players respond with tactical decisions to drive out the opponent(s) from successful areas and/or escape from unsuccessful ones. One interpretation then from Figures 12.8 and 12.9 might be that team B tries unsuccessfully to leave an unwanted situation. In phase 1, the attacking team (B) has a success rate of 89%, whereas the defending team (A) has 87% success, indicating that this particular constellation is not significantly advantageous for team B. As such, team B might look to change attacking behaviour by changing formation from, say, type 4 to type 2 (phase 2) although this formation yielded less success than the previous one. This change in attacking formation for team B, moreover, results in a changed defensive formation for team A from type 5 to type 3 (phase 3). These changes in the last two phases advantages team A at the expense of team B. Of course, additional interpretation of the specific team formations in respect of game context is required for possibly identifying future optimized game behaviours. For now, therefore, this type of interpretation must remain speculative but it nonetheless serves to demonstrate how repeated patterns identified by neural network analysis as tactical invariants could usefully be applied in future sports practice.

In brief, neural network analysis of game behaviour offers the prospect for knowledge advancement when data are reduced to kernel information comprising formation types (or playing constellations). This analytical technique permits detection of tactical behavioural patterns not available to more traditional statistical methods, all the while retaining key information for purposes of statistical analyses if desired. Moreover, patterns such as those from Figure 12.8 can be detected by a second-level network, if required. For complex pattern recognition the inherent ability of 'fuzzification' helps the net to recognize patterns from other tactical formations, even if they should be disturbed by randomness and/or variation. A combined approach using networks and tools like SOCCER offers a productive combination of qualitative pattern recognition and quantitative statistical analysis.

Summary

In this chapter, we have presented consideration of sports games as self-organizing systems on the basis of coupled oscillator dynamics. Relative phase was introduced as a metric for investigating the behavioural dynamics of both net games (e.g. tennis and squash) and invasive games different (e.g. basketball and football), with in-phase and anti-phase in some instances representing attractor states for game behaviours at the expense of other possible phase relations. The notion of behavioural perturbations serving to destabilize the system from these phase attractions was introduced and considered important for game description. Moreover, the presence of behavioural perturbations in game sports has been validated from visual inspection although their predicted corresponding associations with relative phase variability await future demonstration for the most part. Beyond considerations of perturbations, relative phase and transitions between phase attractors, artificial neural networks were introduced as a means of identifying game structure from large datasets using football data as example. As with earlier demonstrations using relative phase, various unique phase structures (playing configurations) were identified by the neural networks, together with time-dependent phase changes indicating the underlying game dynamics. In closing, the approaches outlined in this article go some way to describing and explaining the behavioural structure of sports games and their underpinning dynamics.

References

Beetz, M., Kirchlechner, B. and Lames, M. (2005) Computerized real-time analysis of football games. *IEEE Pervasive Computing*, 4 (3): 33–9.

Bourbousson, J., Sève, C. and McGarry, T. (2010a) Space-time coordination dynamics in basketball: Part 1. Intra- and inter-couplings among player dyads. *Journal of Sports Science*, 28: 339–47.

Bourbousson, J., Sève, C. and McGarry, T. (2010b) Space-time coordination dynamics in basketball: Part 2. The interaction between the two teams. *Journal of Sports Science*, 28: 349–58.

Cordes, O., Siegle, M., Stöckl, M., Durus, M., Beetz, M. and Lames, M. (2011) Kopplung von Mannschaften, Mannschaftsteilen und Spielern im Fußball – Berechnung mit Hilfe der relativen Phase, in D. Link and J. Wiemeyer (eds) *Sportinformatik trifft Sporttechnologie*. Hamburg: Czwalina, pp. 186–90.

deGuzman, G. C. and Kelso, J. A. S. (1991) Multi-frequency behavioural patterns and the phase attractive circle map. *Biological Cybernetics*, 64: 485–95.

Frencken, W., Lemmink, K. Dellemann, N. and Visscher, C. (2011) Oscillations of centroid position and surface area of soccer teams in small-sided games. *European Journal of Sport Science*, 11: 215–23.

Frencken, W. G. P. and Lemmink, K. A. P. M. (2008) Team kinematics of small-sided soccer games: a systematic approach, in T. Reilly and F. Korkusuz (eds) *Science and Football VI*. London: Routledge, pp. 161–6.

Grunz A., Memmert D. and Perl J. (2009) Analysis and simulation of actions in games by means of special self-organizing maps. *International Journal of Computer Science in Sport*, 8: 22–37.

Grunz, A., Endler, S. Memmert, D. and Perl, J. (2011) Netz-gestützte Konstellations-Analyse im Fußball, [Net-based constellation analysis in soccer] in Link and Wiemeyer (eds) *Schriften der Deutschen Vereinigung für Sportwissenschaft, vol. 217*. Hamburg: Czwalina, pp. 111–15.

Haken, H. (1993) *Advanced Synergetics: Instability Hierarchies of Self-organizing Systems and Devices*. New York: Springer.

Haken, H., Kelso, J. A. S. and Bunz, H. A. (1985) Theoretical model of phase transitions in human hand movements. *Biological Cybernetics*, 51: 347–56.

Hughes, M., Dawkins, N., David, R. and Mills, J. (1998) The perturbation effect and goal opportunities in soccer. *Journal of Sports Sciences*, 16: 20.

Jörg, D. and Lames, M. (2009) Perturbationen im Tennis – Beobachtbarkeit und Stabilität, in M. Lames, C. Augste, O. Cordes, Ch. Dreckmann, K. Görsdorf and M. Siegle (eds) *Gegenstand und Anwendungsfelder der Sportinformatik*. Hamburg: Czwalina, pp. 86–96.

Kelso, J. A. S. (1984) Phase transitions and critical behaviour in human bimanual coordination. *American Journal of Physiology: Regulatory, Integrative and Comparative Physiology*, 15: R1000–4.

Kelso, J. A. S. and Jeka, J. J. (1992) Symmetry breaking dynamics of human multilimb coordination. *Journal of Experimental Psychology: Human Perception and Performance*, 18: 645–68.

Kelso, J. A. S., Buchanan, J. J. and Wallace, S. A. (1991) Order parameters for the neural organization of single, multijoint limb movement patterns. *Experimental Brain Research*, 85: 432–44.

Kelso, J. A. S., Holt, K. G., Rubin, P. and Kugler, P. N. (1981) Patterns of human interlimb coordination emerge from the properties of non-linear, limit cycle oscillatory processes: theory and data. *Journal of Motor Behaviour*, 13: 226–61.

Lames, M. (1991) *Leistungsdiagnostik durch Computersimulation: Ein Beitrag zur Theorie der Sportspiele am Beispiel Tennis*. Frankfurt: Harry Deutsch.

Lames, M. and Walter, F. (2006) Druck machen und ausspielen: Die relative Phase und die Interaktion in den Rückschlagsportspielen am Beispiel Tennis. *Spectrum der Sportwissenschaften*, 18 (2): 7–24.

Lames, M., Ertmer, J. and Walter, F. (2010) Oscillations in football – order and disorder in spatial interactions between the two teams. *International Journal of Sports Psychology*, 41 (4 Supplement): 85–6.

McGarry, T. and Franks, I. M. (1996) In search of invariant athletic behaviour in competitive sport systems: An example from championship squash match-play. *Journal of Sports Sciences*, 14: 445–56.

McGarry, T. and Walter, F. (2012) Sport competition as a dynamical self-organizing system: example from the movement coordination kinematics of squash players. *International Journal of Motor Learning and Sport Performance*, 2: 59–67.

McGarry, T., Anderson, D. I., Wallace, S. A., Hughes, M. and Franks, I. M. (2002) Sport competition as a dynamical self-organizing system. *Journal of Sports Sciences*, 20: 771–81.

McGarry, T., Khan, M. A. and Franks, I. M. (1996) Analyzing championship squash match-play: in search of a system description, in S. Haake (ed.) *The Engineering of Sport*. Rotterdam: Balkema, pp. 263–9.

McGarry, T., Khan, M. A. and Franks, I. M. (1999) On the presence and absence of behavioural traits in sport: an example from championship squash match-play. *Journal of Sports Science*, 17: 298–311.

Meijer, O. G. (2001) An introduction to the history of movement science, in M. L. Latash and V. Zatsiorsky (eds) *Classics in Movement Science*. Champaign, IL: Human Kinetics, pp. 1–57.

Memmert, D. and Perl, J. (2009a) Game creativity analysis by means of neural networks. *Journal of Sports Sciences*, 27: 139–49.

Memmert, D. and Perl, J. (2009b) Analysis and simulation of creativity learning by means of artificial neural networks. *Human Movement Science*, 28: 263–82.

Palut, Y. and Zanone, P. S. (2005) A dynamical analysis of tennis players' motion: concepts and data. *Journal of Sports Science*, 23: 1021–32.

Perl, J. (2001) DyCoN: Ein dynamisch gesteuertes Neuronales Netz zur Modellierung und Analyse von Prozessen im Sport, [A dynamically controlled neural network for modelling and analysis of processes in sport] in J. Perl (ed.) *Sport and Informatik VIII*. Köln: Strauß, pp. 85–98.

Perl, J. (2008) Modelling, in P. Dabnichki and A. Baca (eds) *Computers in Sport*. Southampton: Wit Press, pp. 121–60.

Perl, J. and Memmert, D. (2011) Net-based game analysis by means of the software tool SOCCER. *International Journal of Computer Science in Sport*, 10 (2): 77–84.

Schmidt, R. C., Carello, C. and Turvey, M. T. (1990) Phase transitions and critical fluctuations in the visual coordination of rhythmic movements between people. *Journal of Experimental Psychology: Human Performance and Perception*, 16: 227–47.

Siegle, M. and Lames, M. (2013) Modeling soccer by means of relative phase. *Journal of Systems Science and Complexity*, 26: 14–20.

Travassos, B., Araújo, D., Vilar, L. and McGarry, T. (2011) Interpersonal coordination and ball dynamics in futsal (indoor football). *Human Movement Science*, 30: 1245–59.

Travassos, B., Araújo, D., Duarte, R. and McGarry, T. (2012) Spatiotemporal coordination patterns in futsal (indoor football) are guided by informational game constraints. *Human Movement Science*, 31 (4): 932–45.

Part 3

Complexity sciences and sport performance

13 Ecological dynamics as an alternative framework to notational performance analysis

Luís Vilar, Carlota Torrents, Duarte Araújo and Keith Davids

Practitioners and sports scientists have been always seeking to identify key factors or characteristics that can distinguish between successful and less success-ful players and teams (Nevill *et al.* 2009; Reilly *et al.* 2000). Quantitative analysis of performance provides coaches with additional information that describes performance in detail beyond that which they can access through recall of personal observations (Borrie *et al.* 2002). Such critical information allows coaches to improve performance during matches and practice, through the improvement of feedback in an appropriate form (Franks 1997).

Traditional performance analysis have sought to understand performance by identifying the behaviours that are important for a given sport (Lames and McGarry 2007). Notational analysis techniques have described the performance tendencies of players and teams, and strengths and weaknesses in specific performance situations in a range of sports (e.g. playing long or spreading wide during transitions phases in association football). This methodology has sought for performance indicators that helped to characterize successful and unsuccess-ful performance and creating awareness among players and coaches of how individual players can influence team patterns (Hughes and Franks 2004; McGarry 2009).

Performance indicators are variables that can be categorized as scoring indica-tors (e.g. goals, baskets, winning shots, errors, the ratios of winners to errors and goals to shots) or quality indicators (e.g. turnovers, tackles, passes/ball posses-sion; Hughes and Bartlett 2002). Performance indicators are often ranked through the use of statistical procedures, such as factor analysis and multiple regressions, according to their influence on sport outcome. In addition, performance indica-tors may also be considered by their combinatory temporal relationships, typically recorded in a discrete sequential fashion to operationalize patterns of play of each team. For example, analysts have been also considering the sequen-tial actions of players within the same team. By recording discrete action frequencies in a number of games in a sequential 'who[did]–what–where–when' fashion, researchers have identified teams' temporal patterns of play (Borrie *et al.* 2002; McGarry 2009). This sequential analysis also allows the analysis of inter-relationships between performance variables. Temporal patterns are able to reveal those aspects of social interaction that are not immediately observable, detecting the hidden structures underlying an interactive situation, such as a game (Anguera 2005; Anguera and Jonsson 2003; Fernandez *et al.* 2009).

To provide meaningful insights to researchers about successful performance, indicators must be highly correlated with any associated outcomes (i.e. winner, error or neutral outcome; Hughes and Bartlett 2002), which has not been always the case (McGarry 2009). For example, one of the most intriguing indicators of team performance in association football has been the style of play (e.g. 'direct play' or 'possession play'), measured by the number of passes that a team takes to score a goal (Franks *et al.* 1990; Grehaigne 1999; Hughes and Franks 2005; Hughes *et al.* 1988). Although high-level practitioners have emphasized the use of longer passing sequences as a means of scoring goals, notational analysts have reported that the strike ratio of goals from shots is better for 'direct play' than for 'possession play' (Hughes and Franks 2005).

The presumed correspondence of this finding to competitive outcomes remains unclear, owing to a lack of a theoretical understanding of how to interpret the data. This discrepancy suggests that neglecting the constraining influence of information from the performance environment, such as the active role of opponents in shaping players' actions and decision making, may fail to provide understanding on successful performance. By omitting reference to the *why* and *how* of performance that underlie the structure of recorded behaviours, which would define their functional utility, notational analysis has been shown to be somewhat reductionist (Glazier 2010; McGarry 2009). These facts point to the need for descriptive analysis, such as that provided by notational techniques, to be complemented with a sound theoretical rationale that explains sport performance at the player–environment scale of analysis. In this chapter, we present ecological dynamics as a reliable framework for the analysis of performance in team sport, since it recognizes the 'degeneracy' (inherent adaptive flexibility in achieving successful performance outcomes) of players, including sports teams. This framework provides an understanding of how players perform successfully, by using information from their environment, and explains how the same successful performance outcomes can emerge from different movement or tactical patterns (a phenomenon also known as motor equivalence).

Ecological dynamics approach to performance analysis

From an ecological dynamics perspective, performers and teams are neurobiological and social neurobiological systems, respectively, in which patterns emerge from the interaction of their many degrees of freedom or constraints, through a process of self-organization (Kauffman 1993; Warren 2006). Self-organization in complex neurobiological systems is not a random or completely 'blind' process in which any pattern can result; rather, it is influenced by surrounding informational and physical constraints and intentions of a performer (Seifert and Davids 2012). Constraints are features that surround a complex system and reduce the number of configurations that are available to it as it interacts with the performance environment (Davids *et al.* 2013). Most interest for researchers is to examine how these macroscopic patterns of coordination are constructed, sustained and dissembled, through the continuous exchange of information between the athlete and their performance environment (Araújo *et al.* 2006; Kugler and Turvey 1987).

Ecological dynamics captures the intertwined relationships of the performer and their performance environment through an information-based perspective (Warren 1984; Warren and Whang 1987). This rationale was grounded on James Gibson's (1979) arguments that organisms, including humans, do not necessarily need representations of the world (e.g. knowledge about its properties) to be able to perceive its structure. Rather, the energy flows or arrays that surround individuals as they displace though the performance environment can act as specifying information, allowing individuals to directly perceive the properties of the environment and guide action. For example, the rate of dilation of an approaching ball on the retina of a goalkeeper informs him/her about the time-to-contact remaining before the ball arrives at the catching point. In principle, it is not necessary for the goalkeeper to separately compute either distance or speed of the ball to perceive time-to-contact information, under a constant approach velocity (Lee *et al.* 1983). The perception of specifying informational variables allows the perception of opportunities for action or affordances (e.g. a gap between two defenders promotes a pass to an attacking teammate) offered by the environment with the respect to the individual action capabilities, so that individuals directly perceive what they can or cannot do (Turvey 1992). In addition, individuals were shown to be also able to perceive affordances for others; that is, to identify relations between other performers (e.g. teammates and opponents) and key environmental objects (e.g. the locations of the ball and goal) that others may use to guide their behaviour (Richardson *et al.* 2007; Stoffregen *et al.* 1999). In this sense, ecological dynamics suggests that interpersonal coordination in team sports is grounded in the players' ability to identify the multidimensional spectrum of competitive affordances for themselves and others (both teammates and opponents) and acting adaptively towards acquiring (collective) goals.

When performers act upon affordances, a synergy emerges at the ecological scale, attracting the system towards a stable state of coordination (i.e. an attractor or preferable mode of coordination; Warren 2006). Hypothetically, if neither the individual constraints nor the environmental properties change, behaviour would remain attached to the same specific attractor. However, owing to the complex spatiotemporal relations among performers that characterize team sports, ecological constraints change on a moment-to-moment basis. On one hand, constraints of the individual may change, even though the performance environment may remain static. For example, in a team game like futsal (a type of five-a-side association football played on an indoor court) when a fatigued defender late in performance cannot accelerate quickly enough to intercept a shot that it would have been possible to intercept earlier in competitive performance (Fajen *et al.* 2009). On the other hand, changes may occur in the performance environment while the performer's capabilities remain constant. For example, at any moment in futsal, a goal path may open and a shooting chance may be offered.

Milliseconds later, a defender may move into the line of the ball's trajectory with the goal and a successful shot is no longer possible (Fajen *et al*. 2009). The insta-bility that characterizes the interacting constraints in team sports makes opportunities for action continuously come and go instantaneously, leading to fluctuations in the organizational states of games (e.g. increased variability in the way that attackers and defenders coordinate their actions; Araújo and Davids 2009). When these fluctuations are powerful enough to break the existing balance between performers (i.e. if the equilibrium between attacking and defending play-ers is successfully destabilized), a symmetry-breaking process occurs. That is, a previously stable state of the game transits to a new dynamic state of organization (e.g. an attacker dribbles past a first defender, inducing a second defender to cover and leading to a change in the structure of the defending team; Davids *et al*. 2003).

In summary, ecological dynamics provides explanations about the way in which the interaction between players and information from the performance environment constrains the emergence of patterns of stability (i.e. coordination between performers), variability (loss of coordination between performers) and symmetry breaking in organizational states (i.e. how new patterns of coordination emerge in performance) in such systems (Vilar *et al*. 2012a). This is precisely what sport scientists and coaches need to understand in analyses of team game performance (Araújo *et al*. 2006; Davids *et al*. 1994; Handford *et al*. 1997).

Interpersonal coordination in team sports

In its recent years, ecological dynamics has examined coordination among play-ers in team sports by considering the pattern forming dynamics of attacker–defender sub-systems as a basic unit of investigation (Araújo *et al*. 2004; Davids *et al*. 2006). For example, Araújo and colleagues (2004; 2006) provided empirical data about one-versus-one sub-phases in basketball, showing that the attacker's and defender's displacements were highly coupled. The defender was shown to counteract the movements of the attacker, in order to maintain system symmetry (to prevent the immediate attacker from gaining a positional advantage that allows him/her to score). However, as the attacker approached the location of the basket, critical fluctuations were observed in the dyadic stability and a sudden change in the organization of the system occurred towards one of the two follow-ing possible states: (i) an advantage for an attacker (i.e. the defender may not be able to balance the attacker's actions and the attacker may move past the defender); or (ii) an advantage for a defender (i.e. the attacker was not able to break system symmetry and a defender may intercept the ball). This research provided some understanding about how players continuously coupled their actions to information from their opponent and the location of the target, to acquire a desirable state of coordination that allow them to attain their goals in one-versus-one sub-phases in team sports.

In order to conduct appropriate performance analysis, research should exam-ine the spatiotemporal relations that constrain pattern-forming dynamics in team games players during actual competitive performance, such as an international championship (Vilar *et al.* 2012b). In competitive scenarios, the existence of more than one attacker–defender dyadic system performing simultaneously is a distinct constraint is likely to be a major influence on the inter-player coordination dynamics. In the next section, we discuss some extensive work on performance analysis in futsal, seeking to provide understanding on how players coordinate their actions and attain success by using information from other players (teammates and opponents) and the locations of the goal and the ball.

Exemplar analysis of performance in futsal

Previous research on one-versus-one sub-phases in basketball showed that a phase transition in the attacker's and defender's distances to the basket precipitated a scoring event. However, in the competitive environment of futsal, it could also be suggested that a goal could be scored merely as a consequence of instabilities in a defender's alignment between the goal and an attacker's position (Vilar *et al.* 2012b). In this sense, we recorded ten futsal games between five national teams in the 2009 Lusophony Games and analyzed the displacement trajectories of the four outfield players in 13 sequence of plays that ended in a goal being scored ($N = 52$). We considered the coordination between the distances and angles of the attacker and nearest defender to the centre of the goal (Vilar *et al.* 2012b). To capture stabilities and instabilities in attacker–defender phase relations, as well as phase transitions in a given data sequence, we used relative phase (see Chapter 7).

Analysis of the interpersonal coordination between attackers and defenders in five-versus-five competitive environments in futsal showed that stable patterns of coordination emerged from changes to both players' distances and angles to the goal (Figure 13.1C and 13.1F, respectively). Individual analysis of the coordination between the attacker who scored the goal and the nearest defender showed that the defender seemed to be always closer to the goal than the attacker 5 and aligned with the goal and his direct opponent (Figure 13.1A and 13.1D). In-phase patterns of coordination suggest that while the attacker was in possession of the ball and the defender was between the goal and attacker, the stability of the dyadic system was maintained (Figure 13.1B and 13.1E). However, as the sequence of play evolved towards the goal, the defender's efforts to maintain system stability were often insufficient and critical fluctuations precipitated more than one phase transition. States of system stability showed less duration, providing attacker 5 with opportunity to score a goal. Attacker 5 seemed to have used lateral displacement to increase the angle to the goal relative to the defender's position, while decreasing the distance to the goal, to break system symmetry. This analysis suggested that only when symmetry-breaking processes emerged near the goal and the defenders did not have the collective ability to re-establish dyadic system stability, a goal opportunity presented itself. Leading the systems towards critical regions of instable coordination is suggested to constrain the attackers' ability to create opportunities to score.

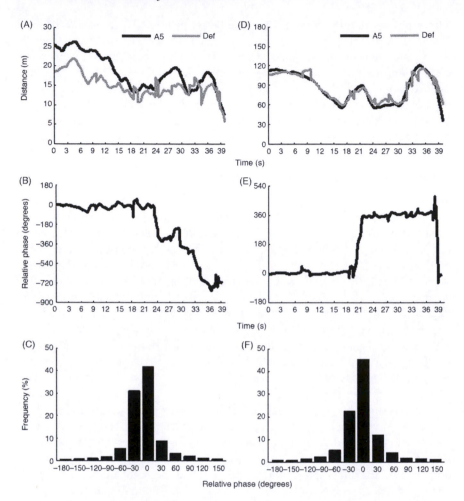

Figure 13.1 The constraint of goal location on coordination processes in dyadic systems presented in decomposed format: (left column) distances of each player to the centre of the goal; (right column) angles of each player to the centre of the goal; (a) and (b) exemplar data from attacker five [A5] and nearest defender [Def]; (A) and (B) exemplar data from attacker five [A5] and nearest defender [D]; (C) and (D) dynamics of the relative phase of the exemplar data from A5 and nearest D; (e) and (f) frequency histograms of the relative phases of all A–D dyadic systems (*n* = 52) (data from Vilar *et al.* 2012a)

However, in futsal, breaking symmetry with the defender does not guarantee *per se* goal scoring. Attackers must shoot the ball and override simultaneously the opposition of the immediate defender and the goalkeeper in order for success to be obtained. To examine the influence of spatial and temporal constraints on shooting performances, we used the model of the required velocity to intercept moving objects (Peper *et al.* 1994). This model suggests that catching a ball is related to the individuals' ability to gear the velocity of the hand to a specified value that ensures that the hand is located at the right place and the right time, regardless of where this might be. Using the same data shown previously, we examined the locations of the ball, the nearest defender and the goalkeeper, from the moment when the ball was shot until it was intercepted or entered the goal, in plays that ended in a defender's interception, in a goalkeeper's save and in a goal. We computed the interception points of the defender and the goalkeeper by recording their shortest distance to the ball's trajectory during the act of shooting. Since we considered the working point from each player, the players' distances to the interception points considered half of the players' shoulder-to-shoulder width (0.40 metres, estimation) and the radius of the futsal ball used in this tournament (0.10 metres). We also calculated the time for the ball to arrive at each player's interception point. Finally, the required velocities of the defender and the goalkeeper to intercept the ball were computed by dividing each player's distance to the interception point by the time for the ball to arrive to each player's interception point (Figure 13.2).

The mean values of the required velocity of the defender to intercept the ball were significantly lower in plays ending in a defender's interception (mean [M] = 3.29, standard error [SE] = 0.39) than in plays ending in a goalkeeper's save (M = 32.16, SE = 10.11) and in plays ending in a goal. This finding suggests that the time taken for the ball to arrive at the interception point was higher than the defender's ability to move to the interception point. That is, the time allowed for

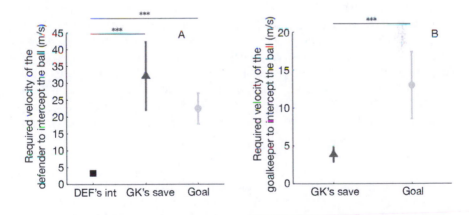

Figure 13.2 Mean values and standard error of the required velocity for intercepting the ball of (A) defender and (B) goalkeeper in shots that ended in a defender's interception, in a goalkeeper's save and in a goal. The represented levels of statistical significance are $P < 0.05$ (*), $P < 0.01$ (**) and $P < 0.001$ (***). Note that the required velocity of the goalkeeper was not measured when the defender intercepted the ball, since it is impossible to compute the goalkeeper's interception point

a defender to close the gap between him and the interception point and to intercept the ball was within the defender's action capabilities. In this sense, to score goals, attackers need to move in order to 'pull' the opponents away from an imaginary line between him and the centre of the goal.

Similarly, the mean values of the required velocity of the goalkeeper to intercept the ball were significantly lower in plays ending in a goalkeeper's save (M = 3.29, SE = 0.39) than in plays ending in a goal (M = 12.97, SE = 4.41). This result suggests that the time for the ball to arrive at the interception point was greater than the time needed for the goalkeeper to arrive at the same point. These data suggest that attackers need to be able to identify an opportunity in the performance environment to shoot the ball without allowing the immediate defender and the goalkeeper to move fast enough to intercept the ball. Such opportunities emerge not only from the information from the performance environment but also from attackers' action capabilities. That is, attackers should scale information they perceive according to their own capabilities. Decisions where, when and how to shoot should always be placed in a performance context and should be guided by the information of both the time for the ball and for the opponents to arrive at potential interception points (Watson *et al.* 2011).

Implications and applications of ecological dynamics perspective on sport analysis and performance

Analyzing performance from an ecological dynamics perspective provides a theoretical rational that explains how reductionist notational analysis may be. To enhance the validity of theoretical interpretations, analysts need to move beyond merely documenting performance statistics to study the emergent interactions between players, in key areas of the field, which underpin success in team sports (Vilar *et al.* 2012a). For example, previous research on shooting performance has investigated independently the placement of the ball in the goal (Alcock 2010; Hughes and Wells 2002; López-Botella and Palao 2007; Morya *et al.* 2004), the velocity of ball flight (Alcock 2010; Kerwin and Bray 2006) and the pitch location of a shot (Alcock 2010; Ensum *et al.* 2000). However, without considering how these variables relate to a defenders' positioning on field and a goalkeeper's positioning in goal and their ability to displace towards possible interception points, researchers will not be able to explain how successful and unsuccessful shots occur during futsal competitive performance. As we have stated in the introduction, sequential analysis has also studied the interaction between variables in sport teams (Johnson 2006), but ecological perspective provides the theoretical framework for identifying the key informational variables of sport success. Its application requires a collective variable to be found that describes the behavioural dynamics of the system. At present, investigation is focused on analyzing the space–time movement trajectories of the ball kinematics, as well as those of the players (Travassos *et al.* 2011).

Ecological dynamics also has major implications for the design of representative training tasks in team sports. The key informational variables that players use to control their performances should be simulated (i.e. represented) in training tasks, allowing them to become better attuned to functionally coupling information and movement during practice (Davids *et al.* 2005). Major implications of these ideas also exist for development programmes in team sports. Instead of deconstructing tasks as repetition drills for learners, coaches should simplify tasks (e.g. by reducing the numbers in teams during small-sided practice games: three-versus-three, five-versus-four or six-versus-four) to facilitate players' performances (Vilar *et al.* 2012a).

Conclusions

In this chapter, we have shown how ecological dynamics provides understanding about how players use information from their performance environment to attain successful performances in team sports. Our programme of research has shown that attackers seek to break symmetry with their nearest opponents, as defenders try to maintain system symmetry by remaining between their own goal and the immediate attacker. Slight changes in player behaviours may induce a symmetry-breaking process in the state of the dyadic systems. In this case, when the defenders do not have the collective ability to re-establish dyadic system stability, a shot at goal may occur. Attackers must perceive the locations of the immediate defender and the goalkeeper and shoot the ball in a specific direction and with a specific velocity that requires the opponents to displace faster than they are able to intercept the ball.

Our results are encouraging and provide evidence that notational analysis based on performance statistics can be too reductionist. Moreover, this approach has potential in areas such as training and programming in team sports, proposing the simplification of tasks instead of deconstructing them. By unveiling the influence of interacting task constraints on the emergent self-organized behaviours of players during performance, ecological dynamics reveals itself as a powerful tool for both researchers and practitioners in sport performance analysis.

Questions for students

1. What are performance indicators? Give some examples.
2. What are affordances? Give one example.
3. What information should attackers use to create opportunities to score?
4. How may ecological dynamics overcome notational analysis limitations? Give one example.
5. What implications does ecological dynamics have for practice?

References

Alcock, A. (2010) Analysis of direct free kicks in the women's football World Cup 2007. *European Journal of Sport Science*, 10 (4): 279–84.

Anguera, M. T. (2005) Microanalysis of T-patterns: analysis of symmetry/asymmetry in social interaction, in L. Anolli, S. Duncan, M. Magnusson and G. Riva (eds) *The Hidden Structure of Social Interaction: From Genomics to Culture Patterns*. Amsterdam: IOS Press, pp. 51–70.

Anguera, M. T. and Jonsson, G. K. (2003) Detection of real-time patterns in sport: interactions in football. *International Journal of Computer Science in Sport*, 2: 118–21.

Araújo, D. and Davids, K. (2009) Ecological approaches to cognition and action in sport and exercise: ask not only what you do, but where you do it. *International Journal of Sport Psychology*, 40 (1): 5–37.

Araújo, D., Davids, K., Bennett, S., Button, C. and Chapman, G. (2004) Emergence of sport skills under constraints, in A. M. Williams and N. J. Hodges (eds) *Skill Acquisition in Sport: Research, Theory and Practice*. London: Routledge, pp. 409–33.

Araújo, D., Davids, K. and Hristovski, R. (2006) The ecological dynamics of decision making in sport. *Psychology of Sport and Exercise*, 7: 653–76.

Borrie, A., Jonsson, G. and Magnusson, M. (2002) Temporal pattern analysis and its applicability in sport: an explanation and exemplar data. *Journal of Sports Sciences*, 20: 845–52.

Davids, K., Handford, C. and Williams, M. (1994) The natural physical alternative to cognitive theories of motor behaviour: an invitation for interdisciplinary research in sports science? *Journal of Sports Sciences*, 12 (6): 495–528.

Davids, K., Glazier, P., Araújo, D. and Bartlett, R. (2003) Movement systems as dynamical systems. the functional role of variability and its implications for sports medicine. *Sports Medicine*, 33 (4): 245–60.

Davids, K., Renshaw, I. and Glazier, P. (2005) Movement models from sports reveal fundamental insights into coordination processes. *Exercise and Sport Sciences Reviews*, 33 (1): 36–42.

Davids, K., Button, C., Araújo, D., Renshaw, I., and Hristovski, R. (2006) Movement models from sports provide representative task constraints for studying adaptive behavior in human movement systems. *Adaptive Behavior*, 14 (1): 73–95.

Davids, K., Araújo, D., Vilar, L., Renshaw, I. and Pinder, R. (2013) An ecological dynamics approach to skill acquisition: implications for development of talent in sport. *Talent Development and Excellence*, 5 (1): 21–34.

Ensum, J., Williams, M. and Grant, A. (2000) Analysis of the attacking set plays in Euro 2000. *Insight: The FA Coaches Association Journal*, 4: 36–9.

Fajen, B., Riley, M. and Turvey, M. (2009) Information, affordances, and the control of action in sport. *International Journal of Sport Psychology*, 40 (1): 79–107.

Fernandez, J., Camerino, O., Anguera, M. T. and Jonnson, F. K. (2009) Identifying and analyzing the construction and effectiveness of offensive plays in basketball by using systematic observation. *Behavior Research Methods*, 41 (3): 719–30.

Franks, I. (1997) Use of feedback by coaches and players, in T. Reilly, J. Bangsbo and M. Hughes (eds) *Science and Football III*. London: E. and F. N. Spon, pp. 267–8.

Franks, I., Partridge, D. and Nagelkerke, P. (1990) *World Cup 90: A Computer Assisted Technical Analysis of Team Performance Technical Report for the Canadian Soccer Association*. Vancouver: University of British Columbia.

Gibson, J. (1979) *The Ecological Approach to Visual Perception*. Boston, MA: Houghton Mifflin.

Glazier, P. (2010) Game, set and match? Substantive issues and future direction in performance analysis. *Sports Medicine*, 40 (8): 625–34.

Grehaigne, J. (1999) Systemic approach and soccer, in M. Hughes (ed.) *Notation of Sport III*. Cardiff: Centre for Performance Analysis, UWIC, pp. 1–8.

Handford, C., Davids, K., Bennett, S. and Button, C. (1997) Skill acquisition in sport: some applications of an evolving practice ecology. *Journal of Sports Sciences*, 15: 621–40.

Hughes, M. and Bartlett, R. (2002) The use of performance indicators in performance analysis. *Journal of Sports Sciences*, 20: 739–54.

Hughes, M. and Franks, I. (2004) Notational analysis: a review of the literature, in M. Hughes and I. Franks (eds) *Notational Analysis of Sport*, 2nd edn. London: Routledge, pp. 59–106.

Hughes, M. and Franks, I. (2005) Analysis of passing sequences, shots and goals in soccer. *Journal of Sports Sciences*, 23 (5): 509–14.

Hughes, M. and Wells, J. (2002) Analysis of penalties taken in shoot-outs. *International Journal of Performance Analysis in Sport*, 2: 55–72.

Hughes, M., Robertson, K. and Nicholson, A. (1988) An analysis of the 1984 World Cup of Association Football, in T. Reilly, A. Lees, K. Davids and W. Murphy (eds) *Science and Football*. London: E. and F. N. Spon, pp. 363–7.

Johnson, J. G. (2006) Cognitive modeling of decision making in sports. *Psychology of Sport and Exercise*, 7 (6): 631–52.

Kauffman, S. (1993) *The Origins of Order: Self-organization and Selection in Evolution*. New York: Oxford University Press.

Kerwin, D. J. and Bray, K. (2006) Measuring and modelling the goalkeeper's diving envelope in a penalty kick, in E. F. Moritz and S. Haake (eds) *Engineering of Sport: Developments for Sports*. New York: Springer Science Business Media, 1: 321–6.

Kugler, P. and Turvey, M. (1987) *Information, Natural Law, and the Self-assembly of Rhythmic Movement*. Hillsdale: Lawrence Erlbaum Associates.

Lames, M. and McGarry, T. (2007) On the search for reliable performance indicators in game sports. *International Journal of Performance Analysis in Sport*, 7 (1): 62–79.

Lee, D. N., Young, D. S., Reddish, P. E., Lough, S. and Clayton, T. M. (1983) Visual timing in hitting an accelerating ball. *Quarterly Journal of Experimental Psychology*, 35 (Pt 2): 333–46.

López-Botella, M. and Palao, J. M. (2007) Relationship between laterality of foot strike and shot zone on penalty efficacy in specialist penalty takers. *International Journal of Performance Analysis in Sport*, 7: 26–36.

McGarry, T. (2009) Applied and theoretical perspectives of performance analysis in sport: scientific issues and challenges. *International Journal of Performance Analysis in Sport*, 9: 128–40.

Morya, E., Bigatão, H., Lees, A. and Ranvaud, R. (2004) Evolving penalty kick strategies: World Cup and club matches, 2000–2002. *Journal of Sports Sciences*, 22: 512–13.

Nevill, A., Holder, R., and Watts, A. (2009) The changing shape of "successful" professional footballers. *Journal of Sports Sciences*, 27 (5), 419–26.

Peper, C., Bootsma, R., Mestre, D. and Bakker, F. (1994) Catching balls: how to get the hand to the right place at the right time. *Journal of Experimental Psychology: Human Perception and Performance*, 20: 591–612.

Reilly, T., Williams, A. M., Nevill, A. and Franks, A. (2000) A multidisciplinary approach to talent identification in soccer. *Journal of Sports Sciences*, 18 (9): 695–702.

Richardson, M., Marsh, K. and Baron, R. (2007) Judging and actualizing intrapersonal and interpersonal affordances. *Journal of Experimental Psychology: Human Perception and Performance*, 33 (4): 845–59.

Seifert, L. and Davids, K. (2012) Intentions, perceptions and actions constrain functional inter- and intra-individual variability in the acquisition of expertise in individual sports. *Open Sports Sciences Journal*, 5 (Suppl 1-M8): 68–75.

Stoffregen, T., Gorday, K., Sheng, Y. and Flynn, S. (1999) Perceiving affordances for another person's actions. *Journal of Experimental Psychology: Human Perception and Performance*, 25 (1): 120–36.

Travassos, B., Araújo, D., McGarry, T. and Vilar, L. (2011) Interpersonal coordination and ball dynamics in futsal (indoor football). *Human Movement Science*, 30: 1245–59.

Turvey, M. (1992) Affordances and prospective control: an outline of the ontology. *Ecological Psychology*, 4 (3): 173–88.

Vilar, L., Araújo, D., Davids, K. and Button, C. (2012a) The role of ecological dynamics in analysing performance in team sports. *Sports Medicine*, 42 (1): 1–10.

Vilar, L., Araújo, D., Davids, K. and Travassos, B. (2012) Constraints on competitive performance of attacker–defender dyads in team sports. *Journal of Sports Sciences*, 30 (5): 459–69.

Warren, W. (1984) Perceiving affordances: visual guidance of stair climbing. *Journal of Experimental Psychology: Human Perception and Performance*, 10 (5): 683–703.

Warren, W. (2006) The dynamics of perception and action. *Psychological Review*, 113 (2): 358–89.

Warren, W. and Whang, S. (1987) Visual guidance of walking through apertures: body-scaled information for affordances. *Journal of Experimental Psychology: Human Perception and Performance*, 13 (3): 371–83.

Watson, G., Brault, S., Kulpa, R., Bideau, B., Butterfield, J. and Craig, C. (2011) Judging the 'passability' of dynamic gaps in a virtual rugby environment. *Human Movement Science*, 30 (5): 942–56.

14 Talent development and expertise in sport

Elissa Phillips, Keith Davids, Duarte Araújo and Ian Renshaw

Complexity sciences have been used to study and explain the rich patterns formed in complex systems such as animal collectives, weather systems, the human brain and movements in team sports, where patterns emerge from seemingly random component trajectories (Bak and Chialvo 2001; Kauffman 1993; Sumpter 2006). From this description, it is clear that an emerging expert performance can be viewed as a complex system, composed of many degrees of freedom on many system levels. The potential for interaction between system components provides the platform for rich patterns of behaviour to emerge as individuals interact with dynamically changing environments. This new perspective reveals that compensatory adaptation in performance achievement occurs as the result of system trade-offs between specificity and diversity of behaviours (Edelman and Gally 2001). These ideas are harmonious with a dynamical systems theoretical perspective on the influence of interacting constraints. This overarching theoretical framework proposes that expert levels of performance can be achieved in diverse ways as individual performers attempt to satisfy the unique constraints on them (Davids *et al.* 2003).

The role of neurobiological degeneracy in expertise acquisition

A brief overview of the strengths and weaknesses of theoretical ideas and empirical methods used in environmental and genetic research on expertise in sport suggests that neither specific approach provides enough explanatory power to account for all the data on expertise in sport. The implicit basis of the deliberate practice perspective is the adage 'all healthy individuals are created equal'. Analysis of the literature on genetic constraints on variability of performance does not support this conclusion but this interpretation of the literature should not be taken to imply that expert performance in sport is biologically predetermined. There is clear evidence rejecting the idea that single gene variants can predispose an athlete to superior performance manifested in a specific domain, without clear and detailed consideration of the performance context (e.g. a gene that is widespread in cricket fast bowlers). Rather, the effects of interacting constraints on acquisition of expertise in sport have been noted since, despite variations in genetic structure, maximal heritability of particular traits includes strong environmental components. Complex neurobiological systems are composed of many interacting parts and levels, which self-organize under constraints (Davids and Baker 2007; Frank *et al.* 2006; Schöllhorn 2003).

One of the main reasons for the failure to identify single gene variants responsible for sport performance has been the inherent degeneracy of athletes considered as neurobiological systems. Degeneracy in this context refers to the ability of structurally different components to be coordinated together to achieve the same behavioural goal (Edelman and Gally 2001). Complex, neurobiological systems have been conceptualized as pleiotropic and degenerate, with huge numbers of degrees of freedom and the distinct ability to adapt to different task and environmental demands (Chow *et al.* 2008; Davids *et al.* 2007b). Pleiotropy concerns the multiple effects of expression of phenotypes or behaviours from one constraint, such as environment and genes, which may have phenotypic effects (Baker and Davids 2006). Pleiotropy provides neurobiological systems with a variety of alternate performance solutions (Davids *et al.* 2007a), while degeneracy refers to the ability of structurally different components to be coordinated together to achieve the same behavioural goal (Edelman and Gally 2001). At the level of gene networks, degeneracy promotes evolutionary fitness by ensuring that genetic diversity supports functional adaptation to variable environments. Genes function in networks and single genes can produce multiple effects, leading to multiple phenotypic expressions. This is why gene expression is an inherently stochastic process (Kaerns *et al.* 2005).

The degenerate relationship between system components and system output in developing experts is important because it implies that there are many different pathways to achieving expert performance. Dynamically varying performance environments interact with the inherent degenerate nature of human movement systems, signalling a new view on the acquisition of expertise in sport. This new perspective reveals that compensatory adaptation in performance achievement occurs as the result of system trades-off between specificity and diversity of behaviours (Edelman and Gally 2001). These ideas are harmonious with a dynamical systems theoretical perspective on the influence of interacting constraints. This overarching theoretical framework proposes that expert levels of performance can be achieved in diverse ways as individual performers attempt to satisfy the unique constraints on them (Davids *et al.* 2003). From this viewpoint, expertise can be defined as the optimal satisfaction of unique, interacting constraints on each individual in specific performance domains. Genetic diversity may be responsible for a small part of training or performance response differences between individuals and only when there is a favourable interaction with important environmental constraints are performance benefits observed. This description of key influences on athletic performance has implications for considering the effects of time spent in practice in sport. Given differences in genetic contributions, performance variations are more likely to assert themselves under intensive practice regimes.

The characteristics of pleiotropy and degeneracy in athletes as complex, neurobiological systems highlight the need for a multidimensional framework (Davids and Baker 2007; Simonton 1999). Expertise attainment in a given skill depends on many additional constraints outside the cognitive domain, including but not limited to genetics, social and physical environment, opportunity, encouragement and the effect of these variables on physical and psychological traits (Wolstencroft 2002). Monodisciplinary approaches to the acquisition of expertise, focusing on effects of genetic or environmental constraints alone, fail to emulate the complementary nature of the relationship between individual, task and environmental constraints (Abbott *et al.* 2005; Beek *et al.* 2003; Davids and Baker 2007). Davids and Baker (2007) lamented the absence of an explanatory framework to examine the interactionist perspective of expertise development in sport and suggested the use of a complex systems framework incorporating key ideas from dynamical systems theory. As we note in the following sections of this chapter, this theoretical approach provides a viable platform for explaining the dynamic relationship between an individual's genetic disposition and the environment and the acquisition of expertise in sport through variable pathways and processes.

Constraints on acquiring expertise

In sports performance contexts, the expression of expertise is limited or shaped by interacting constraints at many system levels. Although numerous constraints might act on any given system, they have been classified into organismic, task and environmental constraints (Newell 1986). The concept of constraints was proposed by Newell (1986) as boundaries or qualities that constrain the interactions of system components. Constraints are the numerous variables that form each individual expert's developmental trajectory. These constraints include individual characteristics such as experience, learning, development, morphology and genes which interact to shape performance and the acquisition of expertise in sport (Davids *et al.* 2008).

It is important to identify the range of constraints on the acquisition of expertise, requiring a multidisciplinary framework of analysis. Given that an individual is born with distinguishing physical characteristics (with a degree of genetic influence), expertise research is concerned with how environmental constraints affect the development of skill and the expression of genotypes.

Performance emerges from the intrinsic dynamics of experts; these preferred coordination tendencies come from the interaction of environmental, task and organismic constraints (including development, experience, genes and learning of each performer; Kelso 1991). Understanding the nature of each individual's intrinsic dynamics is central to understanding how expert performance develops in sport. As individuals progress towards a state of expertise and explore different performance solutions, their intrinsic dynamics will alter and diversify. The learner's ability to adapt to constraints, with dynamic performance solutions, will affect their rate of learning. Learning to perform a new task with dynamics that are similar to a previously learned task can harness an existing landscape of intrinsic dynamics in learners and may provide a more rapid transition to a new required movement pattern. This is the basis of talent transfer. In contrast, acquiring task dynamics which are dissimilar to those of a previously learned task (e.g. tennis and squash movement pattern dynamics) may lead to a longer process of learning because the specific learner's intrinsic dynamics may need to be significantly re-shaped (Renshaw *et al.* 2009).

These ideas in dynamical systems theory have important implications for understanding the development and maintenance of expert performance. Importantly, expertise research on developmental histories, has found both similarities and differences in expert developmental pathways, suggesting that experts can adopt different pathways and strategies as they acquire expertise in athletic performance (Durand-Bush and Salmela 2002; Gould *et al.* 2002; Holt and Dunn 2004). How the intrinsic dynamics of developing experts are continually shaped by genetic and environmental constraints needs to be understood. The effects of environmental constraints on phenotypic gene expression suggests that athletes with what may be perceived as less favourable genetic dispositions may still achieve expert levels of performance given an appropriate skill acquisition environment (Baker and Horton 2004). Alternatively, genetically gifted athletes may fail to achieve expert status without a rich environment for acquiring and practising skills. Rich learning environments do not necessarily imply a need for purpose-built state of the art training facilities. In fact, there is evidence of sporting champions emerging from the most basic learning and performance environments.

To summarize so far, it seems unlikely that a singular common optimal pathway to performance expertise exists because of the degenerate neurobiological system characterizing each individual performer and the effect of interactions between environmental and personal constraints on the intrinsic dynamics of each learner. Expert performers are able to generate different types of functional performance solutions, depending on differences in their intrinsic dynamics (e.g. varying ball speed or type and line and/or length in cricket fast bowling). For example, in cricket fast bowling Pyne *et al.* (2006) examined the relationship between junior and senior high-performance athletes' anthropometric and strength characteristics and bowling speed. They found differences in the variables and strength of correlation of predictors of peak ball speed between age groups and suggested growth and biological maturation largely accounted for greater peak ball speed in seniors. A more comprehensive examination including technical/coordination variants under a variety of tasks' demands such as different delivery types would be needed to gain greater insight into the individual dynamics and movement solutions of such a group (e.g. varying ball speed or type and line and/or length in cricket fast bowling).

The role of metastability in acquiring expertise

Conceptualized as dynamical neurobiological systems, emerging expert athletes exhibit complexity and metastability, owing to the potential for interaction between their subsystems. The inherent degeneracy of neurobiological systems and the nonlinear interactions between system components enable the existence of more than one stable pathway to expertise. This characteristic of dynamical systems is termed *multistability* (Araújo *et al.* 2006; Edelman and Gally 2001; Kelso 1995). Multistable systems can also exhibit metastability when modes of behaviour or performance are weakly stable or weakly unstable (i.e. close to an instability point) and it manifests itself in the switching between modes of organization or structure (Fringelkurts and Fringelkurts 2004; Kelso 2008). The characteristic of metastability has important implications for our understanding of emerging expertise. The rich interactions that can occur between personal, task and environmental constraints can create a fertile 'metastable' region of the performance landscape in which small changes in one constraint can lead to large transitions in system organization. For example, small alterations in experience, practice and/or development, combined with small variations in genetic structure, might induce continuous and abrupt changes (i.e. bifurcations)[1] in the set of possible behaviours available to a developing athlete as these constraints are satisfied. In this way, the whole dynamical landscape of expertise can suddenly change with small variations in responses to constraints impinging on the developing athlete. For example, the emergence of novel actions or responses to performance problems can influence future system behaviours by changing the probability of occurrence of other potentially functional behaviours. These ideas also need to be considered in light of suggestions that critical periods exist for acquisition of skills in developing children. Critical periods have been identified as brief windows of time and space during which a complex system's organisation is most open to modification from external and internal constraints. It has been argued that motor learning can be enhanced when developing athletes are located within these critical periods (Anderson and Ward 2002). These ideas should be interpreted in relation to data tracking the performance trajectories of skilled and less-skilled developing footballers in the UK (Ward *et al.* 2007). These findings suggested that a greater proportion of performance variability in these groups could be explained by the acquisition of skill, in the absence of physical and maturational advantages.

Harnessing the evolutionary strategy of co-adaptation to incur performance paradigm shifts in sport

The challenge for coaches and sport scientists is to identify when individual athletes enter metastable regions or critical periods while developing their expertise levels so that performance paradigm shifts in expertise and skill acquisition might be triggered, as we exemplify in this section. By ensuring exposure to metastable regions of the performance landscape during development, experts can discover new modes of behaviour to satisfy interacting perceptual, affective and task constraints. These new modes of performance are likely to emerge as novel solutions to performance problems as developing athletes co-adapt their responses to challenging constraints imposed by opponents, coaches or performance environments. For example, after the famous 'turn' away from defenders, performed by Johan Cruyff at the 1974 Football World Cup, millions of young players began to imitate and practise the move in training, as coaches directed their search for novel ways to avoid defensive marking.

When self-organizing systems, such as the developing expert, are poised in a state near this region, different types of behaviour (including development pathways) can emerge depending on changes in relevant system control parameters. For this reason, a system poised in the metastable region may enter a critical state which is ready for change. Such states of criticality in complex systems are recognised as 'a global state that is acutely context sensitive' (Van Orden *et al.* 2003, p. 332). Van Orden *et al.* (2003) showed how 'criticality' emerges from a balance between constraints on complex systems. The implication is that a small difference in circumstances can lead to transitions along the expertise pathway for the system. This raises some important issues about attempting to identify future champions. It suggests that sometimes apparently minor changes to individual, task or environmental constraints can result in giant leaps or paradigm shifts in performance. For example, exposing athletes to a minor change in technique, a change of coach, an opportunity to play at a higher level or interaction with a previous champion could be the turning point in a developmental pathway. From a dynamical systems theoretical perspective, these turning points and critical states are likely to be unique to each individual athlete and it may be difficult to identify patterns in the developmental histories of expert performers. This is an area that future talent development research needs to explore in more detail.

In evolutionary theory, the influential role of metastability in organismic change has been observed. Kauffman's (1993) modelling of evolutionary processes from the perspective of spontaneous self-organizing system dynamics has provided valuable insights for understanding how developing experts, viewed as complex, open systems, may undergo transitions along the developmental pathway. According to Kauffmann (1993), evolution occurs as different systems pressurise each other, co-adapting function, structure and organization in the process. In this process, rich and varied patterns of behaviour can emerge as organisms subtly co-adapt their actions in response to a range of specific interacting constraints to achieve specific system outcomes or goals.

Models of evolutionary processes arising from spontaneous self-organizing system dynamics provide valuable insights for understanding the acquisition of expertise (Kauffman 1995). In these models, phase transitions in system behaviour are most prevalent in metastable regions where co-evolving system components compete to modify a system's landscape of behaviours. The co-evolving adaption of system components within critical regions is typically an emergent process because of the evolved coupling between system components. In developing experts, new behaviours and performance levels can emerge out of fluctuations created by interactions between interdependent constituents of the whole performance system. Random interactions between system components can alter into more organized forms of interactions as one key system parameter (a control parameter) changes in value. Fluctuations in a developing system's organization can create instabilities which provide a useful platform to assist transitions in expertise with practice and experience. Near this critical state, inter-actions between system components can become correlated, in a domino effect, capturing global system interactions and leading to a sudden reduction from multiple options to one (a sudden collapse in the critical state). Criticality provides a fertile region for a functional mix of creativity and constraint to emerge in dynamic learning environments. It affords new opportunities for behaviours to emerge which can fit newly arising states of organization during development and skill acquisition. As each individual component in a co-adapting system changes over time, the whole system can move inexorably in the co-created landscape towards a region of self-organizing criticality poised for a transition (Bak and Chialvo 2001). In this respect, variability in a developing athlete can be a useful process to exploit in order to facilitate the transition to a new state of expertise in sport.

To summarize so far, co-adaptation is an evolutionary strategy that has impli-cations for the way that constraints can influence the process of talent development by forcing the developing expert to find new functional perform-ance solutions. It may represent a useful expertise development strategy for practitioners, as different performers and/or technologies attempt to pressurise individuals to seek unique performance solutions. Furthermore, the process occurs naturally as a sport develops (i.e. through technique changes, rule changes or equipment change or as athletes pose each other new performance problems). New solutions to performance problems emerge as talented individuals learn how to assemble creative movement solutions during practice.

The developmental strategy of seeking to move sport performers to a metastable region of their performance landscape might provide a platform to help them create new, more adaptive, modes of action with respect to emerging task and goal constraints of the performance environment. For example, in high jump, early athletes used a scissor technique to jump with the inside leg leading, followed closely by the other leg in a scissoring motion. The scissors action then progressed to the western roll and the Fosbury flop, which represents a good example of the metastable region in the sport of high jumping. The Fosbury flop was a performance solution that emerged coinciding with the use of raised, softer landing areas in modern times. Directing the body over the bar head and shoul-ders first and sliding over on one's back would have likely led to injury without modern landing mats.

Changes to expert movement skill performance in other sports have resulted from advances in equipment design, with these changes interacting with environ-mental constraints of a physical nature. For example, an interesting question concerns why certain types of expertise can be traced to specific cultural groups. In a well-known performance paradigm shift in the sport of football, the first players to 'bend' the trajectory of balls when shooting (adding swerve and dip to flight) were South Americans in the 1960s, rather than European players. This was because, prior to the 1970s, footballs had a leather skin that picked up mois-ture as a game progressed, so during winter games played in the northern hemisphere, the ball increased in mass to almost double its original value. In the generally drier climates of South America the ball did not pick up as much mois-ture and mass, so aerodynamic forces had more influence on the 'lighter' ball, enabling skilled players to acquire expertise in bending and curving ball trajecto-ries. With the advent of waterproof balls in the 1970s, Northern European experts were able to recreate the same effects as their South American counterparts (James 2008). James (2008) also noted recent research observing that the aero-dynamic drag of non-spinning footballs has fallen by as much as 30% over the last 36 years, leading to the ball being able to travel greater distances. These changes in task constraints (e.g. physical characteristics of equipment) have influ-enced the tactical strategies available to teams and consequently re-emphasised the acquisition of specific shooting and long passing skills in players. In other sports, performance paradigm shifts have been created by:

- equipment changes (e.g. the change from bamboo to fibreglass pole vaults leading to the world record increasing from around 4.5 metres to 6.14 metres in a vault by Sergey Bubka in 1993);
- changes to playing surfaces (such as international hockey matches on artifi-cial turf instead of grass), which may explain the ebb and flow of current performance standings and international rankings between countries;
- rule changes, such as the turn-over law in rugby union or the distance of the three-point line in the Olympics versus the US National Basketball Association (NBA). It was argued that the change in this distance (in NBA it is 7.23 metres while at the Olympics it was 6.25 metres) resulted in the all-star American team struggling to score their usual number of three-pointers in the early rounds of the 2008 Olympic Games competition (Thamel 2008).

In elite sport, the drive for success means that performers are being challenged constantly to co-adapt to succeed. This is particularly true of professional tele-vized sports where opportunities to analyze strengths and weaknesses of opponents are enhanced by available television and videotape footage. Through co-adaptation, players need to add new skills or strategies in the off-season in order to continue to challenge opponents with new problems (Cowdrey 1974). Essentially, players have to constantly reinvent themselves or demonstrate an ability to adapt to the strategies developed by opponents to counteract previously observed strengths. A good example of this adaptation was observed in 2008 in cricket when the use of 'switch hitting' by Kevin Pietersen (an English batsman) was first formalized. He developed a strategy of changing his stance (from his typically right-handed position) as a bowler in the process of delivering a ball, by 'jumping' into a left-handed stance in order to overcome the restrictive field placements of opponents in one-day cricket.

Finally, co-adaptation is a process which occurs intra-individually as well as inter-individually, as different subsystems within an individual athlete self-organ-ize in relation to each other. For example, an athlete's cognitive subsystem might constrain their action system and vice versa in a co-adaptive manner. For exam-ple, after World War II, in the sport of athletics the sub-four-minute mile was viewed by many as an impossible dream. However, once Roger Bannister broke the record in 1954, it was almost immediately broken again by John Landy, who improved his personal best from 4.02.1 minutes to 3.57.9 minutes. Interestingly, Landy had been the favourite to become the first athlete to break the four-minute barrier, having run 4.02 six times in the 15-month period prior to Bannister breaking the record. Landy suggested that the first time he ran 4.02 was unexpected and was performed without any pressure. He remarked: 'Once I was aware of what I could do, I was always under pressure. I was under pressure externally and internally and I think that made a lot of difference' (North 2004).

The idea of subsystems co-adapting to constraints imposed by other subsystems of the body is influential in a dynamic systems analysis of motor development across the lifespan (Thelen 1995). For example, during children's motor development, dynamic systems analysts emphasize the idea that specific behaviours may not have yet appeared in developing children, because specific subsystems act as system 'rate limiters' and are 'lying in wait' for another critical subsystem to reach a critical level (e.g. changes in the muscle-to-fat ratio in infants to enable upright postural control). In the performance of specific sports, various subsystems could be critical to the performance development in athletes, such as strength, speed, mobility or game understanding as a result of numerous experiences. John Landy's experience suggests that, in some athletes, a major constraint on performance might be imposed by the cognitive subsystem acting as a rate limiter in the form of psychological effects of prior expectations or motivation on performance.

The role of movement variability in successful co-adaptation

From a dynamical systems perspective, expertise acquisition can be construed as a noisy, nonlinear process, in which, counterintuitively, system variability can be functional. In this process, it is important to note that subsystems can change over differing timescales. The concept of rate limiters which shape the trajectory of expertise acquisition in individuals places into sharp focus the need for theoretical frameworks to capture differences in rates of growth and development in young athletes. An important point to note in the development of talent is the different timescales associated with various subsystems of each performer. A developing athlete viewed as a complex system can transit to a new state of organization (e.g. expertise) when the behaviour of important subsystems suddenly become mutually entrained. Through this process of entrainment, like co-adapting biological organisms seeking to optimize their relative 'fitness' on an evolutionary landscape, important subsystems can become dependent on what is occurring in other key subsystems.

A phase transition in the expertise levels of athletes might therefore be shaped by a change in the relationship between an athlete's subsystems. This change may emerge as a result of development, experience and practice/training and might push the whole system to a state of non-equilibrium (i.e. the region of metastability). In nonlinear dynamics, if a developing system is driven to the edge of its current basin of attraction, the probability of a new state of organization emerging (e.g. a new level of expertise) increases, owing a breaking of symmetry in the initial system structure. This occurrence exemplifies the process of 'self-construction' that Kauffmann (1993) defined in systems that evolve over time. The interaction between critical subsystems creates a flow of information that drives the athletic system to a desegregation of its components. Expert skill acquisition can be promoted by exploiting metastability tendencies in athletes, by creating diverse learning environments, late specialization (e.g. from approximately 13–15 years of age; Côté *et al.* 2007) into sport and discovery learning processes. The process of 'self-construction' may be harnessed by coaches and athletes to propel learners along different expertise pathways by incurring performance paradigm shifts.

The functional role of variability in expert performance may have an important role to play in expert skill acquisition in sports. For example, Morriss *et al.* (1997) examined the variability of men's javelin throwing in the 1995 world athletics championships. They found that the finalist from the event exhibited a range of movement solutions which was reliant on different upper-body contributions to javelin release speed. The silver medallist demonstrated a predominance of linear shoulder movements (shoulder horizontal flexion and extension), whereas the winner of the event used shoulder rotation movements combined with elbow flexion (which had a velocity of 18% greater than any competitor). The other finalists used variations of these movement patterns, supporting the notion of degenerate movement solutions reliant on the self-organization process (Bartlett and Robins 2008) An interesting aside here is to examine how changes in the specification of the javelin in 1986 led to changes in the optimal throwing technique for javelin throwers. As a result of a desire to develop javelins that landed 'point first' on every throw, the projectile's centre of gravity was moved forward by four centimetres. According to Bartlett and Best (1988), the change resulted in the optimal technique being a 'higher release angle'. They also suggested that the changes would benefit more powerful athletes who could generate high release speeds. Sudden inter-athlete changes in performance levels are probably explained by changes in interacting personal and task constraints.

Methodological implications in expertise research: research and practice

What are the methodological implications for adopting a multi-dimensional theoretical approach to the acquisition of expertise and talent development? One major implication is that a range of methods is needed to examine these processes. While qualitative expertise research has identified unique pathways of development as athletes progress through transitions associated with different developmental stages (Abbott and Collins 2002; Bloom 1985), this concept has not been examined comprehensively for its implications in relation to talent development. Unique pathways to expertise development imply the existence of a range of functional performance solutions as a result of unique interactions of individual, environmental and task constraints during expert skill acquisition. The specific intrinsic dynamics of learners is shaped by previous experiences, individual rate limiters and environmental factors, suggesting that the notion of a general theory of expertise is unrealistic.

Gibson (1979) characterized expertise as the refinement of adaptation to specific environments, achieved by perceiving the key properties of the surrounding layout of the performance environment in the scale of an individual's body and action capabilities. Gibson's ecological approach emphasizes that adaptive human movement is underpinned by a synergetic relationship between a performer and the environment. Gibson (1979) suggested that individuals perceive information by what it offers or demands in terms of an action, creating the concept of affordances. This idea conceptualizes that athletes perceive the performance environment in terms of specific affordances for action. The athlete's behaviour emerges out of the dynamics of this system and the system provides enough information to make adaptive behaviour possible (Duchon *et al.* 1998). This information is picked up and used as information to regulate action in specific performance environments. The acquisition of expertise is domain specific and concerns 'skill adaptation', emphasizing the changing nature of the performer–environment relationship through practice, coaching and competing. It is worth noting that affordances are both subjective and objective. The same affordances may not exist at different levels of performance. For example, a short-pitched delivery from a club fast bowler in the sport of cricket may afford hooking for six for an individual batter but a ball pitched in the same place from an international fast bowler may afford ducking (or a bruised cranium). Additionally, as mentioned earlier, the affordances of restrictive field placements in cricket may have been responsible for the emergence of the switch-hitting response of Kevin Pietersen.

The methodological implication of these ideas in ecological psychology is that practice environments should be high in representative design. Egon Brunswik, the ecological psychologist, originally coined the term *representative design* (Brunswik 1955). Brunswik defended the view that cues or perceptual variables should be sampled from an organism's environment so as to be representative of the environmental stimulation to which it had adapted and which formed the focus of an experimenter's generalization. It has been noted that the term could refer equally to the composition of practice task constraints so that they represent the performance environment which learners are faced with (Araújo *et al.* 2007). The acquisition of expertise is predicated on representative design in sports training programmes and refers to the accurate sampling of the information present in performance environments to be reflected in practice task constraints. For example, the use of bowlers rather than ball machines in cricket batting training means that the batter is able to attune to specifying information from the bowler's actions rather than the less-specifying information available from the bowling machine during practice (Renshaw *et al.* 2007). Obviously, only the former specifying sources of information for regulating action are present in the performance context, which has clear implications for designing representative practice tasks.

Representative practice task design ensures that developing individuals can gain expertise in picking up affordances for action in performance environments. However, it should be noted that the training activities of athletes in performance and learning environments, designed by coaches, can lead to substantial changes in an athlete's abilities to perceive and act. This pedagogical activity results in a constant interaction of abilities and affordances over time, leading to dynamic relationships between the individual and practice and performance environments, with new self-organizing behaviours emerging (Chemero 2008). Developing experts will become sensitive selectively to the performance environment (their niche) relative to the things that they can do. Therefore, the design of this environment is critical in influencing the development of the performer's ability to perceive and act. Affordance and abilities causally interact, as changes in abilities will lead to changes in the layout of available affordances, which will change the way abilities are exercised in real-time action (Chemero 2008).

The critical decision for coaches when working with talented young performers is when to expose them to practice and competitive environments that are representative of a new performance level. For example, it is clearly worthwhile for talented young performers to spend a percentage of training time working with senior players to gain exposure to the constraints on performance imposed by highly skilled competitors. However, it would still be prudent for these developing athletes to continue to play against peers in their own age group to maintain levels of confidence and motivation (Côté *et al.* 2007). Clearly, deciding when to expose the developing performer to this higher performance level is a complex decision for the practice of coaching, since it creates instability to allow the performer opportunities to adapt their skills but may threaten his or her self-confidence (Abbott *et al.* 2005).

Nonlinear dynamics, expertise in sport and talent development pathways

Since expertise has a multi-dimensional basis with a range of constraints impinging on its acquisition, the implication is that talent development programmes need to have a multi-dimensional framework. There are a number of multi-dimensional models of talent development (Abbott *et al.* 2005; Simonton 1999), which have conceptualized talent as a nonlinear process, predicting that there is a range of developmental trajectories and timescales that eventually result in the achievement of sporting expertise. These models have criticized traditional talent identification programmes for overemphasising the role of early identification and the role of physical and structural variables (such as physical dimensions, weight and height) and not accounting for variations in maturation rates of adolescents owing to the presence of performance rate limiters (Abbott *et al.* 2005).

Conceptualizing expertise acquisition as a complex system has numerous implications for talent development programmes. From this viewpoint, the aim of talent development is to aid individuals in gaining the expertise needed to satisfy the unique constraints impinging on them in specific performance environments. To achieve this aim, talent development programmes should aspire to promote the transition of individuals into a metastable region of the perceptual–motor landscape. This can be achieved by identifying key constraints on each individual and facilitating development by manipulating these constraints to encourage exploration of coordination. This process in expertise acquisition requires a comprehensive understanding of the intrinsic dynamics of each individual. Talent development programmes can harness these nonlinearities by developing strategies to induce phase transitions in individual performers. This aim might be best achieved by understanding how to force individuals into the metastable region of the perceptual–motor landscape of practice where a strategy of co-adaptation can underpin the emergence of creative behaviours (typical of the profile of expert performers in line with the findings of Durand-Bush and Salmela (2002). The implication of this approach for coaches is to incorporate tasks that promote adaptability and creativity in performers. In cricket, this aim could be achieved by carefully designing games that require batters to explore the boundaries of their skill set. For example, an approach to promote co-adaptation by players could involve setting up a practice task where the batter and bowler are on the same team and the field is split into eight zones but only six fielders are provided. The aim for the bowler is to bowl the ball so that the batter can hit into these 'free' zones. The fielding captain can vary these empty regions to challenge the batter to hit to areas where they may have a weaknesses. Despite the counterintuitive decision to have the batter and the bowler on the same team, this task requires bowlers to learn to bowl to force the batter to hit where they want them to, an essential skill at higher levels of performance. The batter is forced to be adaptable, since, even if the delivery is not 'perfect' for the required shot, they have to improvise and assemble a functional motor solution. The advantages for the fielding captain are the need to work out the strengths and weaknesses of opponents. This example highlights how nonlinear pedagogy can be used to great effect to force co-adaptive behaviours in learners as long as the design of game tasks are based on grounded principles of the game (e.g. Renshaw *et al.* 2007). It has been argued that traditional models need to be adjusted to consider the different rates of development of potentially talented athletes (Abbott *et al.* 2005). Subsystem behaviours shape an individual athlete's intrinsic dynamics. Because of variations in athletes' intrinsic dynamics, individual rates of skill acquisition are likely to progress at different time scales (Liu *et al.* 2006). Talent development models need take into account the different rates of learning and growth and maturation processes experienced by individuals on their pathway to expertise (not least it must take into account the relative age effect to maximize the available talent; Cobley *et al.* 2009). These different rates of learning can be influenced by key constraints which act as 'rate limiters' causing systems to find new coordination solutions (Handford *et al.* 1997). Rate limiters can be defined as system controllers; they are components or systems which limit the development of an individual in sport for example (Thelen and Smith 1994). In this instance, children's strength in key muscle groups may act as a rate limiter that inhibits them from demonstrating the skills that they have acquired already through practice and experience in sport. The complexity of neurobiological systems and associated rate limiters requires future research to adopt multidisciplinary methods to capture the nature of expert skill acquisition in sport.

Some current models of talent development are harmonious with these theoretical ideas, although their tenets are not necessarily predicated conceptually on these insights. For example, Simonton (1999) proposed that talent emerges from multidisciplinary, multiplicative and dynamic processes and is likely to operate as an intricate system beyond the scope of the polar nature–nurture debate. He pioneered mathematical equations to model the potential components that contribute to talent development. These components were weighted by relevance and included reference to genetic dispositions (e.g. height or endurance capacity), environmental (e.g. social and familial support) and developmental constraints. Subsequently the model was described as emergenic and epigenetic, comprising components that interact and change with time (Simonton 1999). The emergenic aspect proposes that potential talent consists of multiple components, including all physical, physiological, cognitive and dispositional traits that facilitate the manifestation of superior expertise in a specific domain. Beyond individual differences, Simonton's (1999) model captures the dynamics of epigenetics. Epigenetics is seen in the diverse components that make up talent that slowly appear and differentiate over time in an individual and ultimately depend on underlying neurological, muscular, cultural, skeletal, social, psychological, physiological and environmental variables (Obler and Fein 1988). However, they emerge gradually during the course of long-term interactions between the internally developing organism and appropriate environmental constraints (Simonton 1999). This system is complicated, as it includes the evolutionary interaction of components, therefore any examination of talent development that uses this model needs to be holistic, impartial and sophisticated (Simonton 1999). Although this mathematical model is a useful starting point for sport scientists since it attempts to operationalize key concepts such as multidisciplinary talent development practices and multiple developmental trajectories towards potential expertise (Abbott *et al.* 2005), it lacks theoretical power as it is not conceptualized within a theoretical framework. This weakness could be mediated by including dynamical systems theory as a viable rationale for talent development as an emergenic and epigenetic process. Furthermore, on a practical level, adopting Simonton's (1999) model may be extremely difficult as its efficacy is predicated on identifying all components that contribute to expertise in any one specific sporting domain. Identification of every component is essential because as the model is said to be multiplicative, a score of zero for any one factor means that expertise cannot be achieved.

Vaeyens *et al.* (2008) provided an insightful model of talent identification capturing the dynamic nature of talent and its development, focusing on potential for development and inclusion rather than early identification. Such a model can be strengthened with a dynamical system theoretical approach using concepts discussed previously, including metastability, nonlinearity, co-adaptation and degeneracy. The interaction of constraints within neurobiological systems means the intrinsic dynamics of each learner will result in unique pathways to expert performance in sport. Degeneracy of individuals will result in individualized performance solutions as interacting constraints are optimally satisfied when striving for acquisition of expertise in sport. In support of this view, qualitative sports expertise research has found differing developmental factors to be important to elite athletes. For example, Baker *et al.* (2005) examined the early sport involvement of elite ultra-triathletes and found early sport specialization was not a requirement for acquiring expertise. This observation has been supported by research into elite swimmers, who found early specialization was related to less time on the national team and an earlier end to their careers compared with swimmers who specialized later (Barynina and Vaitsekhovskii 1992). Although, the idea of multilateral development has many strengths and early specialization many potential pitfalls, early specialization may be an appropriate strategy for some potential experts. For example, it could be argued that early specialization is necessary to reach 'legend' status in a sport, given that this was the pathway of a number of individuals such as Tiger Woods, Sachin Tendulkar and Venus and Serena Williams. These different pathways would depend on the individual and also the chosen sport. Sports which emphasize physiological constraints rather than technical constraints require very different expertise sets, for example (e.g. ultra-marathon running compared with clay-pigeon shooting).

The notion of optimal movement solutions for a specific performance task, generalizable to all sport performers, is inappropriate, given the complex and degenerate nature of neurobiological systems (Glazier and Davids 2009). Characteristics such as complexity, pleiotropy and degeneracy make it challenging to identify a common optimal movement solution for all performers, requiring a remodelling of movement behaviour in dynamic performance contexts. Dynamical systems researchers have suggested that common optimal movement patterns probably do not exist and that variability is an intrinsic feature of skilled motor performance, providing flexibility to adapt performance in dynamic environments (Glazier *et al.* 2003). As Sutton (2008) identified, any specific skilled action is based on 'flexible intelligent action in real time that requires attention to the continuous coupling of perception and action, and the mutually modulatory dynamics operating between brain, body and world' (p.770).

These findings provide some challenges for talent identification programmes that emphasize physical and test performance measures as a major criterion for referencing expertise in sport (see the earlier section on 'Results of research with quantitative methodologies'). Abbott *et al.* (2005) noted several major problems associated with identifying potential athletes solely on current physical and performance measures. Underpinning these concerns was the nonlinear process of development and the difficulty of predicting changes in genetically and environmentally driven variables, which were often unstable. Typically, identification of talent has focused on discrete performance measures with limited task representativeness. As such, these measures have revealed limited information about an athlete's potential and adaptability in the competitive environment (Morris

2000). Abbott *et al.* (2005) suggested that talent identification processes should be focused on the future performance capacity of athletes, rather than current performance measures and highlighted the importance of future research on the factors that underpin successful development towards one's potential (Simonton 1999). However, assessing future performance capacity must take into account the current intrinsic dynamics of each individual in order to identify the current relative position on the developmental pathway. Predicting ultimate performance capacity becomes an even more complex issue when one tries to predict what a sport will look like in five to ten years' time, as technological advances are continually changing the nature of sports. Elite-level sport is moving fast and is evolving continually, owing to rule changes, new training methods and perform-ance strategies. What is clear from this discussion is the need for talent identification and development programmes to provide flexible learning environ-ments that produce performers who have the capacity to adapt to constant change, within a context of expertise.

Conclusion

Complex systems theory is an appropriate functional framework for expert performance research because it can address questions that other frameworks do not have the language and tools to pose. This chapter has discussed several concepts with important implications for expertise and talent development researchers, including the concepts of self-organization under constraints; emer-gence; metastability, creativity; and degeneracy, stabilities and instabilities over different timescales. These ideas on the dynamic interactions between genes and environment and the functional role of degeneracy in the human nervous system require a multidisciplinary theoretical perspective to explain the acquisition of expertise in sport. Within this overarching theoretical framework, it has been argued that the same performance outcomes can be achieved in diverse ways as individual performers attempt to satisfy the unique constraints on them (Davids *et al.* 2003). Genetic diversity may be responsible for a small part of training or performance response differences between individuals and only when there is a favourable interaction with important environmental constraints are performance benefits observed. Phenotypic expression of behaviour might be best understood at the level of individual interactions with key environmental and task constraints. This is particularly relevant for researchers considering effects of time spent in deliberate practice in sport, since there is often little mention of genetic constraints on the acquisition of expertise. Given differences in genetic contribu-tions, performance variations are more likely to assert themselves under intensive practice regimens.

The acquisition of expertise is domain specific and is about adaptation to the environment through satisfying unique constraints which impinge on each devel-oping expert. Expertise acquisition emphasizes the changing nature of the performer–environment relationship through development and gaining experi-ence through training, practice, coaching and competing. A comprehensive examination of expertise involves identifying the intrinsic dynamics of each individual and the specific rate limiters and constraints which shape their behaviour. Each individual athlete comes to a performance context with a particular set of intrinsic dynamics that has already been shaped by genes, development and early experiences. Individualized pathways to expert performance are expected because of the uniqueness of these dynamics constraints.

Note

1   Abrupt changes in the organization of a system are called bifurcations or branchings, since typically they signify changes in the number of possible action modes available.

References

Abbott, A., Button, C., Pepping, G.-J. and Collins, D. (2005) Unnatural selection: talent identification and development in sport. *Nonlinear Dynamics, Psychology, and Life Sciences*, 9 (1): 61–88.

Abbott, A. and Collins, D. (2002) A theoretical and empirical analysis of a 'state of the art' talent identification model. *High Ability Studies*, 13 (2): 157–78.

Anderson, G. S. and Ward, R. (2002) Classifying children for sports participation based upon anthropometric measurement. *European Journal of Sport Science*, 2 (3) 11: 1–13.

Araújo, D., Davids, K. and Hristovski, R. (2006) The ecological dynamics of decision making in sport. *Psychology of Sport and Exercise*, 7 (6): 653–76.

Araujo, D., Davids, K. and Passos, P. (2007) Ecological validity, representative design, and correspondence between experimental task constraints and behavioral setting: comment on Rogers, Kadar, and Costall (2005) *Ecological Psychology*, 19 (1): 69–78.

Bak, P. and Chialvo, D. R. (2001) Adaptive learning by extremal dynamics and negative feedback. *Physical Review E*, 63 (3): 031912; doi: 10.1080/17461390200072301

Baker, J. and Davids, K. (2006) Genetic and environmental constraints on variability in sport performance, in K. Davids, S. J. Bennett and K. Newell (eds) *Movement System Variability*. Champaign, IL: Human Kinetics, pp. 109–29.

Baker, J. and Horton, S. (2004) A review of primary and secondary influences on sport expertise. *High Ability Studies*, 15 (2): 211–28.

Baker, J., Côté, J. and Deakin, J. (2005) Expertise in ultra-endurance triathletes early sport involvement, training structure, and the theory of deliberate practice. *Journal of Applied Sport Psychology*, 17 (1): 64–78.

Bartlett, R. and Robins, M. (2008) Biomechanics of throwing, in Y. Hong and R. Bartlett (eds) *Handbook of Biomechanics and Human Movement Science*. New York: Routledge, pp. 285–95.

Bartlett, R. M. and Best, R. J. (1988) The biomechanics of javelin throwing; a review. *Journal of Sports Sciences*, 6: 1–38.

Barynina, I. I. and Vaitsekhovskii, S. M. (1992) The aftermath of early sports specialization for highly qualified swimmers. *Fitness and Sports Review International*, 27 (4): 132–3.

Beek, P. J., Jacobs, D. M., Daffertshofer, A. and Huys, R. (2003) Expert performance in sport: views from the joint perspectives of ecological psychology and dynamical systems theory, in J. L. Starkes and K. A. Ericsson (eds) *Expert Performance in Sport*. Champaign, IL: Human Kinetics, pp. 321–44.

Bloom, B. S. (1985) *Developing Talent in Young People*. New York: Ballantine.

Brunswik, E. (1955) Representative design and probabilistic theory in a functional psychology. *Psychological Review*, 62 (3): 193–217.

Chemero, A. (2008) Self-organization, writ large. *Ecological Psychology*, 20: 257–69.

Chow, J. Y., Davids, K., Button, C. and Koh, M. (2008) Coordination changes in a discrete multi-articular action as a function of practice. *Acta Psychologica*, 127 (1): 163–76.

Cobley, S., Baker, J., Wattie, N. and McKenna, J. (2009) Annual age-grouping and athlete development: a meta-analytical review of relative age effects in sport. *Sports Medicine*, 39 (3): 235–56.

Côté, J., Baker, J. and Abernethy, B. (2007) Practice and play and the development of sport expertise, in G. Tenenabum and R. Eklund (eds) *Handbook of Sport Psychology*, 3rd edn. *10. Degenerate Brains, Indeterminate Behavior, and Representative Tasks: Implications for Experimental Design in Sport Psychology Research*. New Jersey: Wiley, pp. 184–202.

Cowdrey, M. C. (1974) *Tackle Cricket*. London: Stanley Paul.

Davids, K. and Baker, J. (2007) Genes, environment and sport performance: why the nature–nurture dualism is no longer relevant. *Sports Medicine*, 37 (11): 961–80.

Davids, K., Araújo, D., Button, C. and Renshaw, I. (2007a) Degenerate brains, indeterminate behavior and representative tasks: implications for experimental design in sport psychology research, in G. Tenenbaum and R. Eklund (eds) *Handbook of Sport Psychology*, 3rd edn. *10. Degenerate Brains, Indeterminate Behavior, and Representative Tasks: Implications for Experimental Design in Sport Psychology Research*. New York: Wiley, pp. 224–44.

Davids, K., Button, C. and Bennett, S. J. (2007b) Coordination and control of movement in sport: An ecological approach. Champaign, IL: Human Kinetics.

Davids, K., Button, C. and Bennett, S. (2008) *Dynamics of Skill Acquisition: A Constraints-Led Approach*. Champaign, IL: Human Kinetics.

Davids, K., Glazier, P., Araujo, D., and Bartlett, R. (2003) Movement systems as dynamical systems: the functional role of variability and its implications for sports medicine. *Sports Medicine*, 33 (4): 245–60.

Duchon, A. P., Kaelbling, L. P. and Warren, W. H. (1998) Ecological robotics. *Adaptive Behavior*, 6 (3–4): 473–507.

Durand-Bush, N. and Salmela, J. (2002) The development and maintenance of expert athletic performance: perceptions of World and Olympic champions. *Journal of Applied Sport Psychology*, 14 (3): 154–71.

Edelman, G. M. and Gally, J. A. (2001) Degeneracy and complexity in biological systems. *PNAS: Proceedings of the National Academy of Sciences of the USA*, 98 (24): 13763–8; doi: 10.1073/pnas.231499798 (accessed 10 June 2013).

Frank, T. D., Peper, C. E., Daffertshofer, A. and Beek, P. J. (2006) Variability of brain activity during rhythmic unimanual finger movements, in K. Davids, S. J. Bennett and K. Newell (eds) *Movement System Variability*. Champaign, IL: Human Kinetics, pp. 271–6.

Fringelkurts, A. A. and Fringelkurts, A. A. (2004) Making complexity simpler: multivariability and metastability in the brain. *International Journal of Neuroscience*, 114: 843–62.

Gibson, J. J. (1979) *The Ecological Approach to Visual Perception*. Boston: Houghton Mifflin.

Glazier, P. S. and Davids, K. (2009) Constraints on the complete optimization of human motion. *Sports Medicine*, 39 (1): 15–28.

Glazier, P. S., Davids, K. and Bartlett, R. M. (2003) Dynamical systems theory: a relevant framework for performance-orientated sports biomechanics research. *Sportscience*, 7. Available online at www.sportsci.org/2003/index.html (accessed 10 June 2013).

Gould, D., Dieffenbach, K. and Moffett, A. (2002) Psychological characteristics and their development in Olympics champions. *Journal of Applied Sport Psychology*, 14 (3): 172–204.

Handford, C., Davids, K., Bennett, S. and Button, C. (1997) Skill acquisition in sport: some applications of an evolving practice ecology. *Journal of Sports Sciences*, 15 (6): 621–40.

Holt, N. L. and Dunn, J. G. H. (2004) Toward a grounded theory of the psychosocial competencies and environmental conditions associated with soccer success. *Journal of Applied Sport Psychology*, 16 (3): 199–219.

James, D. (2008) The physics of winning: engineering the world of sport. *Physics Education*, 43 (5); doi: 10.1088/0031-9120/43/5/006. Available online at http://iopscience.iop.org/0031-9120/43/5/006 (accessed 10 June 2013).

Kaerns, M., Elston, T. C., Blake, W. and Collins, J. J. (2005) Stochasticity in gene expression: from theories to phenotypes. *Nature Reviews Genetics*, 6: 451–64.

Kauffman, S. (1995) *At Home in the Universe: The Search for Laws of Complexity*. London: Viking.

Kauffman, S. A. (1993) *The Origins of Order: Self-organization and Selection in Evolution*. New York: Oxford University Press.

Kelso, J. A. S. (1991) Anticipatory dynamical systems, intrinsic pattern dynamics and skill learning. *Human Movement Science*, 10: 93–111.

Kelso, J. A. S. (1995) *Dynamic Patterns: The Self-organization of Brain and Behavior*. Cambridge, MA: MIT Press.

Kelso, J. A. S. (2008) An essay on understanding the mind. *Ecological Psychology*, 20: 180–208.

Liu, Y.-T., Mayer-Kress, G. and Newell, K. M. (2006) Qualitative and quantitative change in the dynamics of motor learning. *Journal of Experimental Psychology: Human Perception and Performance*, 32 (2): 380–93.

Morris, T. (2000) Psychological characteristics and talent identification in soccer. *Journal of Sports Sciences*, 18 (9): 715–26.

Morriss, C. J., Bartlett, R. M. and Fowler, N. (1997) Biomechanical analysis of the men's javelin throw at the 1995 world championships in athletics. *New Studies in Athletics*, 12: 32–41.

Newell, K. M. (1986) Constraints on the development of coordination, in M. G. Wade and H. T. A. Whiting (eds) *Motor Skill Acquisition in Children: Aspects of Coordination and Control*. Amsterdam: Martinus Nijhoff, pp. 341–60.

North, S. (2004) Landy took it all in his stride and is still making the running. *Sydney Morning Herald*, 1 May. Available online at www.smh.com.au/articles/2004/04/30/1083224590040.html (accessed 10 June 2013).

Obler, L. K. and Fein, D. (1988) *The Exceptional Brain: Neuropsychology of Talent and Special Abilities*. New York: Guilford Press.

Pyne, D. B., Duthie, G., Saunders, P. U., Petersen, C. A. and Portus, M. R. (2006) Anthropometric and strength correlates of fast bowling speed in junior and senior cricketers. *Journal of Strength and Conditioning Research*, 20 (3): 620–6.

Renshaw, I., Oldham, A. R., Golds, T. and Davids, K. (2007) Changing ecological constraints of practice alters coordination of dynamic interceptive actions. *Journal of Sport Sciences* 7 (3): 157–67.

Renshaw, I., Davids, K., Chow, J. and Shuttleworth, R. (2009) Insights from ecological psychology and dynamical systems theory can underpin a philosophy of coaching. *International Journal of Sport Psychology*, 40 (4): 540–602.

Schöllhorn, W. I. (2003) Coordination dynamics and its consequences on sport. *International Journal of Computer Science in Sport*, 2: 40–6.

Simonton, D. K. (1999) Talent and its development: an emergenic and epigenetic model. *Psychological Review*, 106 (3): 435–57.

Sumpter, D. J. T. (2006) The principles of collective animal behaviour. *Philosophical Transactions of the Royal Society B: Biological Sciences*, 361: 5–22.

Sutton, J. (2008) Batting, habit and memory: the embodied mind and the nature of skill. *Sport in Society*, 10 (5): 763–86.

Thamel, P. (2008) Poor 3-Point Shooting Can't Stop U.S. Basketball Team. *New York Times*, 12 August: D2. Available online at www.nytimes.com/2008/08/13/sports/olympics/13games.html (accessed 10 June 2013).

Thelen, E. (1995) Motor development: a new synthesis. *American Psychologist*, 50 (2): 79–95.

Thelen, E. and Smith, L. B. (1994) *A Dynamic Systems Approach to the Development of Cognition and Action*. Cambridge, MA: MIT Press.

Vaeyens, R., Lenoir, M., Williams, A. M. and Philippaerts, R. M. (2008) Talent identification and development programmes in sport: current models and future directions. *Sports Medicine*, 38 (9): 703–14.

Van Orden, G. C., Holden, J. G. and Turvey, M. T. (2003) Self-organization of cognitive performance. *Journal of Experimental Psychology: General*, 132 (3): 331–50.

Ward, P., Hodges, N. J., Starkes, J. L. and Williams, M. A. (2007) The road to excellence: deliberate practice and the development of expertise. *High Ability Studies*, 18 (2): 119–53.

Wolstencroft, E. (2002) *Talent Identification and Development: An Academic Review*. Edinburgh: Sportscotland.

15 Creativity in sport and dance

Ecological dynamics on a hierarchically soft-assembled perception–action landscape

Robert Hristovski, Keith Davids,
Duarte Araújo, Pedro Passos, Carlota Torrents,
Alexandar Aceski, and Alexandar Tufekcievski

Innovative and creative goal-directed behaviours in complex neurobiological systems, such as apes and birds, has been studied extensively (see, e.g. Reader and Laland 2001; Taylor *et al.* 2010) and involves the discovery of novel patterns of behaviour by an organism. There has not been the same focus on creative behaviour in sport, although much research in sport sciences and pedagogy has been aimed at improving athletic performance. Traditionally, performance optimization methods have been implemented to identify the set of movement parameters that might maximize competitive outcomes for specific elite athletes (e.g. Bartlett 2007). However, as in the case of Dick Fosbury, the elite high jumper, sometimes exploration of novel movement patterns can not just improve performance but actually push it to a new, higher level.

Such advances occur, not by optimizing model parameters of an existing well-established technique but by construction of new coordination patterns. This creative advance can resolve problems with a previous technique, shape performance outcomes and enrich movement culture, making specific sports more diverse and more aesthetically attractive. On the other hand the sociocultural influence on the performer or the team put strong constraints of nonspecific and specific kind (for more on this issue see Hristovski *et al.* 2011). The changes in socioculturally induced nonspecific task constraints, like the type of tool used or environment on which is acted upon, may be instrumental in eliciting innovative performer–environment relations (e.g. Bril *et al.* 2005). On the other hand, specific social influences, i.e. imitation of extant performer–environment relations, are constraining athletes to comply with these movement forms within the sociocultural milieu. However, complying with extant movement forms is just the opposite from creativity defined as *process of exploration and production* of novel and functional behaviour. Drazin *et al.* (1999) and Sternberg and Lubart (1996) provide detailed explanations of these two basic types of creative behaviour, respectively.

Inventions of novel performance solutions occur regularly in sport and have been well documented in activities like track and field, exemplified by the

'O'Brien' (or rotational) technique in shot put or the 'straddle' and 'Fosbury flop' techniques which replaced more traditional and less successful 'scissors' and 'eastern cut-off' high-jump techniques. In the last few decades alone in gymnastics, 14 novel technical elements have appeared. Yet despite this process, creativity in sport performance has seldom been the subject of systematic research, revealed by the absence in sport science of established theoretical rationales for studying and explaining creative behaviour. In the following text, we present a model of creative behaviour in sports and dance and some new empirical results based on the ecological dynamics approach (Araújo et al. 2006).

Multistability as a prerequisite for creativity in neurobiological systems

The multitude of solutions or states available in complex performer–environment systems is a consequence of the wealth of potential nonlinear couplings available between system components (or between system agents in sports teams as social neurobiological systems (e.g. Challet et al. 2000). Degeneracy, pleiotropy and multistability exemplify performer–environment properties that support such nonlinearity and complexity. In short, degeneracy means that different structural components may be assembled to satisfy the same task goal constraints and pleiotropy means that the same structural component can have a role in satisfying different task goals. Multistability (see Chapter 1 and 2 for definition) is a prerequisite for an important property of complex systems metastability; i.e. the capacity to possess numerous functional, coexistent pattern-forming propensities (e.g. Bressler and Kelso 2001; Kello et al. 2008). It is a prerequisite, since metastable dynamics can exist only in systems which have more than one attracting states under the same longer-term constraints. In such systems, the behaviour can dwell for some time in the vicinity of the attractor or attractive point and then switch to another one. The monostability of linear systems does not allow such metastability. This property of performer–environment systems, allows system states (*qua* performance solutions) to be soft-assembled, emerging under specific constellations of boundary conditions as constraints. These system states are not preformed but emerge under interacting constraints, basic principles that underpin the constraints-led perspective on skill acquisition in sport (Davids et al. 2008; Davids et al. 2013; Davids et al. 2003; Araújo et al. 2004, 2006; Davids et al. 2005; Chow et al. 2006; Newell 1986).

The distinctive configurations of constraints between learners, based on a platform of system degeneracy and pleiotropy, are manifested in how each individual attempts to satisfy specific task constraints during practice. Inventing a new technique or a movement form (i.e. coordination) is always defined as being in the coordination stage of learning, which can be afterwards, through practice, made more functional (for more detailed discussion, see Hristovski et al. 2012). The invented coordination, of course, may be supported and contextualized by already-stabilized skills. Individual creativity is a product of the interactions of three nonlinear properties: cause–effect nonproportionality, parametric (constraint) control and multistability in complex systems (for definitions, see Chapter 1 and 2; Hristovski *et al.* 2009). Within these interactions, nonlinear pedagogy (e.g. Chow *et al.* 2006) frames the individuality of learning pathways and individual creation of performance solutions for a given movement task. Based on these arguments, we next outline a nonlinear, complex systems model of creativity in sports and physical activity.

Ecological dynamics on a hierarchically soft-assembled potential landscape: a model outline

The empirically-based, hierarchical structure of human movement variability (see e.g. Chow *et al.* 2008) provides an *explanation* of the behavioural characteristic of creativity within the framework of statistical mechanics of disordered systems; i.e. systems with many different but *ordered* states, particularly the replica symmetry-breaking framework first developed by Parisi (e.g. Parisi 1979). The hierarchical structure of movement variability implicates a rugged landscape with many nested metastable minima (Hristovski and Davids 2008), within the global basin of attraction. For clarification, one such landscape is depicted for fixed task constraints in Figure 15.1.

The main idea behind this model is the absence of any simple symmetries of potential order parameters (see Chapter 1 and 2) governing discrete and whole body movements. In other words, in principle, it is hard to relate two or more actions through simple symmetry transformations. For example, in the HKB

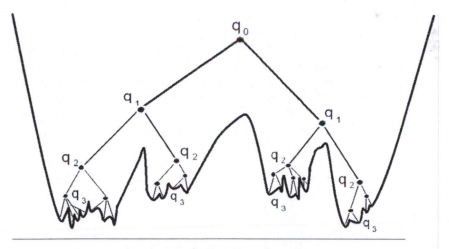

performer – environment configurations

Figure 15.1 Schematic (i.e. one-dimensional) presentation of the corrugated hierarchically soft-assembled potential landscape with two confining barriers on both sides (reproduced with kind permission from *Nonlinear Dynamics, Psychology and Life Sciences*, Springer)

(Haken, Kelso and Bunz) model (Haken *et al.* 1985), the relative phase order parameter exhibits mirror (change of the sign) symmetry, which allows one to relate a set of patterns; i.e. values of the order parameter, with those symmetries. However, a set of whole-body movements/postures or multiarticular discrete movements in sport or dancing, generally, cannot be related by simple symmetries and their rearrangements. Hence, the relatedness of any set of discrete and whole-body movements may be made by the so-called overlap order parameter q, which measures the mutual correlation of this kind of actions. It can be defined as a cosine of the angle between two random vectors, i.e. *replicas*, in real or formal space of any finite dimension (e.g. Domany *et al.* 2001). Under absolutely relaxed constraints, one may expect that these replicas are totally uncorrelated and their average correlation is $<q> = 0$. We can say that the system is replica symmetrical. Any replica, i.e. performer–environment configuration, can emerge. However, under constraining influences of the task, properties of the individual performer and the environment, this symmetry and ergodicity is broken and clusters of correlated actions arise (for detailed examples, see Hristovski *et al.* 2011, 2012). Some similar replicas, i.e. configurations, are more likely to occur and some are unlikely. Constraints break system symmetry, produce a phase transition and also create ergodicity breaking high barriers on the both sides of the potential landscape, confining all available actions within the internal space (Figure 15.1). It can be observed that the action landscape *soft-assembles* under specific constraints configurations.

These correlated clusters form a hierarchical landscape. Actions lying in one attractor basin (see Chapter 1 for definition), separated by smaller barriers are more correlated than those separated by higher barriers. Thus, we can define order parameters at each level, with those defining lower levels depending on increasingly subtle constraints. These order parameters form a tree-like structure. Note that, while slowly changing (i.e. quasi-stationary) interacting constraints, are forming the deterministic structure of the landscape (see Figure 15.1 and the previous text), there is also a need of stochastic agitation force within the performer–environment system, mainly contributed by the interaction between performer's intention to move and the unpredictable and quickly changing physical and information constraints, which are the driving force of reconfigurations. Hence, both the deterministic structure *and* the stochastic drive interact in reconfiguring the systems dynamics. The exploratory dynamics within this landscape, may be seen as a hopping of the system from one basin to another or equivalently as a *random walk on a tree*. The *hopping* or the random walk has a meaning of reconfigurations within the system that are taking place. Hopping over larger barriers means larger reconfigurations and vice versa.

This modelling shows how *exploration* is a requisite of creative behaviour; i.e. inventing novel or innovating extant movement forms and actions with respect to the extant sociocultural milieu (for details see Hristovski *et al.* 2011). Without it, a complex neurobiological system cannot find novel functional behavioural solutions. In Hristovski *et al.* (2011), exploratory breadth Q was defined as being equal to the average escape probability over all possible state basins of attraction (see Saxton 1996), $Q = W_e$. Escape probabilities for each movement mode are defined as $W_e = 1 - W_c$, where W_c is the conditional probability of staying inside the same attractor (Hristovski *et al.* 2009). In other words, W_c measures the trapping strength of the attractor; i.e. the probability of being able to achieve the same performance outcomes sequentially. The larger the average escape probability W_e, the larger the exploratory breadth Q of the system and vice versa. In general, it can be said that: *for any performer–environment system containing a large amount of degrees of freedom, there always exists a set of constraints which maximizes the functional action versatility, i.e. exploratory breadth, defined as maximum action entropy* (see e.g. Hristovski *et al.* 2006; Pinder *et al.* 2012). A more thorough exposition of this model and an experimental example of novel action emergence in martial arts can be found in Hristovski *et al.* (2011) and Hristovski *et al.* (2012).

In the following section, we further illustrate how this theoretical model provides an analysis of movement exploration structure and dynamics applied in context of dance improvisation. The general predictions of a hierarchical structure and softly assembled dynamics were preliminarily tested. A conceptual model of creativity in team sports within the general framework of dynamical systems is also presented.

How creative behaviours emerge under ecological constraints in dance and team sports

Creative behaviour in contact improvisation dance: a soft-assembled hierarchy model analysis

Contact improvisation is a form of dance where contact points between and movements of partners constrain each other's subsequent movements. What are the creative aspects of contact improvisation? Contact improvisation may be thought of as a bank of emergent human movement forms and an expression of continuous *exploration* and *discovery* of idiosyncratic postures and actions supported by immediate affordances; i.e. opportunities for action. It is used systematically as a *dance research method* for identifying innovative set choreography. The invented novel forms of movement, being themselves creative products, could afterwards be stylized and put to a further use. These properties of contact improvisation make it a highly creative activity satisfying both, the *process* and the *product* definitions of creativity as a phenomenon (for these definitions, see (Drazin *et al.* 1999; Sternberg and Lubart 1996). This characteristic of contact improvisation fits nicely within the general approach in our experiments for discovering the dynamical, perception–action landscape of sport/dance performers which involves probing system activity by letting it evolve autonomously under specific task constraints manipulations over a period of time.

Here, we describe some results of an analysis of a typical contact improvisation session lasting 450 seconds under no special instructional constraints, except those provided by the contact with the partner, i.e. visual and haptic information, and the force of gravity. Sequences of actions/postures were analyzed to determine their complex dynamical characteristics. Actions/postures were defined on a coarse-grained scale containing 52 movement/posture components, such as support/contact characteristics and directions and planes of motion of body segments according to established observational methodology (see Torrents *et al.* 2010; Castañer *et al.* 2009). To the active components a value of 1 was ascribed and to the inactive components a value of 0. Hence, a binary matrix was formed with a time resolution of 1 second. Each 1-second window was defined as a 52-component binary vector representing the action configuration during the same time interval. Reconfigurations, i.e. mutations, of action patterns were calculated as Hamming distances between any two binary vectors. For example, the change of one component of the vector from 1 to 0 or vice versa has a Hamming distance equal to 1. Hence, the Hamming distance actually measures the height of the potential barrier between two configurations. Overlap order parameter q was used to determine the structure of the potential landscape of the dancer and its dynamic properties. The overlap was defined in two intrinsically related association measures: as a cosine similarity and as a Pearson correlation between two binary configuration vectors. A hierarchical principal component analysis (HPCA) was performed on the data using the second measure (for the plausibility of using principal component analysis on binary variables, see Joliffe 2002, p. 339), with the aim of detecting the possible nested attractor basin structure of the dancer's action landscape. In order to determine not only the structure of dancer's complex movement patterns but also their exploratory dynamics, the dynamic overlap $q_d(t)$ was calculated as an average cosine autosimilarity of the overlap between configurations with increasing time lag.

The HPCA initially revealed 25 principal components. Seven primary principal components accounting for 81.3% of the total variance were taken into account. The first, the fifth, the sixth and the seventh principal component were weakly but significantly correlated $<q> = 0.401 \pm 0.02$. The other 18 principal components contained statistically rare and short-lived reconfigurations having a role of fluctuations. This structure is interesting in itself. While the dominant dynamics were confined within the seven principal components, the reconfiguration space was with significantly higher dimension. This gives a picture of lower-dimensional global dynamics connected by high-dimensional quick reconfigurations. Seventeen movement–posture components had very high scores on these seven principal components. Consequently, the dynamics were saturated predominantly by these *emergent* movements-posture patterns.

The secondary level consisted of two principal components containing the seven primary principal components as substructure. Hence, the HPCA procedure reduced the dancer's dynamics dimensionality from 449 configuration vectors to the two slowest collective variables (order parameters) containing seven faster variables, each of which was formed by even faster movement/posture configuration vectors. The median dwell time of these configuration vectors was 5.4 seconds. This structure revealed a metastable dynamics in a soft-assembled hierarchy of collective variables with different characteristic time scales (for intuitive understanding, see Figure 15.1). The global and the slowest collective variable consisted of degrees of freedom such as foot–floor surface support, support of the partner with lower and upper limbs and the trunk-torso-back-pelvis surfaces. They were present, with only quick interruptions, over the whole observation timescale. This persistent collective variable formed the global basin of attraction and continually constrained the faster degrees of freedom such as a change in the direction of movement, lateral or forward flexion of the trunk, arm movements, and so on. These degrees of freedom under constraining influence of the slow collective variable formed shorter-lived metastable states (local basins of attraction) on the lower hierarchical level. In other words, the slowest collective variable formed rather persistent pinning surfaces between partners, nucleuses, around which more quick movement motifs were created.

In the upper panel of Figure 15.2, one can see a zoomed example of metastable dynamics of the first 35 seconds, where the action system of a dancer transits from one local metastable configuration attractor basin to another, meanwhile dwelling inside one of them for several seconds. These four principal components extracted from the first 35 time-ordered configurations were correlated $<q> = 0.64 \pm 0.05$ and belonged to a secondary global confining attracting basin (secondary principal component). At each moment, several opportunities for action coexist, owing to informational constraints from the partners and the floor, the gravity and the abundance of nonlinearly coupled degrees of freedom within the system of dancers. Which one of these coexistent propensities will become a temporary solution, i.e. a creative product, depends on subtle and quick information, i.e. fast perceptual-motor degrees of freedom and decisions dressed with randomness, e.g. who will lead and who will follow in the immediate future interval. Aside from their common motive to move, randomness is a crucial part of the dynamics because partners do not deterministically guide each other, i.e. with perfect probability ($P = 1$). Each temporary posture or movement solution is a creative product embedded within the creative exploration dynamics. Hence, 'exploratory' or 'process' and 'product' properties of creative behaviour are becoming obvious (Drazin *et al.* 1999; Sternberg and Lubart 1996).

The darkest areas of the centre panel of Figure 15.2 correspond to maximum overlap q values of certain configurations with the certain principal component and represent the locally attracting configurations. The increasing lightness in the conturogram signifies a lower overlap and represents the local attracting basin around the attractor configurations. One can notice that from the darkest areas (local potential minima) going outwards the lightness increases, reaching in some areas the lightest grey colour, which represents saddles or barriers of the potential landscape. Looking at the lower panel of Figure 15.2, where Hamming distances count the number of reconfigurations or mutations that have occurred, we see that those lighter shaded areas correspond to the intervals of reconfigurations of the action system of the dancer. Hence, reconfigurations correspond to crossing over the potential barriers (saddles) between two metastable minima.

The evolution of the cosine autosimilarity, i.e. the average dynamic overlap $<q_d(t)>$, is given in Figure 15.3. If the dancers stayed in one posture during whole

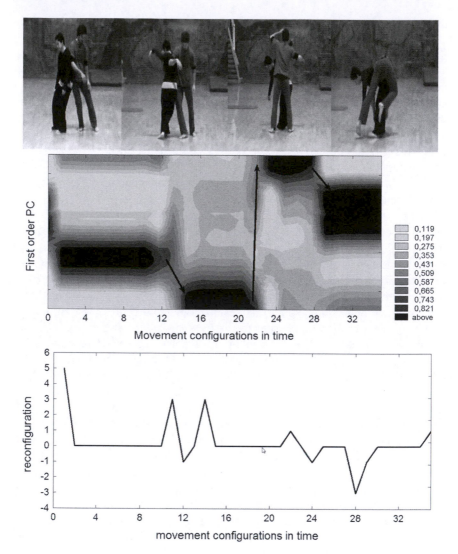

Figure 15.2 (Top) snapshots of the four metastable states of dancers for the first 35 seconds of improvisation; (middle): overlaps *q* of the four metastable body configurations with principal components (axis *Y*) and pathway of their dynamics. Overlap values are given in the legend on right; (bottom): reconfigurations are given as nonzero Hamming distances of the dancer's action system; after some reconfigurations take place, the action system relaxes and dwells in a state where no further reconfigurations occur for some time; i.e. zero reconfiguration; this process represents the metastable attractor configurations (movement/posture pattern)

observation time lasting seven minutes, the average dynamic overlap would be a constant equal to one; i.e. $<q_d(t)> = 1$ for all time lags (see the dashed line on Figure 15.3). On the other hand, if during the performance, the dancers were exploring distant configurations of the whole state space (a case of unbroken ergodicity), the average dynamic overlap $<q_d(t)>$ would drop to zero exponentially fast for the observation time of seven minutes (see the dotted curve on Figure 15.3). Neither of these cases was obtained in the observed performance. The fact that the relaxation of $<q_d(t)>$ was *not* exponential, means that there was no single characteristic time of the dynamics. In other words, the dynamics contains a distribution of relaxation times and thus a distribution of attractor basins of different depth (barriers of different height), which is consistent with the predictions of the model of soft-assembled hierarchy explained briefly previously. According to the model, Figure 15.3 can be interpreted in the following way. The dancer explores subsequent movement configurations, which are correlated; i.e. lying within a local basin of attraction defined by the correlated principal component substructure and makes, on average, small gradual reconfigurations. On average, after longer times, s/he hops into attractor basins which are less correlated with previous ones; i.e. moves within another set of principal components. These reconfigurations with time accumulate and bring the dancer far enough from a certain initial configuration. That is why the dynamical overlap $<q_d(t)>$ decreases for the first 35 time lags, forming the initial relaxation dynamics. The linear fit in log–log plot of this initial relaxation was $\beta = -0.203$; with explained variance $R^2 = 0.977$. This variable roughly shows the *rate of exploration* of the system. One can see that even movement configurations separated by 20 seconds possess overlaps larger than 0.5. However, on average, movement configurations separated in time by more than 35 seconds show a constant average overlap of approximately $<q_d(t)> = 0.45$. This is the value of the

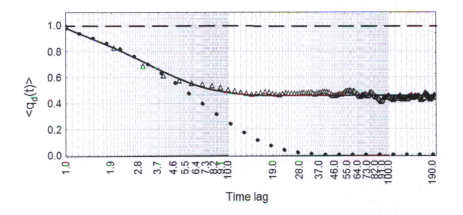

Figure 15.3 The profile of the average dynamic overlap $q_d(t)$ for different time lags; its dynamics proceed on three timescales (from seconds to several minutes) and does not converge to zero during the observation time scale

average overlap of all the dancer's movement configurations that emerged within the seven-minute contact improvisation. In other words, this is the self-overlap value of the superbasin of attraction confining all of the metastable valleys of movement configurations captured by the hierarchical principal component structure. Since the dynamic overlap forms a plateau at values far from zero, the system does not explore arbitrarily distant movement configurations (ergodicity is broken on the observational time scale of seven minutes), because the slowest collective variable (see the previous discussion), confine the emergent metastable opportunities for action and, consequently, the movement dynamics, in a relatively large but limited region of performer–environment state space. Nevertheless, the plateau value $<q_d(t)> = 0.45$, shows a relatively high exploratory; i.e. creative fluency of the system. The fact that the dynamical overlap, during the observation time of seven minutes, did not decrease to zero means that the global relaxation (equilibration) time of the slowest, order parameters (secondary principal components) diverged (did not go to zero) and the system was in a nonequilibrium state. This means that while there was an equilibration within the confined region (primary principal components), the space of all possible configurations remained far from being fully explored. Such slow dynamics is consistent with predictions of the previously discussed theoretical model of soft-assembled hierarchical dynamics. The exploratory breadth of dancer's movement system Q (see previous section) defined as an average escape probability from a certain configuration was $Q = 0.37$, showing a significant exploratory capacity under relaxed constraints.

   In this section we have shown how exploratory, i.e. process and product aspects of creative behaviour can be analyzed within the model of soft-assembled hierarchy. The creative process unfolds on more time scales, owing to the hierarchical structure of the perception–action landscape. The soft-assembled hierarchical landscape model predicts also other interesting phenomena, such as aging: the more time the learner spends in a confined and thus correlated region of the landscape, the less responsive s/he becomes to a change. Based on the obtained consistency of the experimental results with respect to the predictions of the theoretical model, we further hypothesize that, together with Q, the slope of initial relaxation β and the value of the $<q_d(t)>$ plateau, are good candidates for assessing the creative capacity of performer–environment systems under different types and strengths of constraints (for details see Hristovski *et al.* 2011). Future work is needed to test other predictions of the model.

Conceptual modelling of creative behaviour in team sports: the need to play within critical regions of interpersonal distance

Attackers' interactions aim to actively explore space–time windows that emerge because of defender displacements. On the other hand, defender displacements aim to cover the possible paths to goal, which demands high levels of interpersonal coordination among the players in defence. However, space–time windows will only emerge if the attackers' movements are powerful enough to disturb the defenders' interpersonal coordination and, to do that, attackers' actions must be performed within short distances of attacker–defender interpersonal distance (Passos *et al.* 2008).

Thus, sudden changes in the attacker–defender structural organization can only happen when the attacker–defender systems moved towards regions of very short interpersonal distances, where the contextual dependency among players emerge, characterizing the performance region as critical. Within these critical regions, the players' contextual dependency moves the system from equally poised options to a single option, that emerges under the influence of task and environmental constraints. In other words, within these critical regions, creativity occurs as ongoing performance solutions emerge and are annihilated, until a sudden change occurs where a single, i.e. creative solution, emerges (Passos *et al.* 2009). In this sense, within critical regions, *exploratory* metastable behaviour emerges as a precursor to the *creative product*, i.e. the single solution. Hence, both the exploratory and product phase of creative behaviour exist (Drazin *et al.* 1999 and Sternberg and Lubart 1996). The players' contextual dependency creates local information that originates at a specific moment in time and space where a gap in the defensive system emerges and the attackers exploit it to move closer to the goal or even score. This process underlines the notion that creativity in team sports is based upon a self-organization mechanism that only occurs within critical regions.

Creativity in team sports is sustained by the nonlinear interactions among players, which enable nonproportional, abrupt and unpredictable environment for the opponents. As in any other social system, the way that each player interacts with others in the neighbourhood of play influences the behaviours of players within the same team and this is a requisite to disturb the actions of opponents (Fajen *et al.* 2009). From an attacker's perspective, the decisions of the ball carrier and support players are based on the perceptions that they have created of the defenders' relative positioning, running-line trajectories and proximity to each other (Passos *et al.* 2008). On the other hand, the decision making of defenders depends on the perception that they have of the ball carrier's actions as well as the behaviours of the support players (Passos *et al.* 2008). These variables include interpersonal distances, the speed and running-line trajectories that contain important information concerning the attackers' ability to perform different actions. These variables contain information that are perceived by the players and specify the action possibilities of each opponent or teammate (Gunns *et al.* 2002; Weast *et al.* 2011). This is where creativity emerges, with the need for attackers to perform deceptive actions that creates the impression of multiple different possibilities for action. These deceptive actions can also be characterized by intrateam coordination, where attackers perform a set of previous established movements that are intended to open a space–time window against a stable opposing team. This is when creativity is needed again and players need to reorganize, avoiding defenders. This reorganization process is grounded on situational information concerning defenders' relative positions, number, speed and distance to goal (Travassos *et al.* 2011; Cordovil *et al.* 2009; Passos *et al.*

2011). These sources function as task constraints that attackers use to avoid defenders. The reorganization of attackers is grounded on situational information that emerges because of opponent players' nonlinear interactions and is self-organized.

Typically, attacker–defender interactions are characterized with many subtle fluctuations in the attacker–defender balance but also with few abrupt changes in the attacker–defender structural organization, meaning that suddenly the attackers gain an advantage and are in a crucial position to score.

To summarize, in this chapter, we have outlined a model of creative exploration and solution (product) emergence as a soft-assembly of actions under ecological constraints. The obtained structural and dynamical hierarchy of the creative behaviour, consistent with the model predictions, was demonstrated in a contact improvisation dance example. The creative process unfolds on *different timescales*, owing to the hierarchical structure of the perception–action landscape. Hence, creativity is a nested process, both structurally and temporally. The experimental examples provided here are extensions of those in Hristovski *et al.* (2011), where an emergence of a novel punch in martial arts was treated within the framework of the same theoretical model. The role of slowly changing or constant environmental and personal constraints, (i.e. gravity and morpho-anatomical structure in creative exploratory activity) is provided by their slow contextualizing function. Quickly changing and stochastic physical and informational constraints form the base of the unpredictability function in creativity. Through this process they mould the goal-directed activity of complex systems potentially leading to inventions of new movement forms or team actions. By manipulation of these key constraints, athletes structure different types of contexts which eventually lead to soft-assembly of novel forms of actions. In this way, highly motivated athletes, by self-generated experimentation in the full space of constraints, may facilitate the emergence of new and functional action forms.

References

Araújo, D., Davids, K., Bennett, S., Button, C. and Chapman, G. (2004) Emergence of sport skills under constraints, in A. M. Williams and N. J. Hodges (ed.) *Skill Acquisition in Sport: Research, Theory and Practice*. London: Taylor and Francis, pp. 409–33.

Araújo, D., Davids, K. and Hristovski, R. (2006) The ecological dynamics of decision making in sport. *Psychology of Sport and Exercise*, 7: 653–76.

Bartlett, R. M. (2007) Introduction to Sport Biomechanics: Analysing Human Movement Patterns, 2nd edn. London: Routledge.

Bressler, S. L. and Kelso, J. A. S. (2001) Cortical coordination dynamics and cognition. *Trends in Cognitive Sciences*, 5 (1): 26–36.

Bril, B., Roux, V. and Dietrich, G. (2005) Stone knapping: Khambhat (India), a unique opportunity? in V. Roux and B. Bril (eds) *Stone Knapping, the Necessary Conditions for an Uniquely Hominid Behaviour*. McDonald Institute Monograph Series, Cambridge: McDonald Institute for Archaeological Research, pp. 53–72.

Castañer, M., Torrents, C., Anguera, M. T., Dinušova, M. and Jonsson G. M. (2009) Identifying and analyzing motor skill responses in body movement and dance. *Behavior*

Research Methods, 41 (3): 857–67.

Challet, D., Marsili, M. and Zecchina, R. (2000) Statistical mechanics of systems with heterogeneous agents: minority games. *Physical Review Letters*, 84 (8): 1824–7.

Chow, J. Y., Davids, K., Button, C., Shuttleworth, R., Renshaw, I. and Araújo, D. (2006) Nonlinear pedagogy: a constraints-led framework to understand emergence of game play and skills. *Nonlinear Dynamics, Psychology and Life Sciences*, 10 (1): 74–104.

Chow, J. Y., Davids, K., Button, C. and Rein, R. (2008) Dynamics of movement patterning in learning a discrete multiarticular action. *Motor Control*, 12 (3): 219–40.

Cordovil, R., Araujo, D., Davids, K., Gouveia, L., Barreiros, J. and Fernandes, O. and Serpa, S. (2009) The influence of instructions and body-scaling as constraints on decision-making processes in team sports. *European Journal of Sport Sciences*, 9 (3): 169–79.

Davids, K., Araújo, D., Shuttleworth, R. and Button, C. (2003) Acquiring skill in sport: A constraints-led perspective. *International Journal of Computer Sciences in Sport*, 2: 31–9.

Davids, K., Renshaw, I. and Glazier, P. (2005) Movement models from sports reveal fundamental insights into coordination processes. *Exercise and Sport Science Reviews*, 33: 36–42.

Davids, K., Button, C., and Bennett, S. (2008) *Dynamics of Skill Acquisition. A Constraints-led Approach*. Champaign: Human Kinetics

Davids, K., Araújo, D., Vilar, L., Renshaw, I. and Pinder, R. (2013) An ecological dynamics approach to skill acquisition: implications for development of talent in sport. *Talent Development and Excellence*, 5 (1): 21–34.

Domany, E., Hed, G., Palassini, M. and Young, A. P. (2001) State hierarchy induced by correlated spin domains in short-range spin glasses. *Physical Review B*, 64: 224–406.

Drazin, R., Glynn, M. A. and Kazanjian, R. K. (1999) Multilevel theorizing about creativity in organizations: a sensemaking perspective. *Academy of Management Review*, 24: 286–307.

Fajen, B., Riley, M. and Turvey, M. (2009) Information, affordances and the control of action in sport. *International Journal of Sport Psychology*, 40: 79–107.

Gunns, R. E., Johnston, L. and Hudson, S. M. (2002) Victim selection and kinematics: a point-light investigation of vulnerability to attack. *Journal of Nonverbal Behavior*, 26 (3): 129–58.

Haken, H., Kelso, J. A. S. and Bunz, H. A. (1985) Theoretical model of phase transitions in human hand movements. *Biological Cybernetics*, 51: 347–56.

Hristovski, R., Davids, K. and Araújo, D. (2006) Affordance – controlled bifurcations of action patterns in martial arts. *Nonlinear Dynamics, Psychology and Life Sciences*, 4: 409–44.

Hristovski, R. and Davids, K. (2008) Metastability and situated creativity in sport. Paper presented at the 2nd International Congress of Complex Systems in Sport, 4–8 November, Madeira, Portugal.

Hristovski, R., Davids, K. and Araújo, D. (2009) Information for regulating action in sport: metastability and emergence of tactical solutions under ecological constraints, in D. Araújo, H. Ripoll and M. Raab (eds) *Perspectives on Cognition and Action in Sport*. New York: Nova Science Publishers, pp. 43–57.

Hristovski, R., Davids, K., Araújo, D. and Passos, P. (2011) Constraints-induced emergence of functional novelty in complex neurobiological systems: a basis for creativity in sport. *Nonlinear Dynamics, Psychology and Life Sciences*, 15 (2): 175–206.

Hristovski, R., Davids, K., Passos, P. and Araújo, D. (2012) Sport performance as a domain of creative problem solving for self-organizing performer–environment systems. *Open*

Sports Science Journal, 5 (Suppl 1-M4): 26–35.

Joliffe, I. T. (2002) *Principal Component Analysis*, 2nd edn. New York: Springer.

Kello, C. T., Anderson, G. G., Holden, J. G. and Van Orden, G. C. (2008) The pervasiveness of 1/f scaling in speech reflects the metastable basis of cognition. *Cognitive Science*, 32 (7): 1217–31.

Newell, K. M. (1986) Constraints on the development of coordination, in M. G. Wade and H. T. A. Whiting (eds) *Motor Development in Children. Aspects of Coordination and Control*. Dordrecht, Netherlands: Martinus Nijhoff, pp. 341–60.

Parisi, G. (1979) Infinite number of order parameters for spin-glasses. *Physical Review Letters*, 43: 1754–6.

Passos, P., Araújo, D., Davids, K., Gouveia, L., Milho, J. and Serpa, S. (2008) Information-governing dynamics of attacker–defender interactions in youth rugby union. *Journal of Sports Sciences*, 26 (13): 1421–9.

Passos, P., Araújo, D., Davids, K., Gouveia, L., Serpa, S., Milho, J. and Fonseca, S. (2009) Interpersonal pattern dynamics and adaptive behavior in multi-agent neurobiological systems: a conceptual model and data. *Journal of Motor Behavior*, 41 (5): 445–59.

Passos, P., Milho, J., Fonseca, S., Borges, J., Araújo, D. and Davids, K. (2011) Interpersonal distance regulates functional grouping tendencies of agents in team sports. *Journal of Motor Behavior*, 43 (2): 155–63.

Pinder, R., Davids, K. and Renshaw I. (2012) Metastability and emergent performance of dynamic interceptive actions, *Journal of Science and Medicine in Sport*, 15 (1): 1–7.

Reader, S. M. and Laland, K. N. (2001) Primate innovation: sex, age, and social rank differences. *International Journal of Primatology*, 22: 787–805.

Saxton, M. (1996) Anomalous diffusion due to binding: a Monte Carlo study. *Biophysical Journal*, 70: 1250–62.

Sternberg, R. J. and Lubart, T. I. (1996) Investing in creativity. *American Psychologist*, 51: 677–88.

Taylor, A. H., Elliffe, D., Hunt, G. R. and Gray, R. D. (2010) Complex cognition and behavioural innovation in New Caledonian crows. *Proceedings of the Royal Society B Biological Sciences*, 277 (1694): 2637–43.

Torrents, C., Castañer,M., Dinušova, M. and Anguera, M. T. (2010) Discovering new ways of moving: observational analysis of motor creativity while dancing contact improvisation and the influence of the partner. *Journal of Creative Behavior*, 44 (1): 45–61.

Travassos, B., Araújo, D., Vilar, L. and McGarry, T. (2011) Interpersonal coordination and ball dynamics in futsal (indoor football) *Human Movement Science*, 30 (6): 1245–59.

Weast, J. A., Shockley, K. and Riley, M. A. (2011) The influence of athletic experience and kinematic information on skill-relevant affordance perception. *Quarterly Journal of Experimental Psychology*, 64 (4): 689–706.

Part 4

Complexity sciences and training for sport

16 Variability in neurobiological systems and training

Chris Button, Ludovic Seifert, David O'Donovan and Keith Davids

Variability in achieving consistent performance outcomes has become increasingly recognized as important in preparing for dynamic performance contexts like sport. Here, we examine the theoretical basis for viewing variability as functional and examine the implications for understanding training for sport in individual and team sports. The issue of a putative optimal movement pattern, common to all learners, is challenged. In this chapter, we describe motor expertise as the capacity to functionally adapt behaviours to satisfy key constraints in order to achieve intended performance outcomes. Darwin, amongst many others, recognized the fundamental value of individual variation and adaptation for the functional behaviour and long-term survival of biological organisms. Similarly, at the timescale of perception and action, success in sport is underpinned by the capacity of athletes to capitalize on their individual strengths and to respond appropriately to different challenges. Indeed, the principles of overload in physical training (i.e. frequency, intensity, duration, type) are built upon biological adaptation through which the human body becomes increasingly prepared to function more efficiently and to produce sufficient energy to attain higher performance goals. The importance of adaptability in motor control was originally raised by Bernstein (1996) when he conceptualized the notion of resourcefulness (i.e. stability and initiative) as an important property of an organism's dexterity (p. 221). Whilst performing a complex coordination pattern may be difficult for a learner in sport, more challenging is its functional adaptation to a specific performance context; i.e. in responding to interacting constraints (task, environmental, or organismic) that continually change over time (Newell 1986). Biryukova and Bril (2002) commented that 'the dexterity is not movements in themselves, but their ability to adapt to external constraints' (p. 65).

A corollary of these theoretical ideas is the acceptance that there is not one optimal pattern of coordination towards which all developing learners should aspire but, instead, that expertise concerns 'individual-constraint coupling' (Seifert *et al.* 2013). Davids and Glazier (2010) postulated that this requisite adaptability of complex movement systems was founded on pertinent neurobiological system properties including *degeneracy*, defined as 'the ability of elements that are structurally different to perform the same function or yield the same output' (Edelman and Gally 2001: 13763). They proposed that evidence of intra-individual movement variability often observed in experts could play a functional role; for instance, it could correspond to several types of movement and/or to the ability to use co-existing modes of coordination (i.e. exploit multi-stability and metastability in complex neurobiological systems). This relationship between multistability and metastability in expert performance illustrates the requisite subtle balance needed between stability and variability in sport perform-ance (Jantzen *et al*. 2008), which arises from the complex interactions between intentions, actions and perceptions of individual performers.

Traditionally, there has been an overriding tendency to define expertise as the capacity to both reproduce a specific movement pattern consistently and to increase the automaticity of movement (Seifert *et al*. 2013). In representational accounts of expertise, movement variability is seen as noise (i.e. an artefact limit-ing the system's processing of data input and output), which should be minimized (Summers and Anson 2009). Interestingly, in recent times, several computational models of control have surfaced, attempting to cast the problem of variability for motor control in a more positive light (i.e. computational modelling, Wolpert *et al*. 2003; optimal control theory, Todorov and Jordon 2002). However, for some time, research from a dynamical systems theoretical orientation has shown that movement system variability is not noise detrimental to performance, error or deviation from a putative expert model, which should be corrected in the begin-ner. Movement system variability instead indicates the functional flexibility needed to respond to dynamic performance constraints (Davids *et al*. 2003). In this context, Schöllhorn *et al*. (2009) have more radically argued for the value of adding noise to the initial conditions of performance to stimulate learning by forc-ing the individual to adapt to varying constraints of the context.

The functional role of variability has been historically overlooked by researchers because of the types of tasks studied (e.g. pursuit tracking) and limi-tations of data collection and analysis tools. For example, Newell and Slifkin (1998) indicated that the magnitude of performance variability has traditionally been assessed by the standard deviation or variance over trials; these statistical indicators attempt to characterize the data distribution and the amount of noise in a single measurement. The standard deviation measure indicates the *magnitude* of variability (i.e. the amplitude, the spatial aspect of the distribution of performance over trials) but not the *structure* of system variability (Newell and Slifkin 1998). Instead, studying the temporal structure of variability by spectral analysis of noise provides information on its deterministic or stochastic nature. In this chapter, we overview empirical research from sports science employing a range of emerging data analysis tools more suited to examining the structure of movement variabil-ity (for a review of variability analysis in medicine, see Bravi *et al*. 2011). As we will demonstrate in a later section, the functional role of movement variability has typically been explored in performance of ball skills. Our aim for this chapter is to extend our breadth of understanding by exemplifying how intra-individual and inter-individual movement variability could play a functional role in a range of physical activities common to sport, such as different forms of locomotion, object manipulation and team invasion games.

Functional movement variability in sport

Gait

Human gait is seemingly characterized by smooth, regular, repeating patterns. The 'control problem' in terms of mechanical regulation of gait is that there are many more muscle actuators involved than independent equations that define the system (Vaughan 1996). In fact, when analyzed in detail, there are notable stride-to-stride fluctuations even under constant environmental conditions (Hausdorff 2007) and these fluctuations seem to be a prominent feature when key parameters such as gait speed and balance are considered (i.e. Jordan *et al.* 2006, 2007; van Emmerik and Wagennar 1996). Hausdorff (2007) suggests that fluctuations in the stride interval exhibit long range, fractal-like correlations similar to those found in heartrate beat fluctuations. Put simply, in the short term, the stride interval is dependent on other nearby cycles but this dependency weakens in a power-law fashion. Interestingly, the fractal scaling underpinning gait dynamics differs significantly for subgroups who exhibit much less stable and effective gait patterns (e.g. infants and the elderly; Hausdorff 2007).

These ideas were demonstrated in a study by Jordan *et al.* (2007) who required participants to walk for 12-minute trials at 80%, 90%, 100%, 110% and 120% of their preferred walking speed. A range of gait-cycle variables was investigated, including the intervals and lengths of steps and strides and the impulse from the vertical ground reaction force profile. Detrended fluctuation analysis revealed the presence of U-shaped long range correlations in gait-cycle variables. The reduced strength of long-range correlations at certain locomotion speeds (100–110%) was interpreted as reflective of enhanced stability and adaptability at preferred speeds (see also Li *et al.* 2005).

Button *et al.* (2010) pointed out that stable attractor states in healthy and pathological gaits are an important, functional feature of stable coordination and intra-individual and inter-individual variability amongst these patterns are discernible with the appropriate analysis tools. It seems that such differences are more likely to be identified when using time-continuous analysis tools (i.e. self-organizing Kohonen maps) rather than summative, discrete statistics (Schöllhorn *et al.* 2002). For example, a number of discernible patterns can be detected from the phase relations of pelvis and thorax segments as gait speed changes (van Emmerik and Wagenaar 1996). Stability analysis of relative phase and range of motion data have also been used to identify hysteresis effects in transitions between stable patterns (i.e. direction of speed dependent).

A particularly distinctive form of gait (i.e. competitive race walking) has also been considered in relation to functional variability. Donà *et al.* (2009) explored the use of functional principal component analysis for assessing and classifying the kinematics of the knee joint in competitive race walkers. Functional principal component analysis was applied bilaterally to the sagittal knee angle data, because knee joint motion is fundamental to race walking technique. Scatterplots of principal component scores provided evidence of athletes' technical differences and asymmetries, even when traditional analysis (mean plus or minus standard deviation curves) was not effective. Whilst there were certain features, such as the absence of a flight phase, that were common for all seven participants, principal components provided indications for the classification of race walkers and identified potentially important technical differences between higher- and lower-skilled athletes (Donà *et al.* 2009).

Bradshaw *et al.* (2007) were also interested in whether skilled athletes showed evidence of functional variability, in this case related to the sprint start. Indeed, high biological movement variability (in comparison with systematic error) was observed for the joint velocities of ten track sprinters. Of particular interest, regression analysis indicated that a decrease in ten-metre sprint time was associated with an increase in the variability of the lead ankle step velocity.

From this brief overview, it is apparent that functional variability manifested as stride-to-stride fluctuations is a consistent feature of several types of gait patterns (e.g. walking, running, sprinting). Movement variability is most noticeable around transitions in speed, which is an underlying feature of all types of gait that contribute to balance and stability. It is relevant to note that only certain kinds of data analysis tools were suited to detecting the functional fluctuations that subserve gait dynamics.

Breaststroke swimming

Whether locomoting on ground, over an object or through aquatic environments, it seems that biological organisms exhibit strong preferences and many global similarities in terms of the cyclical patterns they use to move. In skilled breaststrokers, one cycle is composed of an alternation of propulsions (i.e. arm propulsion during the leg glide; leg propulsion during the arm glide), a brief glide time with the body fully extended and a synchronization of arm and leg recoveries (Chollet *et al.* 2004). In comparison with beginners, during performance, skilled swimmers display a high level of intra-individual coordination pattern variability, exemplified by a high intracyclic knee and elbow angular variability and several modes of arm–leg coordination, depending on swim speed (Seifert *et al.* 2010). Expert swimmers need to organize different coordination patterns for each performance phase. They display an out-of-phase pattern of coordination of their arms and legs during propulsion (i.e. flexion or extension of a pair of limbs while the other pair of limbs is fixed in extension), an in-phase coordination mode during glide (i.e. extension of the arms and legs) and an anti-phase coordination mode during recoveries (i.e. extension of the arms during leg flexion) (Seifert *et al.* 2010; Figure 16.1). In a cycle of 1.5–2.0 seconds, expert swimmers are able to alternate between these three modes of coordination.

In contrast, owing to their different mix of intentions, perceptions and actions, learner swimmers typically demonstrate low intra-individual coordination variability but very high inter-individual coordination variability (Figure 16.1), notably a bi-stability of the arm–leg coordination modes that could lead to several intermediate profiles. The first coordination mode corresponds to an isocontraction of the nonhomologous limbs: that is, the in-phase muscle contraction of the

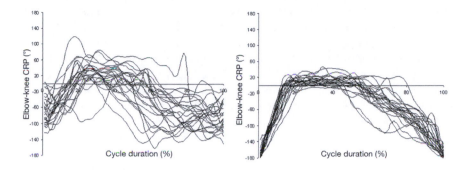

Figure 16.1 Continuous relative phase (CRP) between elbow and knee through a complete cycle for 24 beginners (left panel) and for 24 expert swimmers (right panel), showing lower inter-individual variability for experts

arms and legs (Baldissera *et al.* 1991). One way to enhance system stability is to synchronize the flexion movements of both arms and legs, as well as the extension movements like an 'accordion', supporting emergence of low intracyclic arm–leg coordination variability (Figure 16.1). The accordion mode of coordination corresponds to a superposition of two contradictory actions (Seifert *et al.* 2010): leg propulsion during arm recovery and arm propulsion during leg recovery. It is not mechanically effective and does not provide high swim speed because each propulsive action is thwarted by a recovery action. As observed in other studies of interlimb coordination, this coordination mode appears to be the most stable and the easiest to perform for learners (for an overview, see Kelso 1995).

The second mode of coordination often observed in beginners is the flexion movement of one set of limbs that occurs during the extension of the other set, following the principle of isodirection, which consists of making movements in the same direction (e.g. arms and legs go forward or backward on the longitudinal axis; Baldissera *et al.* 1991). This arm–leg coordination corresponds to a superposition of the propulsive phases of the arms and legs. When the superposition of these two propulsions is complete, the arm–leg coordination pattern resembles the movements of 'windscreen wipers' and shows low intracyclic coordination variability. Finally, although there is bi-stability in the modes of arm–leg coordination of beginning breaststroke swimmers, several combinations of these two modes of coordination may arise for a variety of reasons. From a constraint-led approach, the emergent behaviours of learners are understandable, because they relate to the overarching need to maintain buoyancy, stability and breathing capacity in aquatic environments. These suggestions were supported by a cluster analysis of the movement patterns of 24 beginning swimmers (Seifert *et al.* 2011b). The emergent movement patterns were: (i) stable coordination modes, based on principles of isocontraction and/or isodirection; (ii) indicative of beginners in an exploratory phase with regard to environmental constraints; and (iii) the task constraint or goal of the action 'propel the body forward and fast' imposed by the teacher or coach was perceived differently by beginners. This was because their priority was not just to move forward in the water but also to balance (e.g. to stay in a ventral position), float (e.g. to stay at the water surface) and breathe (e.g. to avoid bringing hands to the chest in order to keep the head above water) and see in the aquatic environment.

In summary, these comparisons between the movement patterns of beginners and expert breaststroke swimmers reveal the influence of different intentional constraints. The findings stimulate a number of interesting practical questions, including: (i) whether beginners should be encouraged to imitate expert swimmers; and (ii), whether coordination patterns observed in beginning swimmers should be considered as 'full of errors' simply because they differ from a putative ideal movement model based on an analysis of expert swimmers. A novice's movement pattern may actually reflect different performance priorities, compared with an expert (i.e. in swimming to maintain buoyancy, rather than the intention of advancing rapidly through the water).

Ice-climbing

The way in which intentions, actions and perception of information guide movement pattern formation has also been shown in a study of ice climbers (Seifert *et al.* 2011a). Ice climbing involves climbing with ice tools in each hand and crampons on each foot on frozen water falls, the properties of which vary stochastically in shape, steepness, temperature, thickness and ice density. Since these environmental constraints are neither predictable or controllable, this task requires successful climbers to use numerous types of movements (e.g. swinging, kicking and hooking actions) and patterns of interlimb coordination (e.g. horizontally, diagonally and vertically located angular positions) during performance by exploiting complex neurobiological system properties of degeneracy and multistability. For instance, climbers could either swing their ice tools to create their own holes or hook an existing hole (owing to the actions of previous climbers or by exploiting the presence of natural holes), supporting the functional role of intra-individual variability. Seifert *et al.* (2011a) examined the performance of beginners and skilled climbers as they climbed a frozen waterfall. They assessed interlimb coordination patterns by using the angle between the horizontal line and the displacement of the heads of the left- and right-hand ice tools for the upper-limb coordination. Lower-limb coordination patterns corresponded to the angle between the horizontal line and the displacement of the left and right crampons (Figure 16.2).

When both groups of climbers climbed an ice fall with a quasi-vertical slope (range between 80–90 degrees), beginners showed low levels of intra-individual movement and interlimb coordination variability, as they varied their upper-limb and lower-limb coordination patterns much less frequently and extensively than the experts. As in the study of the novice breaststroke swimmers, Seifert *et al.*

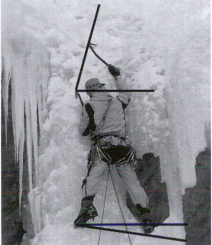 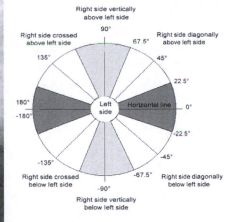

Figure 16.2 Angle between horizontal, left limb and right limb (left panel); modes of limb coordination as regards the angle value between horizontal, left limb and right limb (right panel). The angle between the horizontal line and the left and right limbs was positive when the right limb was above the left limb and negative when the right limb was below the left limb

(2011a) observed patterns of movement that were indicative of the intentions idiosyncratic to this group. Beginners mostly used horizontally and diagonally located angular positions (since limb anchorages are at the same level for the horizontal angle, the arms or legs appear in an in-phase coordination mode). This highly stable behaviour resembled climbing up a ladder and led them to maintain a static 'X' body position with arms and legs extended or with arms flexed and legs extended, corresponding to a freezing of the degrees of freedom of the motor system. Owing to their lack of attunement to information from properties of the ice fall, novices tended to swing their ice tools and kick with their crampons more frequently than experts, in patterns synonymous with achieving deep anchorages, instead of exploiting existing holes in the ice fall. Like the novice breaststrokers, the novice ice climbers tended to prioritize stability and security of posture in interacting with environmental constraints, rather than speed and efficiency of movement.

Conversely, expert ice climbers showed high intra-individual movement and coordination pattern variability as they exploited affordances in the specific ice-fall properties. The efficient individual–environment coupling of the experts was probably predicated on neurobiological system degeneracy (Edelman and Gally 2001), since they varied the types of movement and the interlimb coordination modes they exploited to achieve their task goals. Indeed, the multistability of their complex movement systems allowed them: (i) to swing the ice tools and to kick the crampons in many different ways – in horizontal, diagonal, vertical and crossed angular positions (for instance, crossing the arms is not a natural action but it enabled experts to exploit information and hook existing holes in the ice fall); and (ii), to hook the ice tools into already existing holes (i.e. exploiting information on the shape of the ice fall) and to place the crampons in the holes previously made by their own ice tools, instead of using repetitive ice-tool swinging and crampon kicking as observed in beginners.

As in swimming, an individual's behaviours relate to differentiated intentions and perception of the task and environmental constraints. Notably, the beginners were functioning independently of the icefall properties, because they were mainly focusing on keeping their equilibrium, with respect to gravity, under control. These observations suggest that manipulation of task constraints by a coach or teacher would enable the beginners to further interact with the icefall properties in a secure learning environment, to balance their independency/dependency to the environmental constraints and to gradually support the emergence of a wider repertoire of movement and multi-stability of coordination patterns (Seifert *et al.* 2011a).

Throwing: Boccia

Goal-directed throwing actions typically need to balance the requirements of speed and accuracy and the manipulation of task goals is a powerful constraint on emergent throwing patterns. For example, in throwing tasks, the alteration of target location simultaneously imposes constraints on both movement speed (and by extension movement force) and accuracy. Variability in movement kinematics has been demonstrated in throwing tasks including javelin (Bartlett *et al.* 1996), basketball (Button *et al.* 2003), underarm (Kudo *et al.* 2000) and overarm throwing (Wagner *et al.* 2012) and a Frisbee®-throwing task (Yang and Scholz 2005).

This body of work confirms that kinematic variability is influenced by task constraints. In precision throwing tasks, the relative invariance in inter-trial spatial release points (Hirashima *et al.* 2002) of thrown objects and decreases in kinematic variability closer to object release (Wagner *et al.* 2012) point to the observed variability in joint parameters serving a functional purpose. For example, increased variability in distal joints like the elbow and wrist probably compensate for variations in proximal joints like the shoulder, in that individuals can use a number of joint configurations to maintain desired sets of release parameters (e.g. height, speed, and angle) to satisfy various task constraints.

Compensatory variability has also been observed in a three-dimensional kinematic analysis of athletes with motor system disorders, such as cerebral palsy. Cerebral palsy is a clinical term summarizing a group of non-progressive conditions arising from damage to the brain during early development. Individuals with cerebral palsy display obvious movement difficulties in performing tasks of everyday living, typically showing longer, slower movements, with disturbed speeds and trajectories, particularly at the elbow, wrist, and fingers (Jaspers *et al.* 2009).

Boccia is a precision throwing sport in the Paralympics, similar in nature to lawn bowls or the French game of pétanque. It is played indoors on a firm, flat surface, where the aim of the game is to land six balls closer to the target ball than the balls thrown by an opponent. The sport requires a high degree of muscle control, concentration and tactical awareness. O'Donovan *et al.* (2011) recorded the kinematics of four cerebral palsy athletes who had competed at the Paralympics. In this study, the athletes were required to throw to four different distances (three metres, five metres, seven metres and nine metres). Three-dimensional movement analysis showed that the athletes displayed kinematic variability comparable to typically developed persons but in the context of distinctly individual movement patterns arising from the organismic constraints imposed by their type of cerebral palsy. Adopting an underarm, typically pendulum-like throwing style, all four athletes produced relatively invariant ball release locations, despite systematically adjusting key release parameters (primarily adapting release angle and speed to changes in target distance) to modify the distance thrown. Distal joints (e.g. elbow and wrist) typically showed increased relative variability compared with proximal joints (e.g. shoulder), indicating that kinematic variability is necessary to adapt to task constraints and preserve release parameters in throwing (Figure 16.3).

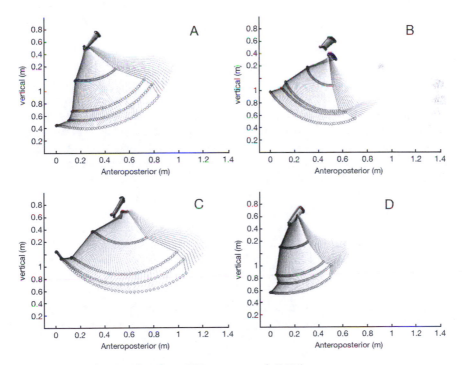

Figure 16.3 Trajectory plots from O'Donovan *et al.* (2011)

Southard (2002) showed that unskilled participants demonstrated highly coupled coordination between the wrist and elbow during overarm throwing for speed, whereas experts exploited a less rigidly coupled joint synergy to transfer energy from biomechanical sequencing. Skilled throwers were able to flexibly and robustly adapt to changes in target size and position, as reflected by less frequent coordination changes compared with lower-skilled throwers and scaling of preferred movement patterns (Bartlett *et al.* 2007). That being said, even skilled performances show intra- and inter-individual differences, indicating that, even in homogenous groups such as elite athletes and people with disabilities, there is no optimal coordination solution for any given task (Glazier and Davids 2009).

Team invasion games: Association football (soccer)

In comparison with precision-throwing actions, movement variability is much more obvious, even to the untrained observer, in team invasion games such as soccer. Rapid technological developments in player tracking systems now provide movement analysts with an intriguing opportunity of measuring the coordination dynamics between teams and players in competition. For example, Frencken *et al.* (2011) measured player positions at 45 Hz in small-sided games used in training. Two measures were proposed as candidate collective variables: a position representing the average position of the players in the team and some measure of the dispersion or spread of the team. The most robust average position is the team centroid, calculated from the mean of the players' positions. Frencken *et al.* (2011) report strong positive correlations for the team centroids of the outfield players across each entire game. Hence, teams as a whole moved together (in-phase coordination) across the course of a game. Indeed, the analysis by Lames *et al.* (2010) of different sports team centroids indicates that similar principles may underpin the collective organization of teams in invasion games.

Duarte *et al.* (2012) also found a strong symmetrical relation between the centroids of the two teams in three-a-side soccer games. Importantly, as the play proceeded to critical moments (i.e. when a final pass was made to a shooter) the distance between the team's centroids decreased. The authors interpreted this feature as a necessary loss in stability between the teams before a decisive moment, such as a shot or a turnover in possession. The surface area of the teams was highly variable, although the attacking team typically covered a greater area of the pitch. Therefore, it seems that either the surface area of the teams in small-sided games does not capture the coordination dynamics well (see also Frencken *et al.* 2011) or that stable states of play are not a common feature of small-sided games.

Various measures can be used to express the dispersion of sports teams. For example, Bourbousson *et al.* (2010) used a 'stretch index' to define the average distance of the players in a basketball team from the team centroid. Moura *et al.* (2012) analyzed player trajectory information from eight Brazilian First Division Championship matches involving 16 different teams. From visual inspection of the graphs for pairs of teams in all games and throughout each game, they considered that the two teams' Frobenius norms (average interpersonal distance for all outfield players), showed anti-phase relationships, whereas the team surface areas did not. Both dispersion measures indicated that, when a team lost possession, the team dispersion decreased; when a team gained possession, the dispersion increased. Additionally, teams had greater Frobenius norms and surface areas defending when a shot was made on their goal than when they tackled ($P < 0.01$). When attacking, teams had greater Frobenius norms and surface areas when they were tackled than when they shot at goal. Hence, compression of both the defending and attacking team's Frobenius norm and surface area was beneficial to performance in those plays.

Clearly, the movement patterns of individual players in a soccer match are coupled with the movements of teammates and opponents. These functional groupings allow a defending team to protect their goal whilst also permitting the attacking side to probe for space and time to shoot. Nested beneath the level of grouped actions in competitive football sits a layer of individual player variability, the unpredictable nature of which contributes to the exciting, dynamic nature of the world's most spectated sport (Bartlett *et al.* 2012).

Team invasion games: Field hockey

Although field hockey has received much less consideration than association football in the sports science literature, interesting data have recently been reported by Brétigny *et al.* (2011) concerning inter-individual variability. The aim of this study was to determine coordination profiles for the field hockey drive. Nine elite female players accustomed to different playing positions (i.e. defenders, midfielders and attackers) were asked to play drive shots typical of a game situation. The high standard deviation values in joint kinematics were indicative of inter-individual variability; that is, several drive solutions. Cluster analysis of the upper-body kinematics identified two distinct profiles among the nine expert players. For the two profiles, the global coordination pattern of movement was in-phase for the right arm and out-of-phase for the left lead arm, suggesting a segmental sequencing. This interlimb organization represents the deep layer of the movement and stayed unchanged across the different field roles. Conversely, the task constraints and, more particularly, the temporal pressure typically encountered at each field role, affected the superficial layer of the movement (i.e. kinematic parameters). Notably, the initial phase of the drive movement (represented by the backswing) was not universal but, conversely, a ground for technical profiles. Players achieved a compromise between: (i) long total and relative backswing durations, which permit adaptations to task constraints and increase drive amplitude to provide great velocity to the ball but which also increase the risks of opponents' interceptions; (ii) short total and relative backswing durations, which are a real advantage in contexts of temporal pressure as the preparation time is shortened but which can be detrimental in terms of adaptation and ball velocity.

It was suggested that the short-grip drive was very useful in contexts of temporal pressure (Bretigny *et al.* 2011). As the hands are placed lower on the stick shaft, the lever arm is shorter, resulting in smaller overall amplitudes and shorter durations in comparison with the classic field-hockey drive. Preparation time (backswing and downswing) is thus reduced, with no loss in ball velocity. This stick-holding technique seems best adapted by midfielders and forwards. Several participants played these roles and formed the 'temporal-effectiveness group'. They had shorter drives and smaller overall amplitudes. The velocity variables, especially ball velocity, were not as high but drive rapidity gave them an important advantage in the context of temporal pressure. The performance level did not differ among these two groups but the task constraints from one field role to another varied greatly, leading to different expert profiles. Similar to the golf swing, for which two weight transfer styles were identified (Ball and Best 2007), expert field-hockey drive performance has no universal solution. The participants were able to exploit the stability and variability of their expert movement patterns to functionally adapt to dynamic task constraints (exemplified by the exploitation of the short grip drive in some performance circumstances).

Summary and practical implications

In this brief review of functional movement variability in sport, it has been demonstrated that both inter- and intra-individual variability is an inherent feature of performance across the broad continuum of expertise. The enhanced focus on variability in movement at an individual level has resulted from changes in theoretical influences in the literature on motor control and from advances in data collection and analysis techniques. The existence of inter-individual variability implies that there is no optimal movement pattern for a given activity and that movement expertise is a reflection of the performer's ability to adapt to dynamic constraints. Intra-individual variability shows us that an individual must reciprocally link their actions with relevant environmental information to consistently achieve performance outcomes. Characterizing learners as complex, biological systems promotes awareness by practitioners that a learner's coordination solutions are the products of self-organization and that periods of movement variability (or instability) should be valued as part of the learning process (Chow *et al.* 2007).

To encourage acquisition of functionally relevant coordination solutions performer–environment interactions should be manipulated through altering relevant task, environmental and performer constraints. Thereby, constraints operate on different timescales, which has important implications for the practitioner's judgment of the learner's rate of progress. When learning a new coordination pattern, more permanent behavioural changes take longer to appear than immediate adaptations to task constraints during practice. Practitioners should understand that some behaviours might represent transient adaptations to immediate task constraints imposed during practice, which interact with organismic constraints related to developmental status (Seifert *et al.* 2013).

A struggling learner can be viewed as a system that is temporarily trapped in a stable attractor state that does not correspond well with a behavioural solution satisfying task demands. As Davids *et al.* (2008) suggest to practitioners, a strategy of perturbing the movement system may be necessary to help the learner to let go of previous movement experiences. Techniques such as altering task constraints like rules, space, equipment and number of opponents are useful ways to induce variability in movement and encourage exploration for alternative information sources and movement solutions. Note that the learner may need additional encouragement and reassurance at this important stage, as performance could fluctuate as a consequence of the perceptual-motor reorganization.

In this chapter, we have demonstrated the value of employing individualized analyses in research on movement to gain a clearer picture of how performers exploit variability. As more studies employ methods such as coordination profiling and cluster analysis, researchers are becoming increasingly convinced that varied movement trajectories emerge from the interplay among the specific task, environmental and organismic constraints unique to each situation. This is particularly apparent within sport, where such factors change frequently and unexpectedly. As we have demonstrated, expert performers are increasingly recognized as having an ability to continually adapt their techniques as perceptual demands change. The mechanisms by which humans progress to this level of control as a function of learning or relearning provide a fruitful focus for future research.

References

Baldissera, F., Cavalleri, P., Marini, G. and Tassone, G. (1991) Differential control of in-phase and anti-phase coupling of rhythmic movements of ipsilateral hand and foot. *Experimental Brain Research*, 83: 375–80.

Ball, K. A. and Best, R. J. (2007) Different centre of pressure patterns within the golf stroke I: cluster analysis. *Journal of Sports Sciences*, 25: 757–70.

Bartlett, R., Muller, E., Lindinger, S., Brunner, F. and Morriss, C. (1996) Three-dimensional evaluation of the kinematic release parameters for javelin throwers of different skill levels. *Journal of Applied Biomechanics*, 12 (1): 58–71.

Bartlett, R., Wheat, J. and Robins, M. (2007) Is movement variability important for sports biomechanists? *Sports Biomechanics*, 6 (2): 224-43.

Bartlett, R., Button, C., Robins, M., Dutt Mazumder, A. and Kennedy, G. (2012) Analysing team coordination patterns from player movement trajectories in soccer: methodological considerations. *International Journal of Performance Analysis in Sport*, 12 (2): 398–424.

Bernstein, N. A. (1996) On dexterity and its development, in M. Latash and M. T. Turvey (eds) *Dexterity and its Development*. Mahwah, NJ: Lawrence Erlbaum Associates, pp. 1–244.

Biryukova E, and Bril, B. (2002) Bernstein et le geste technique. *Revue d'anthropologie des Connaissances*, 2: 49–68 [French].

Bourbousson, J., Seve, C. and McGarry, T. (2010) Space-time coordination dynamics in basketball: Part 2. The interaction between the two teams. *Journal of Sports Sciences*, 28: 349–58.

Bradshaw, E. J., Maulder, P. S. and Keogh, J. W. (2007) Biological movement variability during the sprint start: performance enhancement or hindrance? *Sports Biomechanics*, 6: 246–60.

Bravi, A., Longtin, A. and Seely, A. J. E. (2011) Review and classification of variability analysis techniques with clinical applications. *Biomedical Engineering Online*, 10: 90; doi: 10.1186/1475-925X-10-90. Available online at www.biomedical-engineering-online.com/content/10/1/90 (accessed 12 June 2013).

Bretigny, P., Leroy, D., Button, C., Chollet, D. and Seifert, L. (2011) Coordination profiles of the expert field hockey drive according to field roles. *Sports Biomechanics*, 10: 339–50.

Button, C., MacLeod, M., Sanders, R. and Coleman, S. (2003) Examining movement variability in the basketball free-throw action at different skill levels. *Research Quarterly for Exercise and Sport*, 74 (3): 257–69.

Button, C., Moyle, S. and Davids, K. (2010) Comparison of below-knee amputee gait performed overground and on a motorized treadmill. *Adapted Physical Activity Quarterly*, 27: 96–112.

Chollet, D., Seifert, L., Leblanc, H., Boulesteix, L. and Carter M. (2004) Evaluation of the arm-leg coordination in flat breaststroke. *International Journal of Sport Medicine*, 25: 486–95.

Chow, J. Y., Davids, K., Button, C., Shuttleworth, R., Renshaw, I. and Araújo, D. (2007) The role of nonlinear pedagogy in physical education. *Review of Educational Research*, 77: 251–78.

Davids, K. and Glazier, P. (2010) Deconstructing neurobiological coordination: the role of the biomechanics-motor control nexus. *Exercise and Sport Science Reviews*, 38: 86–90.

Davids, K., Glazier, P., Araújo, D. and Bartlett, R. M. (2003) Movement systems as dynamical systems: the role of functional variability and its implications for sports medicine. *Sports Medicine*, 33: 245–60.

Davids, K., Button, C. and Bennett, S. J. (2008) *Dynamics of Skill Acquisition: A Constraints-Led Approach*. Champaign, IL: Human Kinetics.

Donà, G., Preatoni, E., Cobelli, C., Rodano, R. and Harrison, A. J. (2009) Application of functional principal component analysis in race walking: an emerging methodology. *Sports Biomechanics*, 8 (4): 284–301.

Duarte, R., Araújo, D., Freire, L., Folgado, H., Fernandes, O. and Davids, K. (2012) Intra- and inter-group coordination patterns reveal collective behaviors of football players near the scoring zone. *Human Movement Science*, 31 (6): 1639–51.

Edelman, G. M. and Gally, J. A. (2001) Degeneracy and complexity in biological systems. *Proceedings of the National Academy of Sciences of the USA*, 98: 13763–8.

Frencken, W., Lemmink, K., Delleman, N. and Visscher, C. (2011) Oscillations of centroid position and surface area of soccer teams in small-sided games. *European Journal of Sport Science*, 11: 215–23.

Glazier, P. S. and Davids, K. (2009) The problem of measurement indeterminacy in complex neurobiological movement systems. *Journal of Biomechanics*, 42 (16): 2694–6.

Hausdorff, J. M. (2007) Gait dynamics, fractals and falls: finding meaning in the stride-to-stride fluctuations of human walking. *Human Movement Science*, 26 (4): 555–89.

Hirashima, M., Kadota, H., Sakurai, S., Kudo, K. and Ohtsuki, T. (2002) Sequential muscle activity and its functional role in the upper extremity and trunk during overarm throwing. *Journal of Sports Sciences*, 20 (4): 301–10.

Jantzen, K. J., Oullier, O. and Scott Kelso, J. A. (2008) Neuroimaging coordination dynamics in the sport sciences. *Methods*, 45: 325–35.

Jaspers, E., Desloovere, K., Bruyninckx, H., Molenaers, G., Klingels, K. and Feys, H. (2009) Review of quantitative measurements of upper limb movements in hemiplegic cerebral palsy. *Gait and Posture*, 30 (4): 395–404.

Jordan, K., Challis, J. H. and Newell, K. M. (2006) Long range correlations in the stride interval of running. *Gait and Posture*, 24: 120–5.

Jordan, K., Challis, J. H. and Newell, K. M. (2007) Walking speed influences on gait cycle variability. *Gait and Posture*, 26: 128–34.

Kelso, J. A. S. (1995) *Dynamic Patterns: The Self-Organization of Brain and Behavior*. Cambridge, MA: MIT Press.

Kudo, K., Tsutsui, S., Ishikura, T., Ito, T. and Yamamoto, Y. (2000) Compensatory coordination of release parameters in a throwing task. *Journal of Motor Behavior*, 32 (4): 337–45.

Lames, M., Erdmann, J. and Walter, F. (2010) Oscillations in football: order and disorder in spatial interactions between the two teams. *International Journal of Sport Psychology*, 41: 85–6.

Li, L., Haddad, J. and Hamill, J. (2005) Stability and variability may respond differently to changes in walking speed. *Human Movement Science*, 24 (2): 257–67.

Moura, F. A., Martins, L. E. B., Anido, R. D., De Barros, R. M. L. and Cunha, S. A. (2012) Quantitative analysis of Brazilian football players' organisation on the pitch. *Sports Biomechanics*, 11: 85–96.

Newell, K. M. (1986) Constraints on the development of coordination, in: M. G. Wade and H. T. A. Whiting (eds) *Motor Development in Children: Aspects of Coordination and Control*. Dordrecht, Netherlands: Martinus Nijhoff, 341–61.

Newell, K. M. and Slifkin, A. B. (1998) The nature of movement variability, in: J. P. Piek (ed.) *Motor Behavior and Human Skill: A Multidisciplinary Perspective*. Champaign, IL: Human Kinetics, pp. 14–60.

O'Donovan, D. P. (2011) Kinematics of throwing in paralympic boccia athletes with cerebral palsy. Unpublished Masters thesis, University of Otago. Available online at: http://otago.ourarchive.ac.nz/handle/10523/2009

Schöllhorn, W. I., Nigg, B. M., Stefanyshyn, D. J. and Liu, W. (2002) Identification of individual walking patterns using time discrete and time continuous data sets. *Gait and Posture*, 15: 180–6.

Schöllhorn, W. I., Mayer-Kress, G., Newell, K. M. and Michelbrink, M. (2009) Time scales of adaptive behavior and motor learning in the presence of stochastic perturbations. *Human Movement Science*, 28: 319–33.

Seifert, L., Leblanc, H., Chollet, D. and Delignières, D. (2010) Inter-limb coordination in swimming: effect of speed and skill level. *Human Movement Science*, 29: 103–13.

Seifert, L., Wattebled, L., L'Hermette, M. and Hérault, R. (2011a) Inter-limb coordination variability in ice climbers of different skill level. *Education and Physical Training in Sport*, 1: 63–8.

Seifert, L., Leblanc, H., Herault, R., Komar, J., Button, C. and Chollet, D. (2011b) Interindividual variability in the upper-lower limb breaststroke coordination. *Human Movement Science*, 30: 550–65.

Seifert, L., Button, C. and Davids, K. (2013) Key properties of expert movement systems in sport: an ecological dynamics perspective. *Sports Medicine*, 43 (3): 167–78.

Southard, D. (2002) Change in throwing pattern: critical values for control parameter of velocity. *Research Quarterly for Exercise and Sport*, 73 (4): 396–407.

Summers, J. J. and Anson, J. G. (2009) Current status of the motor program: revisited. *Human Movement Science*, 28: 566–77.

Todorov, E. and Jordan, M. I. (2002) Optimal feedback control as a theory of motor coordination. *Nature Neuroscience*, 5 (11), 1226–35.

van Emmerik, R. E. A. and Wagenaar, R. C. (1996) Effects of walking velocity on relative phase dynamics in the trunk in human walking. *Journal of Biomechanics*, 29 (9): 1175–84.

Vaughan, C. L. (1996) Are joint torques the Holy Grail of human gait analysis? *Human Movement Science*, 15 (3): 423–43.

Wagner, H., Pfusterschmied, J., Klous, M., von Duvillard, S. P. and Müller, E. (2012) Movement variability and skill level of various throwing techniques. *Human Movement Science*, 31 (1): 78–90.

Wolpert, D. M., Doya, K. and Kawato, M. (2003) A unifying computational framework for motor control and social interaction. *Philosophical Transactions of the Royal Society of London*, 358: 593–602.

Yang, J.-F. and Scholz, J. P. (2005) Learning a throwing task is associated with differential changes in the use of motor abundance. *Experimental Brain Research*, 163 (2): 137–58.

17 Individual pathways of change in motor learning and development

Yeou-Teh Liu and Karl M. Newell

Individual differences are observed in motor learning and development; however, studies typically analyze the averaged data over groups of participants. Based on the ergodic theorem of mathematics, it is clear that the processes of human motor learning and development are non-ergodic as reflected in non-stationarity and heterogeneity. Given this, it is necessary to analyze the intra-individual data to unravel the characteristics of the change processes. We present a landscape model of multiple timescales as a framework to describe the individual pathways of change in motor learning and development from a dynamical systems perspective. Examples of individual differences, including those in the context of sport skills, are provided from the evolving attractor landscape of multiple timescales.

Motor learning and development are individual but related processes that are reflected in changes of motor ability. Studies of motor learning and development typically examine the motor performance of groups of people over a period of time in order to observe changes due to the learning/development processes. Although individual differences have been acknowledged in the motor skills acquisition literature (e.g. Ackerman 1987; Fleishman 1978), these differences are often masked, if not eliminated entirely, by way of averaging data over the group (Liu *et al.* 2006).

One general assumption of averaging data is that the individual differences that appear in the motor performance are from the incidental random-like movement variability that does not reflect the stable performance of the participants. In this view, averaging over the participants will minimize or eliminate this individual noise-like variability and allow the general trend of learning and development to be revealed more robustly. The results from analyzing the averaged data, however, may only reflect a constructed learning trend of a group of participants, because the individual learning characteristics tend to be lost in the averaging process. Moreover, averaging learning data can produce a general performance trend that is *not* present in the data of any participant. Thus, the challenge is to identify the individual characteristics of interest to be analyzed before averaging the performance data.

In this chapter, we focus on the individual pathways of change in motor learning and development from a dynamical systems perspective. We use an epigenetic landscape model as the theoretical framework for examining the performance change at the individual level. We outline parallels in sport to the individual differences identified in a dynamical systems approach to laboratory experiments. Our approach limits itself to individual difference phenomena that are related to the dynamics of the behaviour – we do not draw on individual differences in motor learning and development that have been interpreted by information processing frameworks (Ackerman 1987; Fleishman 1978).

Motor learning and development processes are non-ergodic

Human motor learning and development systems are considered to be reflections of deterministic and stochastic processes. From the classic ergodic theorems of mathematics, any measurable stochastic processes have to meet the stationary and homogeneous conditions to guarantee that the inter-individual structure and the intra-individual structure of the processes are equivalent, so that the result of an analysis from one structure can be generalized to the other (Molenaar 2004). A non-ergodic process does not have an a priori relationship between the inter-individual structure and the intra-individual structure, making the inference from individual to group data challenging.

The stationary condition for a Gaussian stochastic process implies a constant mean and higher-order (moment) measures without a trend or periodicity. In motor learning and development, however, the mean function and variance are typically changing over the learning/development sequence (e.g. Adams 1952), hence violating the stationary condition of ergodicity. The homogeneous condition dictates that each individual in a sample population possesses the *same* dynamics of change. When the condition of homogeneity is violated, the result obtained from the group analysis may not be applicable at the individual level. Motor learning and development reflect the product of the evolving individual interacting with the many contexts of the environment to realize the task demands. Studies have shown different individual patterns of learning that are due to individual differences (e.g. Liu *et al.* 2006).

Thus, motor learning and development processes tend to be non-stationary and heterogeneous within the observable conditions or groups, leaving them non-ergodic in nature in the technical sense (Molenaar 2004). This is because motor learning and development by definition are characterized by the change of behaviour over time and, therefore, by definition are non-ergodic. It follows that it is necessary to analyze the intra-individual data (for example, the time series of individual performers) to unravel the characteristics of these processes.

The likelihood of individual pathways of change in motor learning and development will be magnified in the performance of certain motor tasks, including sport tasks. This is because there is degeneracy of the perceptual-motor system in realizing task goals. That is, the same task goal can be met with different solutions of movement coordination and control. We postulate that the nature of the particular sports skill influences the number of potential solutions as reflected in within and between subject variability. Intuitively, it would seem that the maximal performance tasks of sport (e.g. weight lifting, track and field) will tend to have fewer viable solutions than other tasks, such as soccer and the mid-range passing of the ball in the context of the game. This task-related difference in the potential range of movement solutions will influence the presence of individual differences in the pathways of change in motor learning and development.

Multiple processes of performance change

The studies of motor learning and development, although they may focus on different populations (adults vs. children and elderly) and different tasks (phylogenetic vs. ontogenetic movements), share the common goal of characterizing behavioural change over time. In addition to the comparative paradigm where pretest and post-test are performed and analyzed to examine the change of behaviour, the learning (performance) curve has also been a focus of research attention. For nearly two decades, the predominant description was the 'power law' function (Newell and Rosenbloom 1981), which covered a range of task outcomes and context domains but considered to be the single function that characterized learning behaviour (see Heathcote *et al.* 2000; Newell *et al.* 2001). In fact, many forms of mathematical functions have been proposed to account for the different shapes of performance curves over time (see Mazur and Hastie 1978; Thurstone 1919; Welford 1987). These different shapes of performance curves may be due to different task constraints that were imposed on the performers and reflect different levels of change, such as continuous scaling improvement of the task or discontinuous jumps between coordination patterns.

Additionally, the adaptive phenomena such as warm-up, fatigue, inhibition and noise which were frequently observed in the learning curve data but usually discarded or ignored for analysis also contribute to the overall change of performance in learning and development. These adaptive features in performance are also most obvious to the teachers and coaches but are often misinterpreted in terms of their role within learning. The different levels of learning and development, as well as the adaptive phenomena observed during the performance sequences, reflect the multiple contributions of the evolving set of dynamical subsystems to learning and development, each with its own changing time scale. The power function that is considered to be scale free (infinite timescales) could be the result of the averaging processes over different learning curves (individual learners) and/or over different segments of learning curves (Newell *et al.* 2001).

Dynamical systems and landscape metaphor of change

The use of an evolving landscape as a metaphor to describe the behavioural change in learning and development can be traced back to Waddington's (1957) epigenetic landscape. Waddington was interested in the genetic expression of the embryo and the landscape model was a metaphor for considering the dynamics of developmental growth and change. In Waddington's landscape model, the elevations of the landscape depict the stability of each developing behaviour (Figure 17.1). The two axes perpendicular to the vertical axis of elevation represent the

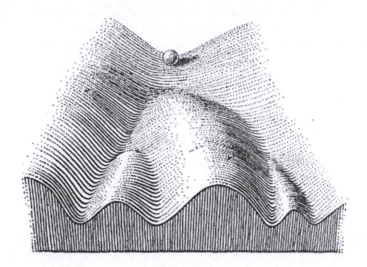

Figure 17.1 Waddington's (1957) schematic of the epigenetic landscape

emergence of particular activities along the developmental time. For example, the only stable pattern of an infant at birth might be the 'lying down with arms and legs curled' pattern. Additional stable patterns emerge later on in the infant's motor development sequence, such as lying in the prone position with chin up and then sitting and crawling. Although no specifics of the landscape were provided in Waddington's model, a dynamical systems interpretation of the epigenetic landscape has been outlined for the case of prone progression in infants (Newell *et al.* 2003).

The concept of the landscape model is individually based. The landscape of motor behaviour describes the ability to perform different motor activities and the height of the landscape at each activity location specifies the stability of the performance. For example, in the HKB (Haken-Kelso-Bunz) model of the finger oscillation tasks, while the 0-degree in-phase and 180-degree anti-phase relations are both stable at low frequencies, only the in-phase relation will remain stable and be observed when frequency is increased to cross the threshold for transition (Figure 17.2). However, the specific value for the threshold is individually dependent; that is, the value of b/a in Figure 17.2, where the concave shapes at ± 180 degrees dissolve into a convex shape, depends on the specific performer.

In the landscape example of Figure 17.2, the elevations of the landscape determine the stability regions in the landscape and the motor performance follows the descending slope toward the nearby fixed-point attractor. If, now, the task is to perform a 90-degree relative phase, under the current landscape structure of Figure 17.2, there is no attractor at the 90-degree region; therefore, a restructuring of the landscape to form a 'well' at the 90-degree area is required. Learning a

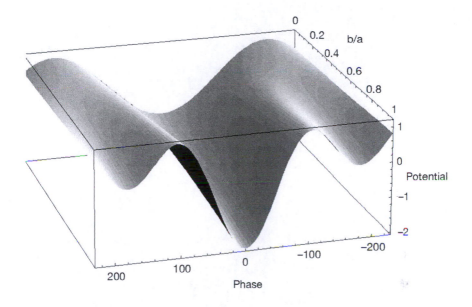

Figure 17.2 The landscape dynamics of the basic equation of the HKB (Haken-Kelso-Bunz) model (Haken *et al.* 1985), with the same parameters as in Kelso (1995, Figure 2.7)

new coordination pattern, such as oscillating two fingers in 90-degree relative phase, would be modelled as changing the motor landscape (see Zanone and Kelso 1997). From the dynamical systems approach, new coordination learning involves a phase transition (Liu *et al.* 2006) and, although sufficient practice usually leads to a transition to the new coordination pattern, the number of practice trials (practice time) required to induce a transition is not constant among individual learners.

Figure 17.3 shows the hypothetical landscape change for the 90-degree relative-phase learning (Newell *et al.* 2009). The top panel of Figure 17.3 depicts the landscape at the beginning stage of the 90-degree relative-phase learning where, although the trajectory from initial position C shows a temporarily stable target pattern of 90-degree relative phase, the trajectories from all initial positions still tend toward the stable in-phase pattern. Continuing practice results in further change in the layout of the landscape. The middle panel of Figure 17.3 shows the landscape at transition where selected initial positions will tend to the stable 90-degree relative phase target pattern but the majority of the initial positions still converge to the in-phase pattern. The landscape continues to deform with further practice and the probability of converging to the stable 90-degree relative phase from any initial position is greatly increased. Practice contributes to the change of landscape and the change of landscape creates a new stable coordination pattern.

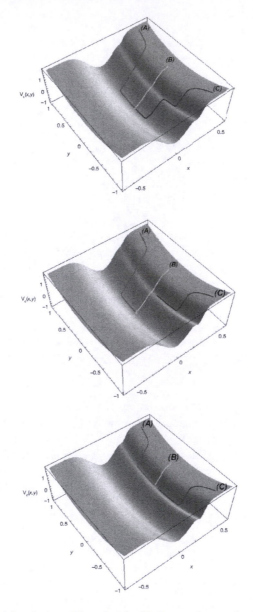

Figure 17.3 (a) Landscape of learning the 90-degree phase task of the HKB model; at the beginning of practice (C = 0.4) only temporary stabilization of the target phase x0 = 0.25 can be achieved when starting from special initial conditions close to C; (b) right at the transition (C = 0.425) the target phase x0 = 0.25 shows one-sided stability: initial conditions close to C will be attracted to the new attractor. Note that, in this situation, the system is very sensitive to noise perturbations; (c) after sufficient practice (C = 0.525), all initial conditions close to the target attractor x0 = 0.25 will converge to the fixed point (reproduced from Newell *et al.* 2001)

Averaging masks the individual learning processes

The existing structure of the motor landscape determines the ability to perform particular coordination patterns (whether there is an attractor at the particular location); performing a particular coordination pattern will also modify the structure of the motor landscape. When the current landscape conforms to the required coordination pattern of the target task, the learning curve usually shows improvement on the precision and/or stability of the performance and the learning dynamics may be modelled as approaching to a fixed-point attractor (Newell *et al.* 2009). Theoretically, the dynamics close to the fixed point show an exponential function that provides a single timescale as the basis of improvement rate. However, if the learning curves are averaged among different individual learners, it is likely that the resulting improvement rate does not capture any individual's learning rate. The exponential nature of the learning curve is also lost in the averaging process.

Within the class of fixed-point-attractor learning, although the dynamics of learning can be approximated by an exponential function, there may be other dynamics involved in the process. Based on the frameworks of multiple timescales of learning and development, a two-timescales landscape model of a sensory–motor learning task has been established to examine the co-existing adaptation and learning dynamics (Newell *et al.* 2009). The two-timescale model of adaptation and learning was derived from a decomposition of the performance dynamics into separate adaptation and learning processes.

Figure 17.4 shows the graphical illustration of the two-timescale model. The fast timescale, indicating a large change of performance level, describes the adaptation phenomenon that is observed at the beginning of each practice session. The slow timescale, on the other hand, representing the small changes over time, reflects the persistent change of learning. Other processes of different timescales, such as fatigue/inhibition, may also be identified and included to make the model more comprehensive (e.g. Newell *et al.* 2010). These different processes dominate different parts of the practice sequence and will be masked if averaging over the sequence of trials is implemented in data processing. The contemporary work in neuroscience has also shown multiple processes to memory consolidation that each have their own timescale of change on the performance dynamics (Kandel 2006; Shadmehr and Holcomb 1997; Tse *et al.* 2007). The averaging technique has been widely practised in the processing of learning data. However, the analyses based on averaged data do not reflect well the characteristics of the individual learning performance.

Self-organization in learning and development

Practice is one of the most important factors in motor skill learning. Through practice, learners try to produce the target movement under the organismic, environmental and task constraints (Newell 1986). Practice sessions provide the opportunity for the learners to organize the movement systems and perform the

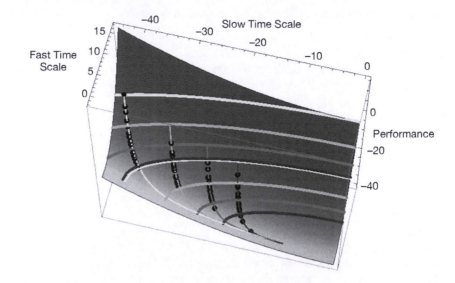

Figure 17.4 A two-timescale landscape model associated with Snoddy's (1926) score
data (black dots) as elevation levels. The four clusters correspond to the
four practice sessions. The *x* behavioural variable corresponds to the slow
timescale (shallow dimension), whereas the *y* variable corresponds to the
fast timescale (steep dimension)

target movement repeatedly, the movement subsystems interact with one another
en route to the equilibrium state of the system. Consequently, the emergent movement performance reflects the results of self-organization process of the complex
dynamical systems.

Self-organization is a characteristic of the complex dynamical systems where
the subsystems within and between levels interact with one another without
central/external commands. Individuals learning to perform a new coordination
pattern tend to undergo the self-organization processes. For example, in the study
of learning to ride a pedalo (Chen *et al.* 2005), subjects practised 350 trials of
pedalo task over seven days. The participants were only informed about the goal
of the pedalo task, which was to ride a designated distance as fast and as smooth
as possible, no additional instruction as to how to ride the pedalo was given. The
participants had to organize their movement systems during practice trials to learn
the task.

The results of data analyses showed that, although the movement time and
movement smoothness measures indicated a practice-day effect (improvement
over seven days), the principal components analysis on the individual participants
showed that different participants had a different number of principal components
before and after seven days of practice and the variance accounted for by these
components was also different. These data indicate that participants all improved
their pedalo performance with practice but the movement coordination patterns

and the way the movements were changed was not the same for each individual participant. These results suggest that individual learners underwent self-organization process during practice in order to meet the requirement of the task dynamics. The interaction between the movement systems and the instrument (pedalo) and within the movement subsystems are the processes of self-organization.

Individual differences and the landscape model of multiple timescales

There are multiple levels of analysis to human movement that evolve over time. The learning of tracing a particular shape (start tracing), learning to produce a specific relative phase (90 degree) or the lifetime evolution of the postural and locomotion patterns can all be captured with the landscape model. The general idea is that the shape of the landscape (that is, the elevation and slope of each relevant location of the landscape that represents a particular quality of special interest) describes the stability of the movement performances. The different levels of analyses are reflected in the different timescales of the landscape models and these landscapes are continuously evolving.

As noted previously, learning and development are individual processes and the individual differences have been observed and reported in various relevant literatures. Based on the landscape metaphor of movement learning and development, the individual differences may come from two sources: the initial state and the rate of deformation. If the individual differences reside in the initial state, there is a 'well (attractor)' that exists in the hypothetical movement landscape of the performer, it is the incidental choice of the initial attempt that differentiate the outcome performances (see Newell and McDonald 1992). For example, in a motor learning study where the combined spatial and temporal feedback were given to the learners to improve the mirror tracing task, the results of the cluster analysis identified three groups of different initial strategies – the movement time group, the spatial error group and the mixed group (King *et al.* 2012). Although the final performances among the three groups did not show any significant differences, these different initial strategies were sustained throughout the subsequent exploration of the perceptual work space (Figure 17.5).

For the type of differences where the source comes from the rate of landscape deformation, it is assumed that, for the individual learner, the elevation is high at the location of the landscape where the target movement is specified; the change of the landscape is required to invoke the transition of the movement dynamics. In addition to the structure of the landscape at the initial stage of learning, the 'hardness' of the landscape also contributes to the rate of change of the landscape. In a rollerball learning study, where participants were asked to learn to accelerate a top encapsulated in a seven-centimetre diameter spherical shell, seven days of practice were given to all the participants to learn the task (Liu *et al.* 2006). Among the eight successful participants who learned to accelerate the rollerball by the end of the experiment, the number of trials used to reach the criterion of

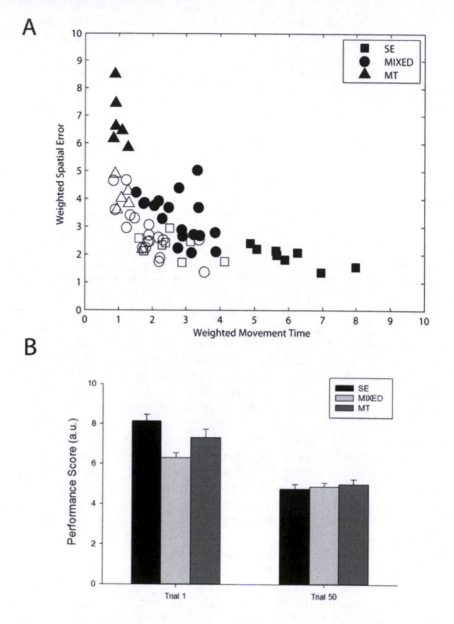

Figure 17.5 Initial and final performance of the mirror tracing task; (A) breakdown of one-dimensional performance score measure into movement time and spatial error (movement time) components. Filled and open symbols indicate outcome score on trial 1 and trial 50, respectively. Triangle, circle and square symbols reflect movement time (MT), mixed (MIXED) and spatial error (SE) group assignment (see text for detailed explanation); (B) performance score on trial 1 and trial 50 as a function of group; error bars indicate standard error

success ranged from 10 to 300. There were three participants who did not reach the goal of learning to accelerate the rollerball within seven days of practice.

There are additional examples of individual differences in the learning literature, as well as in practical situations such as athletic training, skill learning and infant motor development (e.g. Chow *et al.* 2008). The landscape model of multiple timescales provides a theoretical framework for systematically examining the source and the influence of individual differences in motor learning and development.

Individual differences are ubiquitous in every aspect of human performance. This feature is especially significant in the processes of learning and development. Not only in the data analysis procedure in research, where learning and development data are often treated as a group, in practical settings such as activity classes and sports training, skills and performances are also taught and evaluated under a group criterion. The multiple processes of change provide a base for understanding the source of individual differences. The challenge for teachers and coaches is to identify and recognize the consequences of these processes to better assist the development of motor skills.

Concluding comments

We have shown in this chapter that the motor learning and development processes are non-ergodic (Molenaar 2004). Therefore, it is necessary to analyze the intraindividual data of motor learning and development in order to reveal the characteristics of these processes. We have also used the landscape model of multiple timescales from dynamical systems theory (Newell *et al.* 2001) as the framework to emphasize the importance of examining the individual pathways of learning and development in motor behaviour. Over 100 years of research on human motor behaviour have mostly analyzed learning data over groups of participants. In the light of the individual nature of the learning and development of movement, further research should examine the individual pathways of learning and development to obtain a better understanding of these processes and contribute to the theories and practices of related fields.

Acknowledgements

This paper was supported in part by NSF grant 0848339.

References

Ackerman, P. L. (1987) Individual differences in skill learning: an integration of psychometric and information processing perspectives. *Psychological. Bulletin*, 102: 3–27.

Adams, J. A. (1952) Warm-up decrement in performance on the pursuit rotor. *American Journal of Psychology*, 65: 404–14.

Chen, H.-H., Liu, Y.-T., Mayer-Kress, G. and Newell, K. M. (2005) Learning the pedalo locomotion task. *Journal of Motor Behavior*, 37: 247–56.

Chow, J. Y., Davids, K., Button, C. and Rein, R. (2008) Dynamics of movement pattern-ing in learning a discrete multiarticular action. *Motor Control*, 12: 219–40.

Fleishman, E. A. (1978) Relating individual differences to the dimensions of human tasks. *Ergonomics*, 21: 1007–19.

Haken, H., Kelso, J. A. S. and Bunz, H. A. (1985) Theoretical model of phase transitions in human hand movements. *Biological Cybernetics*, 51: 347–56.

Heathcote, A., Brown, S. and Mewhort, D. J. K. (2000) The power law repealed: the case for an exponential law of practice. *Psychonomic Bulletin and Review*, 7: 185–207.

Kandel, E. R. (2006) *In Search of Memory: The Emergence of a New Science of the Mind*. New York: Norton.

King, A. C., Ranganathan, R. and Newell, K. M. (2012) Individual differences in the exploration of a redundant space-time motor task. *Neuroscience Letters*, 529: 144–9.

Liu, Y.-T., Mayer-Kress, G. and Newell, K. M. (2006) Qualitative and quantitative change in the dynamics of motor learning. *Journal of Experimental Psychology: Human Perception and Performance*, 32: 380–93.

Mazur, J. E. and Hastie, R. (1978) Learning as accumulation: a reexamination of the learn-ing curve. *Psychological Bulletin*, 85: 1256–74.

Molenaar, P. C. M. (2004) A manifesto on psychology as idiographic science: bringing the person back into scientific psychology, this time forever. *Measurement: Interdisciplinary Research and Perspective*, 2: 201–18.

Newell, A. and Rosenbloom, P. S. (1981) Mechanisms of skill acquisition and the law of practice, in J. R. Anderson (ed.) *Cognitive Skills and Their Acquisition*. Hillsdale, NJ: Erlbaum, pp. 1–55.

Newell, K. M. (1986) Constraints on the development of coordination, in M. G. Wade and H. T. A. Whiting (eds) *Motor Skill Acquisition in Children: Aspects of Coordination and Control*. Amsterdam: Martinus Nijhoff, pp. 341–60.

Newell, K. M. and McDonald, P. V. (1992) Searching for solutions to the coordination function: learning as exploratory behavior, in G. E. Stelmach, J. Requin (eds) *Tutorials in Motor Behavior II. Advances in Psychology, Vol. 87*. Amsterdam: Elsevier, pp. 517–32.

Newell, K. M., Liu, Y-T. and Mayer-Kress, G. (2001) Time scales in motor learning and development. *Psychological Review*, 108: 57–82.

Newell, K. M., Liu, Y-T. and Mayer-Kress, G. (2003) A dynamical systems interpretation of epigenetic landscapes for infant motor development. *Infant Development and Behavior*, 26: 449–72.

Newell, K. M., Mayer-Kress, G., Hong, S. L. and Liu, Y. T. (2009) Adaptation and learn-ing: characteristic time scales of performance dynamics. *Human Movement Science*, 28: 655–87.

Newell, K. M., Mayer-Kress, G., Hong, S. L. and Liu, Y-T. (2010) Decomposing the performance dynamics of learning through time scales, in P. C. M. Molenaar and K. M. Newell (eds) *Individual Pathways of Change in Learning and Development*. Washington, DC: American Psychological Association, pp. 71–86.

Shadmehr, R. and Holcomb, H. H. (1997) Neural correlates of motor memory consolida-tion. *Science*, 277: 821–5.

Thurstone, L. L. (1919) The learning curve equation. *Psychological Monographs*, 26: 1–51.

Tse, D., Langston, R. F., Kakeyama, M., Bethus, I., Spooner, P. A., Wood, E. R., Witter, M. P., Witter, M. P. and Morris, R. G. M. (2007) Schemas and memory consolidation. *Science*, 316: 76–82.

Waddington, C. H. (1957) *The Strategy of the Genes*. London: George Allen and Unwin.
Welford, A. T. (1987) On rates of improvement with practice. Journal of Motor Behavior, 19, 401–15.
Zanone, P. G. and Kelso, J. A. S. (1997) The coordination dynamics of learning and transfer: collective and component levels. *Journal of Experimental Psychology: Human Perception and Performance*, 23: 1454–80.

18 A constraints-based approach to the acquisition of expertise in outdoor adventure sports

Keith Davids, Eric Brymer, Ludovic Seifert and Dominic Orth

Previous work has shown that changes in behaviour, as a function of learning, emerge as a consequence of continuous interactions between learners and a performance environment (Chow *et al*. 2011; Davids *et al*. 2008). These interactions, with other individuals and key objects, surfaces and events during learning, need not be the result of programmed, formalized instructions but can occur through unstructured, exploratory activity (Davids *et al*. 2012). As a result of their continuous interactions with the performance environment, learners become adept at exploiting sources of information available as properties of the environment for regulating and changing their behaviours.

Research has also demonstrated several important properties to emerge in nonlinear complex systems under the effect of constraints, including: system *multi-* and *metastability*, *adaptive variability*, *degeneracy* and *attunement to affordances for action* (Araújo *et al*. 2004; Davids *et al*. 2008; Hristovski *et al*. 2006a; Kelso 1995; Seifert *et al*. 2011; Seifert *et al*. 2013). This chapter outlines a constraints-based framework for explaining how these key neurobiological system properties may influence processes of learning and performance in the context of outdoor adventure sports. With reference to current empirical work, we discuss how functional patterns of behaviour might emerge from engagement in outdoor adventure sports.

The constraints-based model focuses on change in individuals over different timescales and is generically suited to the study of learning and performance in a variety of outdoor adventure sports contexts (Brymer and Renshaw 2010, Brymer and Davids 2013). This is because it has a strong focus on the relationship between the individual performer, the task and the environment (social and physical) as the appropriate scale of analysis for understanding behavioural change on different timescales. There is an important and functional role of *movement pattern variability* in supporting the necessary short-term performance adaptations required between and within skilled individuals in outdoor adventure sports and physical activities (Davids *et al*. 2003, 2006). Over the longer timescale of learning, understanding of these complex system properties has signalled that the acquisition of functional performance behaviours does not emerge from repetitive and imitative practice to gradually reduce a perceived 'void' differentiating the behaviours of learners and a putative expert model. Rather, learners' behaviours need to be understood in terms of their functionality in achieving their intentions. For example, in kayaking or canoeing, learners need to discover functional patterns of behaviour that provide stability of the system formed by each individual and the interaction with the boat, the paddle and the water during exploratory practice in safe settings, such as small lakes and slow-moving rivers. More advanced exploratory practice can be undertaken as the ecological constraints of performance are manipulated by a coach exposing learners to more dynamic environmental settings, as might be found in open-water settings, oceans or fast-moving rivers. A constraints-based framework theoretically verifies why there exists no ideal motor coordination solution for any adventure sport, in an absolute sense, towards which all learners should aspire (Brymer and Renshaw 2010).

Different categories of constraints are resources that limit or set the boundaries for the emergence of coordination patterns in human movement systems. For example, personal constraints, relevant to each individual athlete, are structural or functional and refer to characteristics of an individual, such as genes, anthropometric properties, strength, endurance, body shape, fitness level, technical abilities, age, and so on. In adventure sports, psychological factors like beliefs, fear, anxiety, emotional readiness and motivation obviously play a significant role in shaping the way that participants approach a task such as climbing a vertical surface two hundred feet off the ground or paddling through extreme white-water rapids (Brymer and Schweitzer 2013; Brymer and Renshaw 2010). These personal factors play a significant role in determining the responses to outdoor adventure settings adopted by individuals.

Environmental constraints are external to each individual and can be social and physical, reflecting the environmental conditions of a task in outdoor sports (e.g. height, light, temperature, altitude, gravity, climbing tethered by a rope in a group). Outdoor adventure sports are reliant on the natural environment (water, air and land) and environmental and weather conditions represent a major influence on participation and emergent behaviours. For example white-water kayaking depends on water flow in a river: no water, no kayaking (Brymer, Downey and Gray, 2009). Related to this category are task constraints, which include the goal of the task, instructional information, the equipment and the nature of the surface (e.g. texture of rock in climbing, airflow in BASE jumping). Task constraints shape the movement pattern variability exhibited by adventure sport athletes. For instance, functional performance behaviours in rock and ice climbers emerge from their interactions with specific informational properties of a particular rock cliff (i.e. shape, steepness, type of rock, overhang) or a frozen waterfall (i.e. shape, steepness, ambient temperature at the surface, overhang, ice thickness and density of an icefall; Seifert *et al.* 2013). This is because the conditions of the rock and ice (as affordances) are mostly unpredictable when viewed from the ground before the climb.

Constraints and affordances in rock climbing

Complex biological systems, even simple ones without nervous systems, have the capacity to use information to regulate their functional behaviours in complex environments. For example, Reid *et al.* (2012) demonstrated that slime mould, a brainless unicellular organism, functions as a complex system to explore its environment, enhance its spatial awareness and use externalized memory mechanisms to find food or avoid nasty substances. It uses an information regulation system to maintain its functionality. Smaller units of the slime mould oscillate at different frequencies when food is sensed by molecular binding at its outer molecular surface area. Oscillating frequency increases with attraction to an environmental source of information or decreases in the presence of a repellent source. The membrane structure of the organism softens or hardens as a result of increasing or decreasing oscillation frequency to absorb food or repel a substance like salt, respectively. Our work has shown that complex neurobiological systems, with highly structured nervous systems, use similar information detection systems to explore and act in their performance environments. Attunement to affordances is one such exploratory system exploited by complex neurobiological systems.

For example, during the sport of rock climbing, performance is characterized by individuals interacting with various task and environmental constraints. Gravity could be viewed as an environmental constraint because quadrupedal vertical locomotion involving the minimal support of at least one limb is required to prevent falling under the force of gravity. One major climbing task constraint on the fluency of a climber's movements is the interface of limb extremities with the rock cliff surface, since the performer has to maintain body equilibrium on a more or less vertical climbing surface (Bourdin *et al.* 1999; Quaine and Martin 1999), while combining upper- and lower-limb movements to ascend (Sibella *et al.* 2007). Assessment of climbing fluency through analysis of the geometric entropy index from the three-dimensional body centre of mass displacement (Cordier *et al.* 1994; Sibella *et al.* 2007) is a relevant indicator to understand how a climber alternates climbing with time spent maintaining body equilibrium under control in a tripodal position (Bourdin *et al.* 1999). Expert climbers exhibit a low geometric entropy index value since they travel a great distance up a surface slope between each grip hold to maintain energy efficiency (Cordier *et al.* 1994, 1996). A high value of climbing movement fluency suggests a more functional level of individual–environment coupling. For instance, Sibella *et al.* 2007 emphasized the relationship between a lower geometric entropy index and the capacity of rock climbers to move when using fewer than three holds. This observation is known as the 'three-holds-rule': if a rock climber uses a smaller number of holds he/she has to be quick enough to maintain equilibrium on the surface. Conversely, if the number of holds is equal to or greater than three, it is more likely that the rock climber will climb slowly, because his/her equilibrium is always under control (Sibella *et al.* 2007).

Climbers can achieve these different intentional aims by increasing their attunement to affordances to regulate their actions in different climbing contexts. Ecological psychology (Gibson 1966, 1979) proposed that *affordances* are opportunities in the environment that invite actions and experts are more able to functionally exploit them in their behaviour. The implication is that affordances do not exist independently of an individual's perceptions and intentions. In the context of rock climbing, affordances (called 'climbing opportunities' by Boschker *et al.* 2002) imply that the coordination dynamics of action emerge from a mutual coupling of a climber's perceptions and intentions with the specific properties of a climbing surface, such as a rock cliff (i.e. shape, steepness, type of rock). In line with ideas on the important role of affordances, Boschker *et al.* (2002) previously reported how expert rock climbers recalled more information and focused on the functional properties of a climbing wall, neglecting to perceive its structural features. Conversely, in their study, beginners were not able to recall such functional properties of the wall for action and they tended to report almost exclusively the structural features of the holds (Boschker *et al.* 2002).

As environmental properties of the rock cliff are mostly not predictable from the ground, an important challenge is to examine whether and how expert climbers detect information when they proceed to a pre-ascent climbing route visual inspection (i.e. route preview; Sanchez *et al.* 2012) and how they recall climbing surface properties once they are in the ascent (Pezzulo *et al.* 2010) compared the capability of expert and novice climbers to preview and recall the sequences of holds composing easy, difficult and impossible routes. When the climbers were voluntary distracted between the route preview and the recall, they showed that a greater level of movement expertise enabled a better recall of sequences of holds on difficult routes. These findings suggest that route preview-ing on a climbing wall activates a motor, embodied simulation, which relies on the motor competence of the climbers. In this way, Sanchez *et al.* (2012) high-lighted that route previewing did not influence movement output performance but influenced movement form. Notably, climbing fluency was better after a preview of the route, since the climbers made fewer and shorter stops during their ascent. Finally, these findings showed that, with increasing levels of expertise, climbers previewed and recalled perceptual variables that are more functional (i.e. those which can specify actions) under a variety of different performance circum-stances compared to novices who tended to focus and recall structural properties of the climbing environment.

Affordances for ice climbing in skilled and unskilled climbers

The coordination of a climber's actions with the properties of a frozen waterfall are mediated by ice picks for use with the hands and crampons on the feet. The ice fall can vary because key properties are stochastically distributed through the surface. For example, ambient temperature can modify the ice density in certain regions of the ice fall, causing changes to the structure of the surface and the placement of holes for actions, such as hooking with an ice pick and kicking with the crampons. Icefall properties such as these provide affordances for climbers who perceive, use and shape movement opportunities from their own unique perspective. For example, two climbers on the same crag would be working with the same environmental properties but individual differences, such as limb length, body length and emotional regulation, would result in different perceptions and actions emerging during performance. Objectively, a crag might have various climbing affordances but, because of different personal constraints, not all climbers will be able to take advantage of a specific affordance.

Environmental constraints are not under the control of the climber, since this task requires experience at using numerous types of actions (e.g. swinging, kicking and hooking actions) during exploratory behaviour. Patterns of interlimb coordination (e.g. horizontally, diagonally and vertically located angular positions) can also be used to explore functionality of the neurobiological system properties of degeneracy and multistability. For instance, climbers could either swing their ice tools to create their own holes in the surface of the ice fall or hook an existing hole (formed by the actions of the lead climber or exploiting the presence of natural holes). The latter strategy is more energy efficient and requires some expertise in perceiving the affordances of holes for supporting body weight. This conceptualization of skill in ice climbing supports the functional role of intra-individual variability in exploring affordances of icefall properties for action. Research undertaken by Seifert *et al.* (2011) on ice-climbing performance has assessed interlimb coordination patterns by using the angle between the horizontal line and the displacement of the heads of the left- and right-hand ice tools for upper-limb coordination. Lower-limb coordination patterns corresponded to the angle between the horizontal line and the displacement of the left and right crampons (Figure 18.1; Seifert *et al.* 2011).

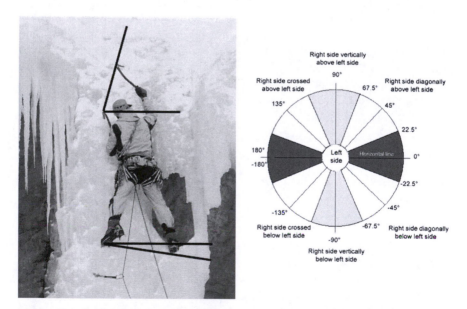

Figure 18.1 (left) Angles identified for the horizontal planes of the left and right limbs in the upper and lower body of ice climbers; (right) modes of limb coordination as regards the angle value between horizontal, left limb and right limb (from Seifert *et al.* 2011)

Unskilled ice climbers showed low levels of intra-individual movement and coordination pattern variability, as they varied their upper- and lower-limb coordination patterns much less frequently and extensively than the experts. Beginners mostly used horizontally and diagonally located angular positions (since limb anchorages are at the same level for the horizontal angle, the arms or legs appear in an in-phase coordination mode). This behaviour resembled climbing up a ladder and led them to maintain a static 'X' body position with arms and legs extended or with arms flexed and legs extended, corresponding to a freezing of the motor system degrees of freedom (Bernstein 1967). Moreover, beginners tended not to hook the ice tool into existing holes in the ice fall but tended to swing the ice tool into or out of the holes. Beginners mainly focused on attaining a deep anchorage on the ice fall for both ice tools and crampons, by numerous episodes of ice-tool swinging and crampon kicking, suggesting that the icefall properties were either not perceived or were not used by them as relevant affordances. While this behaviour might enhance their stability on the ice fall, it also led them to greater levels of fatigue.

These data exemplify how unskilled ice climbers tended to perceive the affordance of an icefall surface as requiring a significant amount of stability with respect to the force of gravity. From a Gibsonian perspective, it was likely that they perceived the icefall surface as 'fall-offable', which led them to typically prioritize stability and security of posture in interacting with environmental constraints, rather than speed and efficiency of displacement up the surface. For novice climbers extending their range of skills in more difficult terrains, psychological factors such as fear and anxiety might interfere with their ability to use affordances that might have been perceived and used when nearer the ground or on simpler surfaces. Use of affordances is often mediated by psychological constraints such as fear in the transition from novice to high-level adventure sport performer (Brymer and Schweitzer 2013; Brymer and Renshaw 2010).

Conversely, in the skilled ice climbers, the frozen waterfall afforded opportunities to hook their ice tools and kick in their crampons. They also tended to show high levels of intra-individual movement and coordination pattern variability, supporting an efficient balance between dependency/independence of their actions from the environment as they exploited affordances in the specific icefall properties. The efficient individual–environment coupling of the experts was probably predicated on the neurobiological property of degeneracy (Davids and Glazier 2010; Edelman and Gally 2001) since they varied the types of movement and the interlimb coordination modes they exploited to achieve their task goals. Indeed, the multistability of their complex movement systems allowed them: (i) to swing the ice tools and to kick the crampons in many different ways (horizontally, diagonally, vertically and in crossed angular positions), exploiting the functionality of intra-individual movement pattern variability. For instance, crossing the arms is not a natural action but it enabled skilled climbers to exploit information and hook existing holes in the ice fall; and (ii), to hook the ice tools into already existing holes (i.e. exploiting information on the shape of the ice fall) and to place the crampons in the holes previously made by their own ice tools, instead of using repetitive ice tool swinging and crampon kicking, as observed in beginners.

From a constraint-based perspective, these behaviours are completely understandable and related to differentiated perceptions of personal (e.g. fear), task and environmental constraints and significantly varying intentions. Beginners tended to function independently of the ice fall's properties for climbing upwards at speed, because their main goal was to keep their equilibrium, with respect to gravitational forces, under control. Manipulation of task constraints under the guidance of a climbing instructor would enable the beginners to further interact with the icefall properties in a secure learning environment, to balance their independence of/dependence on environmental constraints when performing. This pedagogical approach would provide gradual support for the emergence of a wider repertoire of movement by exploiting system multistability in coordinating their actions while allowing novice climbers to come to terms with and move through individual constraints such as fear.

Knowledge of performance environments in outdoor adventure sports

A constraints-based approach also highlights the importance of the role of *knowledge* of the performance environment, which underpins the detection of these affordances to regulate actions (Gibson 1966; Araújo and Davids 2011; Davids and Araújo 2010b). Gibson (1966) proposed that knowledge of the environment is embedded in knowing how to realize an action because it involves perception of affordances used to control action directly (Araújo and Davids 2011; Davids and Araújo 2010b). Expert performers are able to transit functionally between various functional coordination solutions in ice climbing by exploiting system multistability, notably by picking up affordances for action. In contrast, novices tend to pick up and use sources of information that may be only partially functional in a particular performance situation because they do not specify actions. A similar experience occurs in white-water kayaking, where a novice would invariably cross a fast-moving current by using a standard but stable ferry glide, which involves continuous arm work with the paddle and trunk work keeping the boat on edge and at an appropriate angle to the current. The same move by an expert might take one stroke, as the expert is attuned to the nuances of the water. By perceiving and using and even shaping aspects of the current possibly considered too dangerous by the beginner, the expert glides effortlessly across the current using the upstream face of a standing wave. In outdoor adventure sports, knowledge of the environment can also mean the difference between life and death, as the adventurer makes a decision based on an assessment of the environment and about the likely success of an action in partnership with a particular environmental condition (Brymer and Gray 2010).

Related to the notion of performance dependency/independence is the concept of *metastability*, another important property of complex, dynamical movement systems. System metastability emerges when a subtle blend arises between behavioural stability and instability, which research indicates can be exploited to achieve adaptive functional performance goals in sport (Hristovski *et al*. 2006a,b; Pinder *et al*. 2012). The same process is also apparent in outdoor adventure sports. Metastability has been defined as a transient or semi-transient behaviour or a 'dynamically stable' state of system organization (Kelso 1995, 2012, 2012). In a metastable performance region, component tendencies for action independence coexist with tendencies to couple actions with affordances, explaining how rich and varied sequences of goal-directed behaviour can spontaneously emerge in highly dynamic adventure environments. Metastability helps an individual to adapt their motor behaviours to achieve particular performance goals (Chow *et al*. 2011; Hristovski *et al*. 2006a,b; Pinder *et al*. 2012). In a metastable performance region, one or several movement patterns are weakly stable (when there are multiple attractors) or weakly unstable (when there are only attractor remnants) and switching between two or more movement patterns occurs according to interacting constraints.

Movement variability as adaptive skilled behaviour

In sport, traditional approaches to the study of performance and expertise mostly focus on *performance outputs* and their consistent achievement. An important challenge is to pay closer attention to *movement organization* in studying expertise in outdoor adventure sports, since the existence of several expert performance profiles may imply that there actually is no putative expert model of performance towards which all learners should aspire. Ecological dynamics and its emphasis on emergent behaviours under interacting constraints distinguishes variability in movement organization, a healthy sign of adaptive behaviour in indeterminate biological movement systems, from variability in *movement output*, which is synonymous with performance inconsistency and, therefore, less functional (Davids *et al*. 2006).

Research in ecological dynamics has shown that movement system variability is not necessarily noise that is detrimental to performance, error (Newell and Corcos 1993; Newell and Slifkin 1998; Newell 2006) or a deviation from a putative expert performance model that should be corrected in beginners. Considering the functional role of movement variability leads to an exploration of what *adaptive* behaviour means, so that it could be more appropriate to consider the term *adaptability* rather than variability. Adaptability relates to an appropriate ratio between *stability* (i.e. persistent behaviours) and *flexibility* (i.e. variable behaviours; Davids *et al*. 2003; Li *et al*. 2005; van Emmerik and van Wegen 2000; Warren 2006) and is essential to skilled performance in outdoor adventurous sports. Expert behaviour is characterized by stable and reproducible movement patterns that are consistent over time, resistant to perturbations and reproducible, in that a similar movement pattern may recur under different task and environmental constraints. It is not stereotyped and rigid but flexible and adaptive. Even if movement patterns could show regularities and similarities within their structural components, an individual is not fixed into a rigidly stable solution but can adapt a movement pattern in a functional way, as neurobiological complex systems reveal degeneracy (Edelman and Gally 2001). In white-water kayaking, for example, no two rapids are alike; however, there are only a limited number of ways of crossing a fast moving current. The expert is able to adapt (and perhaps merge) the basic processes to fit emergent environmental affordances. In this process, there is a fine line between stability and instability as the expert coordinates extreme boat edge, boat angle, body movement, paddle stroke and mental capacity to decide and act. The expert is able to expend less effort by exploring this fine line between stability and instability, as it take less energy to cross the river when the kayak is in a position of impending instability but there is also a potential cost if the fine line is crossed.

An ecological dynamics model of expertise articulates both stability and flexibility: experts and non-experts each have their stable states and sometimes share the same coordination modes; however, a particularity of expert performance is the capacity for adaptability, i.e. to produce behaviour which is stable when needed and variable when needed. In fact, although human movement systems naturally tend to move toward stable states, as more economical organization modes (Hoyt and Taylor 1981; Sparrow 2000; Sparrow and Newell 1998), stability and flexibility should not be construed as opposites. Flexibility should not be interpreted as a loss of stability but, conversely, as a sign of adaptability (van Emmerik and van Wegen 2000; Warren 2006). From there, Bartlett *et al.* (2007) indicated three functional roles of movement pattern variability: (i) to adapt to interacting constraints; (ii) to facilitate (structural or not) changes in coordination modes and, at the same time, maintaining functional performance through degeneracy or redundancy; and (iii) to reduce the risk of injury.

Mason (2010) has highlighted four avenues for degeneracy in biological systems that could help us to understand how expert individuals functionally adapt their motor behaviours to exhibit high levels of performance outcomes in dynamic outdoor adventure sport contexts. Firstly, 'redundancy can create the opportunity for degeneracy to arise as the function of the original structure is maintained by one copy, while any other copy is free to diverge functionally' (Mason 2010, p. 282). Secondly, degeneracy can occur through *parcellation*, when an initial structure is subdivided into smaller units that can still perform the initial function and can also be functionally redeployed (Mason 2010, p. 282). Thirdly, degeneracy may emerge through a coordinative structure that realises a function in combination. This means that, whether or not a structure is able to perform an initial function independently, another one is available for modification. Lastly, degeneracy may exist when two or more independent structures converge upon the same function. These four avenues for degeneracy emphasize the potential adaptation in human movement systems that coaches and teachers could encourage to emerge in various individual motor responses to satisfy a task.

In white-water kayaking, for example, there are numerous ways of exiting a fast water section of a river to enter a slow moving eddy. If the exit/entry move requires a fast turn then one of the most efficient ways of undertaking this in a kayak is to coordinate boat, body and paddle in such a way that the whole system is potentially unbalanced. In its basic form, many students of kayaking would recognise this move as a bow rudder. The paddler drives for the eddy employs a turning stroke on the opposite side then edges the boat to near imbalance and plants a blade into the eddy at an angle that, if effectively undertaken, ensures balance. If ineffectively undertaken, the move could result in a capsize, which is not recommended on fast-moving rocky rapids. A 'novice' in this situation would most likely err on the side of ensuring that the boat was not edged too far and that the stroke was planted parallel with their feet and a short distance from the boat. The top arm would be securely in front of their head to ensure strength and mini-mize risk of injury. However, the turn speed and precision would not be optimal for a smaller eddy or for turns that require sharp, instant precision. For this reason, an expert would invariably edge the boat to a position that would be unstable on its own but would balance this by varying the position of their body and the planted paddle in the turn. Depending on the environmental context, the expert might even undertake a move where the top hand is behind the head, thus ensuring further system imbalance. The potential downside of this move is that risk of injury is heightened because the system is so far out of balance. If the coor-dination of boat, body and paddle is not finely tuned, injury is possible and capsize is assured.

At an *inter-individual level*, movement pattern variability has been observed both at novice and expert level, suggesting that neurobiological degeneracy is a common property in human motor behaviour. However, degeneracy occurs in different ways as regards to expertise level. Owing to extensive experience in various performance contexts, experts exploit to the fullest their individual prop-erties according to the task demands and the environmental constraints. As stated previously, when the gap existing between the pre-existing movement pattern repertoire of an individual and the task demands is low and/or when the tasks demands are weak, multistability of movement patterns could emerge, giving support for neurobiological degeneracy. For instance, expert climbers regularly use several hand grasping patterns and body positions for a given hold (e.g. crimp, gaston, jug, mono, pinch, pocket, sloper and undercling grasping pattern; bridge, campus, crossover, deadpoint, flag, heel hook, knee bar and mantle body positions; Phillips *et al.* 2012) exhibiting several individual climbing profiles. In contrast, novices tend to demonstrate a basic quadrupedic climbing pattern that resembles climbing a ladder.

Conclusions and implications

A constraints-based framework enables a new understanding of expertise in outdoor adventure sports by considering performer–environment couplings through emergent and self-organizing behaviours in relation to interacting constraints. Expert adventure athletes, conceptualized as complex, dynamical movement systems, pick up affordances for action to regulate adaptive transitions between functional movement behaviours. For example, icefall properties contain affordances that can induce variable motor coordination patterns in expert climbers, whereas beginners use a basic and stable motor organization to achieve the main goal of maintaining body equilibrium with respect to gravity. Movement pattern variability could play a functional role as individuals adapt their behaviours to ecological constraints of performance by exhibiting multistability and metastability. The properties are exploitable by coaches and educators who can use system instability to stimulate creativity and skill acquisition. In this way, expertise relates to the neurobiological property of adaptability, a subtle blend between stability and flexibility, as experts are able to be stable when needed and variable when needed. We highlighted a new emphasis on how novices and experts individually manage motor system degrees of freedom in coordinative structures through redundancy or degeneracy as they structurally adapt system and sub-system organization to achieve functional goals. The main implications for adventure athletes are to identify and manipulate key constraints to perturb and create emergence of appropriate behaviours rather than to encourage the imitation of a single response in reference to a putative ideal expert model. Indeed, imitating so-called 'expert behaviours' could lead to frustration and a prolonged skill-acquisition process, as novices may encounter difficulties in matching the required behaviours. Using a constraint-led approach could lead to the emergence of individualized movement responses directly related to the pre-existing intrinsic dynamics of a performer in outdoor adventure sports.

References

Araújo A. and Davids K. (2011) What exactly is acquired during skill acquisition? *Journal of Consciousness Studies*, 18 (3–4): 7–23.

Araújo, D., Davids, K., Bennett, S. J., Button, C. and Chapman, G. (2004) Emergence of sport skills under constraint, A. M. Williams and N. Hodges (eds) *Skill Acquisition in Sport: Research, Theory and Practice*, 2nd edn. London: Routledge, pp. 409–33.

Bartlett, R., Wheat, J., and Robins, M. (2007) Is movement variability important for sports biomechanists? *Sports Biomechanics*, 6, 224–43.

Bernstein, N. A. (1967) *The Co-ordination and Regulation of Movement*. New York: Pergamon Press Elmsford.

Boschker, M. S. J., Bakker, F. C. and Michaels, C. F. (2002) Memory for the functional characteristics of climbing walls: perceiving affordances. *Journal of Motor Behavior*, 34: 25–36.

Bourdin, C., Teasdale, N., Nougier, V., Bard, C. and Fleury, M. (1999) Postural constraints modify the organization of grasping movements. *Human Movement Science*, 18: 87–102.

Brymer, E. and Davids, K. (2012) Ecological dynamics as a theoretical framework for development of sustainable behaviours towards the environment. *Environmental Education Research*, 19 (1): 45–63.

Brymer, E. and Davids, K. (2013) Experiential learning as an constraint-led process: an ecological dynamics perspective. *Journal of Adventure education and Outdoor Learning*, doi: 10.1080/14729679.2013.789353.

Brymer, E. and Gray, T. (2009) Dancing with nature: rhythm and harmony in extreme sport participation. *Journal of Adventure Education and Outdoor Learning*, 9 (2): 135–49.

Brymer, E. and Gray, T. (2010) Developing an intimate 'relationship' with nature through extreme sports participation. *Leisure/Loisir*, 34 (4): 361–74.

Brymer, E. and Renshaw, I. (2010) An introduction to the constraints-led approach to learning in outdoor education. *Australian Journal of Outdoor Education*, 14 (2): 33–41.

Brymer, E. and Schweitzer R. (2013) Fear is good for your health: a phenomenological understanding of fear and anxiety in extreme sport. *Journal of Health Psychology*, 18 (4): 477–87.

Brymer E., Downey, G. and Gray, T. (2009) Extreme sports as a precursor to environmental sustainability. *Journal of Sport and Tourism*, 14 (2–3): 193–204.

Chow, J. Y., Davids, K., Hristovski, R., Araújo, D. and Passos, P. (2011) Nonlinear pedagogy: Learning design for self-organizing neurobiological systems, *New Ideas in Psychology*, 29: 189–200.

Cordier, P., Dietrich, G. and Pailhous, J. (1996) Harmonic analysis of a complex motor behaviour. *Human Movement Science*, 15 (6): 789–807.

Cordier, P., France, M. M., Pailhous, J. and Bolon, P. (1994) Entropy as a global variable of the learning process. *Human Movement Science*, 13: 745–63.

Davids, K. and Araújo, A. (2010a) The concept of 'organismic asymmetry' in sport science. *Journal of Science and Medicine in Sport*, 13: 633–40.

Davids, K. and Araújo, A. (2010b) Perception of affordances in multi-scale dynamics as an alternative explanation for equivalence of analogical and inferential reasoning in animals and humans. *Theory and Psychology*, 20 (1): 125–34.

Davids K. and Glazier, P. (2010) Deconstructing neurobiological coordination: the role of the biomechanics-motor control nexus. *Exercise Sport Science Reviews*, 38 (2): 86–90.

Davids, K., Araújo, D., Shuttleworth, R. and Button, C. (2003) Acquiring skill in sport: a constraints-led perspective. *International Journal of Computer Science in Sport*, 2, 31–9.

Davids K., Bennett S., and Newell, K. (2006) *Movement System Variability*. Champaign, IL: Human Kinetics.

Davids, K., Button C. and Bennett S. (2008) *Dynamics of Skill Acquisition: A Constraints-led Approach*. Champaign, IL: Human Kinetics.

Davids, K., Araújo D., Hristovski, R., Passos, P. and Chow, J.-Y. (2012) Ecological dynamics and motor learning design in sport, in A. M. Williams and N. Hodges (eds) *Skill Acquisition in Sport: Research, Theory and Practice*, 2nd edn. London: Routledge, pp. 112–30.

Edelman, G. M. and Gally, J. A. (2001) Degeneracy and complexity in biological systems. *Proceedings of the National Academy of Sciences of the U S A*, 98 (24): 13763–8.

Gibson, J. J. (1979) *An Ecological Approach to Visual Perception*. Boston, MA: Houghton-Mifflin.

Gibson, J. (1966) *The Senses Considered as Perceptual Systems*. Boston, MA: Houghton Mifflin.

Hoyt, D. F. and Taylor, C. R. (1981) Gait and the energetics of locomotion in horses. *Nature*, 292: 239–40.

Hristovski, R., Davids, K. and Araújo, D. (2006a) Affordance-controlled bifurcations of action patterns in martial arts. *Nonlinear Dynamics, Psychology, and Life Sciences*, 10 (4): 409–44.

Hristovski, R., Davids K., Araújo, D. and Button, C. (2006b) How boxers decide to punch a target: emergent behaviour in non linear dynamic movement systems. *Journal of Sports Science and Medicine*, 5: 60–73.

Kelso, J. A. S. (1995) Dynamic patterns: the self-organization of brain and behaviour. Cambridge, MA: MIT Press.

Kelso, J. A. S. (2012) Multi-stability and meta-stability: understanding dynamic coordination in the brain. *Philosophical Transactions of the Royal Society B Biological Sciences*, 367: 906–18.

Li, L., Haddad, J. M. and Hamill, J. (2005) Stability and variability may respond differently to changes in walking speed. *Human Movement Science*, 24: 257–67.

Mason, P. H. (2010) Degeneracy at multiple levels of complexity. *Biological Theory*, 5 (3): 277–88.

Newell, K. M. (1986) Constraints on the development of coordination, in M. G. Wade and H. T. A. Whiting (eds) *Motor Development in Children: Aspect of Coordination and Control*. Dordrecht: Martinus Nijhoff, pp. 341–60.

Newell, K. M. and Corcos, D. M. (1993) Issues in variability and motor control, in K.M. Newell and D. M. Corcos (eds) *Variability and Motor Control*. Champaign, IL: Human Kinetics Publishers, pp. 1–12.

Newell K. M. and Slifkin A. B. (1998) The nature of movement variability, in J. P. Piek (ed.) *Motor Behaviour and Human Skill: A Multidisciplinarity Perspective*. Champaign, IL: Human Kinetics Publishers, pp. 143–60.

Pezzulo, G., Barca, L., Lamberti Bocconi, A. and Borghi, A. M. (2010) When affordances climb into your mind: advantages of motor simulation in a memory task performed by novice and expert rock climbers, *Brain and Cognition*, 73: 68–73.

Phillips, K. C., Sassaman, J. M. and Smoliga, J. M. (2012) Optimizing rock climbing performance through sport-specific strength and conditioning. *Strength and Conditioning Journal*, 24 (3): 1–18.

Pinder, R. A., Davids, K. and Renshaw, I. (2012) Metastability and emergent performance of dynamic interceptive actions. *Journal of Science and Medicine in Sport*, 15 (5): 437–43.

Quaine, F. and Martin, L. (1999) A biomechanical study of equilibrium in sport rock climbing, *Gait and Posture*, 10: 233–9.

Reid, C. R., Latty, T., Dussutour, A. and Beekman, M. (2012) Slime mold uses an externalised spatial 'memory' to navigate in complex environments. *PNAS Proceedings of the National Academy of Sciences of the USA*, 109 (43): 17490–4.

Sanchez, X., Lambert, P., Jones, G. and Llewellyn D. J. (2012) Efficacy of pre-ascent climbing route visual inspection in indoor sport climbing, *Scandinavian Journal of Medicine and Science in Sports*, 22: 67–72.

Seifert, L., Wattebled, L., L'Hermette, M. and Hérault, R. (2011) Inter-limb coordination variability in ice climbers of different skill level. *Education and Physical Training in Sport*, 1: 63–8.

Seifert, L., Button, C. and Davids, K. (2013) Key properties of expert movement systems in sport: An Ecological Dynamics perspective. *Sports Medicine*, 43 (3): 167–78.

Sibella, F., Frosio, I., Schena, F., and Borghese, N. A. (2007) 3D analysis of the body center of mass in rock climbing. *Human Movement Science*, 26: 841–52.

Sparrow, W. A. (2000) *Energetics of Human Activity*. Champaign, IL: Human Kinetics.

Sparrow, W. A. and Newell, K. M. (1998) Metabolic energy expenditure and the regulation of movement economy. *Psychonomic Bulletin and Review*, 5: 173–96.

van Emmerik, R. E. A. and van Wegen, E. E. H. (2000) On variability and stability in human movement. *Journal of Applied Biomechanics*, 16: 394–406.

Warren, W. H. (2006) The dynamics of perception and action. *Psychological Review*, 113 (2): 358–89.

19 Skill acquisition and representative task design

Ross A. Pinder, Ian Renshaw, Jonathon Headrick and Keith Davids

Egon Brunswik's (1956) insights have revealed that representative task design is a key concept in understanding the organization of task constraints in experiments, evaluation tests and learning programmes in sport. Representative design implies that these environments need to be predicated on key information sources found in specific performance contexts. Although Brunswik's ideas have, until now, failed to be fully appreciated in a wide range of experimental and behavioural sciences, many of the concepts have begun to be accepted in the study of complex systems in sport (Araújo and Davids 2009; Beek *et al.* 2003; Davids 2008; Dicks *et al.* 2008; Fajen *et al.* 2009; Pinder *et al.* 2011b,c). Here, we discuss the ideas of representative task design and examine its implications for constructing experimental and learning environments in sport. We provide principles for sport scientists, experimental psychologists and pedagogues to recognize the potential application and adaptation of Brunswik's original concepts, with examples from various sports to demonstrate how the model can be applied in practice. We also discuss the role of representative design in supporting the psychology of learning and creating holistic learning environments for learners as complex systems, in addition to considering the integrated emotional engagement of participants for the enhancement of learning and practice task design.

Egon Brunswik's representative design

Traditional research designs in sports science and motor learning have been historically reductionist and systematic in nature (Dhami *et al.* 2004). The traditional distinction between experimental control and 'field' research has been recognized as a false dichotomy, where reductionist approaches are being complemented by functional paradigms of movement coordination considered in humans modelled as complex dynamical systems. This paradigm has been largely supported by theoretical and empirical work from ecological psychology (Brunswik 1956; Gibson 1979). The insights of James Gibson (1979) revealed why specific environments need to be carefully structured and organized so that they maintain functional relations between processes of perception and action during performance. In ecological psychology, there have been recent attempts to mediate the links between Gibsonian and Brunswikian theoretical and methodological approaches (Araújo *et al.* 2007; Kirlik 2009; Vicente 2003), to broaden ecological research and develop cumulative knowledge. Current neo-Gibsonian research into event perception coincides with ideas on organism–environment relationships demonstrated in the lens model (Figure 19.1; Brunswik 1952, 1956), where research is now confronting the problem of uncertainty highlighted by Brunswik's theory of probabilistic functionalism (Kirlik 2009). The integration of Egon Brunswik's and James Gibson's theoretical work provides an advantageous methodological approach for studying complex systems in sport, maintaining the scale of analysis as the performer–environment relationship (Kirlik 2009; Reed 1996; Vicente 2003).

Egon Brunswik proposed the term *representative design* as an alternative to systematic design in the 1950s, advocating that the study of human performance and psychological processes should be at the level of organism–environment interaction. That is, a focus should be maintained on the complex system formed by a sports performer and their performance environment. These ideas proposed that experimental stimuli must be sampled from an organism's (e.g. performer's) natural environment, so as to be representative of the stimuli to which it is adapted and to which experimental data are intended to be generalized (Brunswik 1956). Generalization of findings beyond the constraints of the experiment is highly problematic when studying the adaptability of human movement in dynamic environments (see Chapter 15). There is a need to adequately sample environmental constraints which facilitate the emergence of functional human behaviours based on the informational variables of the specific performance context of interest. In sport, these variables emerge from the interpersonal interactions between performers and between performers and key events, objects and surrounding energy structures present in the performance environment (exemplified by how a soccer player interacts with the ball, the opposition and performers within their own team): the basis of sport as a complex system.

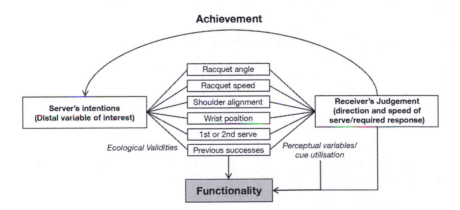

Figure 19.1 The role of Brunswik's lens model in understanding informational variables for complex systems in sport – analysis of a tennis serve (model adapted from Araujo and Kirlik 2008)

Brunswik (1956) concluded that the adequate sampling of situations and problems in psychological experimentation should take precedence over the concerns of population sampling. His ecological approach to cognition (considered here to encompass intentionality, see Searle 1983; Shaw 2001), perception and action was implemented through the theoretical framework of probabilistic functionalism (Hammond and Stewart 2001; Kirlik 2009). Simply stated, this idea signifies that, in sport, performers try to use multiple sources of imperfect information to infer about future events or aspects of the dynamic environment (e.g. the way a rugby defender might use kinematic information from an opponent's movements to predict their attacking intentions). In describing organism–environment interactions, Brunswik (1956) referred to distal variables (remote properties of the environment, such as an opponent's intentions) and proximal variables or cues (information sources directly available, such as vision of an opponent's movements). Importantly, this process is inherently probabilistic, with variables available from the environment providing different levels of *functionality*. Perceptual judgements are based on the inferences of proximal cues (perceptual variables), with different sets of cues available in different environmental conditions. The ability to identify and selectively use informational variables (or in Brunswikian terms, cues) has been considered to be one of the major factors influencing the ability to predict future behaviour of other performers in complex sport tasks (van der Kamp *et al.* 2008; Williams *et al.* 1999). As informational sources differ in their degrees of functionality, they may also vary in the degree to which they are intercorrelated with each other (for example the relationship between multiple limb segments of a tennis server's action).

Importantly, cues must be combined in a context-specific manner, allowing for the development and refinement of robust performer–environment couplings, known as *vicarious functioning*. Owing to the interdependence of the processes of intentionality, perception and action, and the ways in which human movement systems have evolved, the separation of these processes during experimental or learning designs, often in the name of enhancing internal validity, is of major concern (Michaels and Carello 1981; van der Kamp *et al.* 2008). Simulations (e.g. experimental or practice designs attempting to simulate aspects of a performance environment) that decouple the processes of perception and action do not permit perceptual and action subsystems to function, as they have been developed or trained to do in a particular sport performance context, nor do they allow for the same emotional or psychological engagement of an individual with the task. The mutual interdependence between intentionality, perception and action suggests that these processes should be allowed to function in an interdependent manner in an experiment or learning programme (Araújo *et al.* 2007; Pinder *et al.* 2011b; van der Kamp *et al.* 2008). As achievement of an action cannot be defined without reference to the environment, functional systems of an individual (such as ventral and dorsal visual streams, or engagement of the limbic system) are viewed as contributing factors to task goal achievement (Kirlik 2001). In representative design, there is a strong emphasis on the relations between the participant and the environment, which is often neglected in traditional approaches to the study of human behaviour, such as in cognitive psychology (e.g. Dunwoody 2006).

Perceptual motor skill research has all too frequently attempted to focus on the precise (presumed singular) source of information that perceivers putatively use to achieve a specific task outcome (Withagen and van Wermeskerken 2009), assuming that some source of optimal information will be available to the perceiver (Reed 1996). Studies focusing on perceptual learning have now begun to cast doubt over this assumption of information singularity, with a greater emphasis on understanding information plurality when individuals use various informational variables to regulate their actions, changing their use of variables over time (Jacobs *et al.* 2001; Runeson and Andersson 2007; Withagen and Michaels 2005). The use of a variety of perceptual variables to regulate behaviours is supported by a better understanding of neurobiological complexity, especially of system degeneracy, which performers can exploit to contextually adapt their actions under changing task constraints (Davids and Araújo 2010). The perceiver is likely to use a variety of relatively reliable perceptual cues to provide themselves with the required information to support action (Kirlik 2009; Runeson and Andersson 2007). For example, a performer may use a combination of kinematic cues from a baseball pitcher's action, such as wrist position, seam position and shoulder alignment, to predict the speed and angle of the upcoming pitch. The establishment of robust organism–environment relationships (i.e. information–movement couplings), therefore, is analogous to Bernstein's (1967) mastering degrees of freedom problem. Essentially, several different couplings may be available for exploitation in goal-directed behaviour, with learning characterized by the refinement of established information–movement couplings. The lens model (see Figure 19.1) explains how performers cope with complex and dynamically changing environments through exploiting perceptual and motor system degeneracy (Davids 2008); essentially, a pictorial representation of vicarious functioning (see Goldstein 2006).

In considering sport performance as a complex system, the major implication is that practitioners need to ensure that all key informational variables are available in particular experimental and learning environments to allow performers to detect information and perceive affordances for action. Note that *ecological validity* was originally defined as the statistical correlation between proximal cues available in the environment (perceptual variables) and the extent to which they depict the distal criterion state of the environment (see also, Araújo *et al.* 2007; Brunswik 1956; Pinder *et al.* 2011b). This idea is exemplified by the statistical correlation between the presence of an observable kinematic detail of a tennis server's action and the resultant action (e.g. a cross-court serve). The definition of representative design emphasizes the need to ensure that task constraints of experiments represent (i.e. simulate) the particular task constraints of the performance environment that forms the focus of study. In this way, the distinction between ecological validity and representative design is not a trivial issue, as the clarification allows for a more comprehensive and principled approach to studying complex system interactions in sport.

Principles of representative learning design

Brunswik's (1956) concept of representative task design provides a critical framework for the study of intention, perception and action processes in sport (Dicks *et al.* 2008). A key concept of experimental design in the analysis of complex human behaviour is the importance of manipulating task constraints (Araújo *et al.* 2004), which are central to the process of harnessing inherent self-organization tendencies in complex neurobiological systems. In sport, representative design supports the generalization of task constraints in learning designs to the ecological constraints of performance (Araújo *et al.* 2006; Davids 2008), implying that a performer needs to be able to search the environment for reliable information to support and direct action. Learning designs need to be predicated on the ability of performers to use information from the performance environment, which is vital for the acquisition of a functional and efficient relationship between perceptual and motor processes in the control of action (Le Runigo *et al.* 2005). Skill acquisition programmes in sport, therefore, need to be designed to enhance the existing coupling between an individual's intentions and perception and action subsystems. Based on these ideas, it is important for sport practitioners to identify the major ecological constraints of a particular performance environment, especially the informational constraints.

Despite technological and methodological advances, many experimental and practice tasks in the analysis of dynamic human behaviours in sport fail to provide an adequate platform to facilitate the intertwined processes of cognition, perception and action to function as a complex system. For example, Dicks *et al.* (2010) demonstrated significant changes in the detection of information when performers responded under experimental task constraints varying in levels of functional coupling between perception and action processes (see also Farrow and Abernethy 2003). Soccer (association football) goalkeepers were observed to use different information sources under the constraints of video simulations and 'in situ' tasks representative of intercepting a penalty kick in competition. These data demonstrated the need for the analysis of behaviour at an ecological scale of performance (e.g. performers directly interacting with the performance environment), ensuring that task designs allow for the emergence of functional behaviours representative of the performance environment of interest. The presence of this key characteristic of system complexity can be assessed and achieved through the careful manipulation of key task constraints (e.g. informational constraints) during practice and experimentation. The design of learning environments that effectively capture and enhance functional movement responses representative of performance contexts should be constructed using the theoretical principles of representative learning design (Pinder *et al.* 2011b).

Representative learning design (Figure 19.2) provides a principled framework which theoretically captures how insights from ecological dynamics and nonlinear pedagogy approaches can be used to ensure that experimental and practice task constraints are representative of sport performance environments as integrated complex systems (see Renshaw *et al.* 2010). Assessment of representative

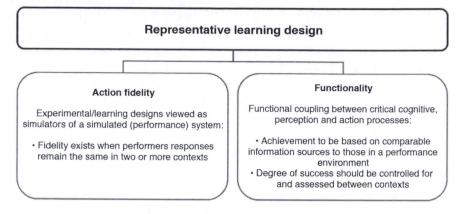

Figure 19.2 Principles for the assessment of representative learning design

learning design in specific practice tasks allows sport scientists to understand the functionality and limitations of particular training environments. Understanding how the complexity sciences can inform representative learning design may provide opportunities to optimize learning programmes in sport and inform use of performance enhancement tools, such as projection technology, during practice. Practitioners should consider both the functionality and action fidelity of a simulation design. This will ensure that the complexity of the performance context is considered and the coupling between key cognitive, perceptual and action processes is maintained. Functionality provides a measure of action achievement and the information on which this level of attainment is based. Considering the functionality of a task ensures that: a) the degree of success between two or more contexts is controlled and compared; and b), participants are able to use comparable information sources for goal attainment and control of movement behaviour between learning/experimental and performance tasks (e.g. by comparing visual search strategies or detection of information between contexts).

Action fidelity (see Stoffregen *et al.* 2003) is a measure of the degree of association between behaviour in two or more contexts, allowing scientists or practitioners to examine whether the actions and decisions of a complex neurobiological system remain the same under experimental or learning designs and their respective performance contexts. Essentially, action fidelity provides information about the fidelity of a performer's actions between the simulator (e.g. a practice situation that is attempting to simulate one or all aspects of a performance environment) and the simulated context (the performance environment of interest). For example, large video simulations are a common research and learning tool in perceptual-motor analysis in sport; however, the concept of simulating aspects of performance should be extended to all practice and learning tasks. Experimental, practice and learning designs can be viewed as simulations of the performance environment of interest (e.g. a ball projection machine simulating aspects of facing a 'live' bowler in performance – also see below). Key measures of behaviour, such as time taken to complete a task and observed movement organisation during action, are suitable variables for assessing action fidelity of simulation environments (Araújo *et al.* 2007). In the next section, we demonstrate how the principles outlined here have and may be used to assess the representative design of practice and learning designs in sport using short examples from empirical findings.

Representative learning design for complex systems in sport

Considering sport performance as an integrated complex system, as outlined throughout this book, can encourage the development of a more representative design for learning, practice and experimental settings. To date, the primary focus of representative (learning) design has been ensuring that links between perception and action processes and the informational variables provided in complex interactions in sports performance are representative. Essentially, up to now, this focus has been on ensuring the presence of specifying information in the external environmental. However, information from within the performer can also act as a constraint, shaping cognitions, feelings and behaviours during learning. In the following section, we build on these ideas and provide examples from external environmental and internal intrinsic dynamics.

The significance of ensuring representative designs for experimental and learning tasks in the analysis and acquisition of skilled human behaviour is exemplified by the use of ball projection machines. Our work has shown that using projection machines with developmental athletes can create significant differences in timing and control of their actions compared to when facing a 'live' opponent (Pinder *et al.* 2011a; Renshaw *et al.* 2007). Junior cricket batters initiated key movements significantly later when playing against a projection machine set to the same speed (approximately equal to 28 metres per second) and with similar ball trajectory characteristics as a ball delivered by a 'live' performer. These delays in movement initiation resulted in significant adaptations in movement organization and reduction in quality of bat–ball contact during interception; similar to findings in tennis (Shim *et al.* 2005). Technologies, such as projection machines, have the potential to change the key ecological (informational) constraints between practice and performance and demonstrate how caution should be taken in designing practice simulations. Practitioners should use complex systems modelling to assess the representative design of such tasks to inform how and when to use technology in learning design, as the removal of key information sources may limit a performer's ability to create robust and functional information–movement couplings required in the performance environment (Pinder *et al.* 2011d).

Analyses of complex human behaviour in invasion sports (e.g. soccer, rugby, basketball) have also demonstrated that sometimes apparently small modifications in task constraints within aspects of the experimental design can lead to substantial and critical changes in the functional and emergent performances of individuals. Analyses of team games sub-phases (e.g. one-versus-one, two-versus-one) have shown that performers are highly attuned to the presence and movements of opponents, regulating movement organization and decision-making behaviours within these complex systems. For example, successful attacking performance in soccer and rugby union has been highly constrained by the relative interpersonal coordination and velocities of opponents (Duarte *et al.* 2010; Passos *et al.* 2008) or simply the presence of defenders (Orth *et al.* 2012). Furthermore, Headrick *et al.* (2012) demonstrated that the emergent attacking strategies of soccer players were influenced by the proximity to goal and the subsequent intentions of both the player in possession and the defender. These findings suggest that for simulations (e.g. practice tasks) to demonstrate fidelity, practitioners should consider the state and context of specific game situations, allow performers to practice *against opponents* in the same areas of the field, as they would in competition, and use standard pitch markings to orient players within those tasks. This is an important issue that is often overlooked in the design of practice tasks, particularly with junior or developmental performers. Subtly, in invasion games such as football, pitch size needs to be carefully considered from the physiological and skill acquisition perspective. For example, while the use of small-sided games is strongly recommended from the viewpoint of nonlinear pedagogy (see Renshaw *et al.* 2010), practitioners need to also carefully consider the player numbers and pitch dimensions in terms of the physiological workloads of players (Hill-Haas *et al.* 2011). Principled frameworks from a complex systems perspective are ideal for understanding the interacting and complex nature of performer–environment relationships and how the careful manipulation of task constraints can lead to substantial changes to other areas or subsystems. Altering the spatiotemporal constraints available to players on the ball is likely to lead to significant qualitative changes in ball reception strategies and the time taken from ball reception to pass initiation. These ideas are discussed in Renshaw *et al.* (2012) where a 'game intensity index' is proposed as a way of controlling and manipulating the time–space available to players. These ideas are important for those studying representative learning design in complex sports tasks and provide some pointers for future research.

Representative design also has significant implications for the identification and development of talent in skill acquisition in sport. The developed principles, based on identifying and manipulating the major constraints during learning, provides a principled basis for the design of performance evaluation tests in talent programmes (Vilar *et al.* 2012), allowing performance and physiological capacities of potential performers to be assessed. Just as experimental and learning designs should be based on the performance context of interest, testing protocols should ensure that the tests exhibit representative design (Araújo *et al.* 2007; Pinder *et al.* 2011b). For example, it has been highlighted how static drills used in the identification of potentially talented performers lack the key informational variables and functionality between perception and action subsystems as they would contribute in competitive performance (Vilar *et al.* 2012), nor do they consider emotional or social aspects of sports performance; in such instances, fundamental relationships between performers and key informational variables of a complex sporting system are jeopardised.

Representative learning design and the psychology of learning

As previously discussed, the concept of representative (learning) design has been outlined primarily in relation to the informational aspects of an environment that provide the context for a performer's action. Another factor to be considered for the design of practice tasks is their interaction with psychological constraints such as emotions, attention, goal orientations and self-efficacy. When sampling complex tasks with the aim of simulating experiences from competition in practice, consideration of the psychological aspects of performance is important in enabling practitioners and sport scientists to design representative learning environments that faithfully replicate interactions between task constraints and individual constraints such as emotions, behaviours and cognitions. From this perspective, the performer is seen as an interconnected system, which suggests that there is a requirement for supporting the emotional and psychological engagement of the individual in practice to simulate the intensity experienced in competitive performance. Learning to cope with emotions created by complex performance environments such as anger, fear, excitement, frustration or anxiety is just as important as learning a technical skill. The development of functional perception–action couplings is intertwined with emotions via vertical integration between the lower emotional (e.g. limbic system) and higher, cognitive systems (cortex). The emotional and psychological engagement of individual performers is an important consideration to further enhance the representative design of practice, learning and experimental tasks, allowing for a more integrated perspective of the learner.

Emotions underpin numerous motivational aspects of learning, 'playing an integral part in shaping mental abilities, processes and skills' (Lewis 2004, p. 221). Additionally, at a neurobiological level, learning is strengthened through emotional engagement in learning activities (Lewis 2004; Tucker *et al.* 2000). Similarly, when individual learners are required to fashion new strategies out of older established stable patterns that have been functional in the past, they have to learn to deal with and understand the accompanying emotional turmoil associated with the high levels of variability that are typically experienced in the cognition–action relationship around these phase transitions (Lewis 2004; Thelen and Smith 1994). Unfortunately, coaches tend to have limited skills and knowledge of how to incorporate psychological skills into learning design for complex systems (Harwood 2008). One way of enhancing a practitioner's ability to implement psychological goals in practice could be to implicitly embed them into the design of practice tasks. For example, Renshaw *et al.* (2012) demonstrated how nonlinear pedagogy could be used to develop autonomy, competence and relatedness; the key components underpinning self-determining behaviour (Deci and Ryan 2002). Deci (1980) defined emotion as:

a reaction to a stimulus event (either actual or imagined). It involves change in the viscera and musculature of the person, is experienced subjectively in characteristic ways, is expressed through such means as facial changes and action tendencies, and may mediate and energise subsequent behaviours.

(Deci 1980: 85)

In essence, emotional activation constrains cognitive processes such as attentional processes by appraising situations as beneficial or harmful (Lewis 2004). Those situations that are identified as significant trigger an emotion and demand cognitive or motor responses. Consequently, exposure to emotionally engaging tasks leads to changes in physiological responses (e.g. heart rate, skin responses), subjective experiences (e.g. what a performer consciously experiences prior to, during and after an event) and specific and individual action tendencies (Vallerand and Blanchard 2000). In effect, as individuals interact in complex and dynamic environments, changes in emotions influence intentions, perceptions and actions. For example, momentary failure in a practice bout in judo may lead to an immediate intention to avoid experiencing failure (avoidance goal orientation) and adoption of a more defensive strategy (Gernigon *et al.* 2004). In essence, an increase in negative emotions such as anxiety owing to short term failure could result in the reduction of performance degrees of freedom (e.g. biasing or narrowing perception; Pessoa 2011) or reducing movement options (Parfitt *et al.* 1990). Conversely, success is more likely to produce positive emotions such as pride and satisfaction (Lewis 2004) and lead to goal orientations that aim to demonstrate competence and lead to more attacking, assertive and aggressive actions (Gernigon *et al.* 2004).

Psychological aspects of performance can also be linked to, and exemplified by Brunswik's lens model. Referring to the example given (Figure 19.1), the previous success and subsequent perceived competence of a performer will influence how they approach a task. Likewise, the context of the task (e.g. first or second serve) can influence whether the actions of the performer tend to approach success (e.g. hit an attacking return on a second serve) or avoid failure (e.g. only try to return the ball back into play on a first serve). In this way, psychological aspects considered above can be viewed as contributing towards the functionality of the practice or learning task design, and an enhancement of the representative design of complex sports interactions.

Emotion and learning in nonlinear pedagogy

Learning something new is an emotionally demanding experience, irrespective of the learner being a complete beginner or an established champion. For the beginner, who is required to construct a new coordination pattern or a champion who has to move away from a successful strategy to adapt to new rules, equipment or clever opponents that are always emerging in complex environments, new learning requires risk-taking that can potentially threaten self-efficacy and create somatic and cognitive anxiety as they struggle to deal with the relative 'failure' that comes with trying to develop something new. As Australian Test cricketer, Ed Cowan (2011, p. 11) eloquently put it when describing how he tried to improve his ability to 'hit' in T20 games (a short version cricket that requires batters to score by regularly clearing the boundary), 'learning "to hit" from scratch meant dealing with the feeling of initial inadequacy'. Clearly, exploration commensurate with becoming less reliant on tried and trusted stable behaviours in search of new, potentially more advantageous, ways could be threatening on a number of levels and requires appropriate psychosocial support from coaches and teachers who understand the multilayered consequences of 'risk' in learning.

Practitioners need to carefully consider the impact of manipulating constraints that lead to performance failure and the consequent search for new solutions. As discussed earlier from a complex systems perspective, moving performers into metastable regions that result in self-organizing phase transitions is accompanied by the creation of emotions that impact on intentions and actions of each individual. High levels of emotion can be used to index transition phases (Lewis 2004) and reflect the competition between new emergent solutions and previously established patterns. In their initial learning design, coaches need to understand that learners will always be attracted to patterns that 'work' and that this would be indexed directly by 'what feels good'. This in turn is shaped by the intentionality of each learner to pursue his/her goals (e.g. to improve, please the coach, demonstrate competence or protect self-worth) as effectively as they can (Lewis 2004). As such, coaches should not only sample the informational constraints on actions of learners but should also predict the likely psychological consequences caused by potentially stressful practice tasks, based on knowledge of each individual learner. On an individual level, because responses are likely to reflect stable cognitive–emotional attractor patterns laid down in earlier phases of development (Lewis 2004), identifying previous learning histories of individuals is an important requirement when programming learning activities. Consequently, coaches might not always want to create high levels of representative learning design in respect of emotional responses for all practice tasks. This process can be carefully controlled if the outlined framework is followed and coaches are able to make principled decisions based on sampling of competition and practice environments.

Conclusions

Egon Brunswik's original insights and concepts have proven to be highly applicable and adaptable (Dhami *et al.* 2004; Wigton 2008). The development of a functional and principled framework in sport demonstrates how sport scientists, coaches and pedagogues can assess and provide representative experimental, testing and learning tasks which maintain, enhance or emphasize the functional and intertwined relationships between performers' perceptions, actions, intentions and emotions. Considering sport performance as an integrated complex system encourages the development of more representative learning, practice and experimental designs, particularly in supporting the role of information in the environment and the emotional and psychological engagement of the individual in practice. While, the role of emotion in learning has been considered by psychologists, we suggest that by considering how emotions couple with intentions, perceptions and actions within a representative learning design may reveal new insights on learning via a nonlinear pedagogy.

Questions for students

1. Choose a sports task (e.g. springboard diving, baseball batting, tennis serving):
   - What are the key perception and action processes which should be maintained in practice to ensure a representative degree of functionality?
   - What measures would allow you to assess the fidelity of action between learning and performance contexts?
2. What are the implications of representative learning design for task decomposition in the learning of complex sports skills?
3. How do representative learning environments support and foster positive psychological experiences in performers?
4. Why is it important to consider emotion in the design of learning tasks?

References

Araújo, D. and Kirlik, A. (2008) Towards an ecological approach to visual anticipation for expert performance in sport. *International Journal of Sport Psychology*, 39: 157–65.

Araújo, D. and Davids, K. (2009) Ecological approaches to cognition and action in sport and exercise: ask not only what you do, but where you do it. *International Journal of Sport Psychology*, 40 (1): 5–37.

Araújo, D., Davids, K., Bennett, S., Button, C. and Chapman, G. (2004) Emergence of sport skills under constraints, in A. M. Williams and N. J. Hodges (eds) *Skill Acquisition in Sport: Research, Theory and Practice*. London: Taylor and Francis, pp. 409–33.

Araújo, D., Davids, K. and Hristovski, R. (2006) The ecological dynamics of decision making in sport. *Psychology of Sport and Exercise*, 7: 653–76.

Araújo, D., Davids, K. and Passos, P. (2007) Ecological validity, representative design, and correspondence between experimental task constraints and behavioral setting: comment on Rogers, Kadar, and Costall (2005) *Ecological Psychology*, 19 (1): 69–78.

Beek, P. J., Jacobs, D. M., Daffertshofer, A. and Huys, R. (2003) Expert performance in sport: views from joint perspectives of ecological psychology and dynamical systems theory, in J. L. Starkes and K. A. Ericsson (eds) *Expert Performance in Sport: Advances in Research on Sport Expertise*. Champaign, IL: Human Kinetics, pp. 321–44.

Bernstein, N. A. (1967) *The Control and Regulation of Movements*. London: Pergamon Press.

Brunswik, E. (1952) *The Conceptual Framework of Psychology*. Chicago, IL: University of Chicago Press.

Brunswik, E. (1956) *Perception and the Representative Design of Psychological Experiments*, 2nd edn. Berkeley, CA: University of California Press.

Cowan, E. (2011) *In the Firing Line: Diary of a Season*. Sydney: NewSouth Publishing.

Davids, K. (2008) Designing representative task constraints for studying visual anticipation in fast ball sports: what we can learn from past and contemporary insights in neurobiology and psychology. *International Journal of Sport Psychology*, 39 (2): 166–77.

Davids, K. and Araújo, D. (2010) The concept of 'organismic asymmetry' in sport science. *Journal of Science and Medicine in Sport*, 13 (6): 633–40.

Deci, E. L. (1980) *The Psychology of Self-Determination*. Lexington, MA: D. C. Heath and Company.

Deci, E. L. and Ryan, R. M. (eds) (2002) *Handbook of Self-Determination Research*. Rochester, NY: University of Rochester Press.

Dhami, M. K., Hertwig, R. and Hoffrage, U. (2004) The role of representative design in ecological approach to cognition. *Psychological Bulletin*, 130 (6): 959–88.

Dicks, M., Davids, K. and Araújo, D. (2008) Ecological psychology and task representativeness: implications for the design of perceptual-motor training programmes in sport, in Y. Hong and R. Bartlett (eds) *The Routledge Handbook of Biomechanics and Human Movement Science*. London: Routledge, pp. 129–39.

Dicks, M., Button, C. and Davids, K. (2010) Examination of gaze behaviors under in situ and video simulation task constraints reveals differences in information pickup for perception and action. *Attention, Perception and Psychophysics*, 72 (3): 706–20.

Duarte, R., Araújo, D., Gazimba, V., Fernandes, O., Folgado, H., Marmeleira, J. and Davids, K. (2010) The ecological dynamics of 1v1 sub-phases in association football. *Open Sports Sciences Journal*, 3: 16–18.

Dunwoody, P. T. (2006) The neglect of the environment by cognitive psychology. *Journal of Theoretical and Philosophical Psychology*, 26: 139–53.

Fajen, B. R., Riley, M. A. and Turvey, M. T. (2009) Information, affordances and the control of action in sport. *International Journal of Sport Psychology*, 40: 79–107.

Farrow, D. and Abernethy, B. (2003) Do expertise and the degree of perception-action coupling affect natural anticipatory performance? *Perception*, 32 (9): 1127–39.

Gernigon, C., d'Arripe-Longueville, F., Delignieres, D. and Ninot, G. (2004) A dynamical systems perspective on goal involvement states in sport. *Journal of Sport and Exercise Psychology*, 26: 572–96.

Gibson, J. J. (1979) *The Ecological Approach to Visual Perception*. Boston, MA: Houghton Mifflin.

Goldstein, W. M. (2006) Introduction to Brunswikian theory and method, in A. Kirlik (ed.) *Adaptive Perspectives on Human–Technology Interaction*. Oxford: Oxford University Press, pp. 10–24.

Hammond, K. R. and Stewart, T. R. (2001) Introduction, in K. R. Hammond and T. R. Stewart (eds) *The Essential Brunswik: Beginnings, Explications, Applications*. New York: Oxford University Press, pp. 3–11.

Harwood, C. (2008) Development consulting in a professional football academy: the 5Cs coaching efficiency program. *Sport Psychologist*, 22: 109–33.

Headrick, J., Davids, K., Renshaw, I., Araújo, D., Passo, P. and Fernandes, O. (2012) Proximity-to-goal as a constraint on patterns of behaviour in attacker-defender dyads in team games. *Journal of Sports Sciences*, 30 (3): 247–53.

Hill-Haas, S. V., Dawson, B., Impellizzeri, F. M. and Coutts, A. J. (2011) Physiology of small-sided games training in football: a systematic review. *Sports Medicine*, 41 (3): 199–220.

Jacobs, D. M., Runeson, S. and Michaels, C. F. (2001) Learning to visually perceive the relative mass of coliding balls in globally and locally constrained task ecologies. *Journal of Experimental Psychology: Human Perception and Performance*, 27 (5): 1019–38.

Kirlik, A. (2001) On Gibson's review of Brunswik, in K. R. Hammond and T. R. Stewart (eds) *The Essential Brunswik: Beginnings, Explications, Applications.* Oxford: Oxford University Press, pp. 238–42.

Kirlik, A. (2009) Brunswikian resources for event perception research. *Perception*, 38 (3): 376–98.

Le Runigo, C., Benguigui, N. and Bardy, B. G. (2005) Perception-action coupling and expertise in interceptive actions. *Human Movement Science*, 24: 429–45.

Lewis, M. D. (2004) The emergence of mind in the emotional brain, in A. Demetriou and A. Raftopoulos (eds) *Cognitive Developmental Change.* New York: Cambridge University Press, pp. 217–40.

Michaels, C. F. and Carello, C. (1981) *Direct Perception.* Englewood Cliffs, NJ: Prentice Hall.

Orth, D., Davids, K., Araújo, D., Renshaw, I. and Passos, P. (2012) Effects of a defender on run-up velocity and ball speed when crossing a football. *European Journal of Sport Science*, iFirst article: 1–8; doi: 10.1080/17461391.2012.696712

Parfitt, G., Hardy, L. and Pates, J. (1990) Somatic anxiety and psychological arousal: their effects upon a high anaerobic, low memory demand task. *International Journal of Sport Psychology*, 26: 196–213.

Passos, P., Araujo, D., Davids, K., Gouveia, L., Milho, J. and Serpa, S. (2008) Information-governing dynamics of attacker-defender interactions in youth rugby union. *Journal of Sports Sciences*, 26 (13): 1421–9.

Pessoa, L. (2011) Reprint of: Emotion and cognition and the amygdala: from 'what is it?' to 'what's to be done?', *Neuropsychologia*, 49 (4): 681–94.

Pinder, R. A., Davids, K., Renshaw, I. and Araújo, D. (2011a) Manipulating informational constraints shapes movement reorganization in interceptive actions. *Attention, Perception and Psychophysics*, 73 (4): 1242–54.

Pinder, R. A., Davids, K., Renshaw, I. and Araújo, D. (2011b) Representative learning design and functionality of research and practice in sport. *Journal of Sport and Exercise Psychology*, 33: 146–55.

Pinder, R. A., Renshaw, I., Davids, K. and Kerhervé, H. (2011c) Principles for use of ball projection machines in elite and developmental sport programmes. *Sports Medicine*, 41 (10): 793–800.

Pinder, R. A., Davids, K. and Renshaw, I. (2011d) Learning design for use of ball projection technologies with different skill levels in ball skill acquisition. Paper presented at the Technologies in Sport Symposium.

Reed, E. S. (1996) *Encountering the World: Toward an Ecological Psychology.* New York: Oxford University Press.

Renshaw, I., Oldham, A. R. H., Davids, K. and Golds, T. (2007) Changing ecological constraints of practice alters coordination of dynamic interceptive actions. *European Journal of Sport Science*, 7 (3): 157–67.

Renshaw, I., Chow, J. Y., Davids, K. and Hammond, J. (2010) A constraints-led perspective to understanding skill acquisition and game play: a basis for integration of motor learning theory and physical education praxis? *Physical Education and Sport Pedagogy*, 15: 117–37.

Renshaw, I., Oldham, A. R. H. and Bawden, M. (2012) Nonlinear pedagogy underpins intrinsic motivation in sports coaching. *Open Science Journal*, 5 (Suppl 1-M10): 88–99.

Runeson, S. and Andersson, I. E. K. (2007) Achievement of specificational information usage with true and false feedback in learning a visual relative-mass discrimination task. *Journal of Experimental Psychology: Human Perception and Performance*, 33 (1): 163–82.

Searle, J. R. (1983) *Intentionality: An Essay in the Philosophy of Mind*. Cambridge: Cambridge University Press.

Shaw, R. (2001) Processes, acts, and experiences: three stances on the problem of intentionality. *Ecological Psychology*, 13 (4): 275–314.

Shim, J., Carlton, L. G., Chow, J. W. and Chae, W. K. (2005) The use of anticipatory visual cues by highly skilled tennis players. *Journal of Motor Behavior*, 37 (2): 164–75.

Stoffregen, T. A., Bardy, B. G., Smart, L. J. and Pagulayan, R. (2003) On the nature and evaluation of fidelity in virtual environments, in L. J. Hettinger and M. W. Haas (eds) *Virtual and Adaptive Environments: Applications, Implications and Human Performance Issues*. Mahwah: Lawrence Erlbaum Associates, pp. 111–28.

Thelen, E. and Smith, L. B. (1994) *A Dynamic Systems Approach to the Development of Cognition and Action*. Cambridge, MA: The MIT Press.

Tucker, D. M., Derryberry, D. and Luu, P. (2000) Anatomy and physiology of human emotion: Vertical Integration of brainstem, limbic, and cortical systems, in J. Borod (ed.) *Handbook of the Neuropsychology of Emotion*. New York: Oxford University Press, pp. 56–79.

Vallerand, R. J. and Blanchard, C. M. (2000) The study of emotion in sport and exercise: Historical, definitional, and conceptual perspectives, in Y. L. Hanin (ed.) *Emotions in Sport*. Champaign, IL: Human Kinetics, pp. 3–38.

van der Kamp, J., Rivas, F., van Doorn, H. and Savelsbergh, G. (2008) Ventral and dorsal contributions in visual anticipation in fast ball sports. *International Journal of Sport Psychology*, 39 (2): 100–30.

Vicente, K. J. (2003) Beyond the lens model and direct perception: toward a broader ecological psychology. *Ecological Psychology*, 15 (3): 241–67.

Vilar, L., Araújo, D., Davids, K. and Renshaw, I. (2012) The need for 'representative task designs' in efficacy of skills tests in sport: a comment on Russell, Benton and Kingsley (2010) *Journal of Sports Sciences*, 30 (16): 1727–30.

Wigton, R. S. (2008) What do the theories of Egon Brunswik have to say to medical education. *Advances in Health Sciences Education*, 13: 109–21.

Williams, A. M., Davids, K. and Williams, J. G. (1999) *Visual Perception and Action in Sport*. London: Routledge.

Withagen, R. and Michaels, C. F. (2005) The role of feedback information for calibration and attunement in perceiving length by dynamic touch. *Journal of Experimental Psychology: Human Perception and Performance*, 31 (6): 1379–90.

Withagen, R. and van Wermeskerken, M. (2009) Individual differences in learning to perceive length by dynamic touch: evidence for variation in perceptual learning capacities. *Attention, Perception and Psychophysics*, 71 (1): 64–75.

Index

accumulated effort 66–7, 70–2, 75–7
action fidelity 178, 324–5
adaptation 44, 47, 65, 77–8, 105, 113,
  115, 117, 120, 136, 176, 241, 242, 245,
  247–9, 251, 253–4, 256–7, 287–8, 299,
  306, 314, 319, 325; biological 277;
  co-adaptation 105, 113, 120, 245,
  247–9, 253–4; compensatory 241–2;
  functional 117, 242, 277; performance
  306; psychobiological 77

adaptive flexibility 117, 230
affordances 181, 231, 237, 251–2, 256,
  265, 283, 306–15, 322; attunement to
  306, 308, 313
aging 270
anti-persistent 74–5, 77
anti-phase 48, 50–3, 113, 208–10, 212–14,
  223, 280, 287, 289, 296; attraction 213;
  behaviour 212; coordination 208, 210,
  213, 280
association football see also soccer 56,
  109, 111, 114, 119, 120, 160, 161, 162,
  167, 171, 214, 229–31, 286–7, 323
attacker-defender dyad 107, 109, 111, 114,
  233
attention 20–1, 25, 27, 31–3, 327
attention focus 66–7, 75–6
attractor 5–9, 13–16, 47, 67–8, 73, 88–9,
  113, 150, 156, 208, 210–11, 223, 231,
  262, 264, 266–9, 279, 289, 293, 296,
  298–9, 301, 313, 239; fixed-point
  attractor 296, 299
attractor landscape 293, 295–9, 303
autocorrelation function 99, 125, 127–30,
  132–5
avatars 182

basin of attraction 5–7, 14–15, 250, 263,
  267, 269–70

badminton 210
baseball 322
basketball 55, 107–9, 114–15, 150–1, 156,
  171, 195, 210, 212, 214, 223, 233, 248,
  284, 286, 325
behavioural pattern 27, 31, 201, 217, 222
bifurcation 7–8, 11–13, 28, 31, 34, 47, 65,
  67, 245, 257; definition 257; pitchfork
  13; saddle-node 13
boccia 284–5
bootstrapping 151
breaststroke swimming 280
Brunswik's lens model 320, 322, 328
Brunswik's probabilistic functionalism
  320–1
Butterworth low-pass filter 166

cognition 18–20, 26, 35, 47, 321, 323,
  325, 327
classification 53–4, 98, 145–7, 149, 154
cluster analysis 146–51, 154–5, 157, 187,
  301
collective variable see also order
  parameter 7–11, 46–8, 54, 65–6, 73, 77,
  79, 106–8, 110–11, 121, 151, 160, 236,
  266, 267, 270, 286
complexity 3–5, 7, 46, 69, 93–4, 98–9,
  142, 151, 175, 179, 195, 241, 244,
  254–5, 262, 322–4; neurobiological
  322; of behavior 5; system 99, 323
compound kinematic variable 161
configurations 137, 141, 217, 220–1, 223,
  269–70; movement 269–70; playing
  217, 220–1, 223; spatial 137, 141
contextual dependency 106, 109, 113, 271
control parameter 8–9, 11–16, 22–3, 32,
  34, 44, 46–7, 55, 66, 78–9, 106–10,
  112, 116, 167–8, 171, 246
constraints 11, 56, 69, 71, 108–10, 112,
  115, 117, 161–2, 175–6, 180–2, 231,

237, 242–8, 250–1, 254, 256, 261–5,
271–2, 282–4, 285, 287–9, 295, 299,
306–8, 310–13, 315–16, 319, 320,
322–3, 325–6; based-model 306;
ecological 161, 231, 265, 307, 316,
323; environmental 11, 71, 242–7, 254,
256, 271, 282–4, 307–8, 310–13, 315,
320; informational 264; interacting 47,
232, 241–3, 246, 255, 262, 264, 277,
313; structural 109; task 56, 69,
108–10, 112, 115, 117, 162, 175–6,
180–2, 237, 245, 248, 250–1, 256,
261–3, 265, 272, 282, 285, 287–9, 295,
299, 307–8, 312, 319, 322–3, 325–6
cooperative effects 20, 65
coordination 19–35, 44–9, 50–2, 54–7,
65–6, 69, 71, 105–15, 120–1, 150, 156,
160–1, 176, 181, 184, 213, 223–33,
270, 326, 280, 282, 284, 286, 295,
299–300, 307, 309–11; attacker-
defender 111; dynamics 19–35, 44–9,
51–2, 54–7, 65–6, 69, 71, 160–1, 213,
223–33, 286, 309; interpersonal 23,
105–10, 114–15, 120, 160, 176, 181,
184, 231–33, 270, 326; interteam 105;
intrateam 105, 271; intrapersonal
113–14; patterns of 24, 28, 44–5, 50,
52, 54–5, 109, 112–16, 150, 156, 160,
176, 209, 231–3, 245, 261, 280, 282,
284, 295, 299–300, 307, 310–11; state
of 107–8, 231–2; variable 21–3, 28,
106–8, 110–11, 121
coordinative structure 31, 46, 56, 105,
314, 316
coupling angle 49–51
coupling tendency 167
creativity 194, 201–5, 247, 253, 256, 261–
3, 265, 270–2, 316; tactical 201–3
cricket 241, 244, 248, 251, 253, 324–5,
329
critical fluctuation 3, 14, 213, 232–3
critical regions 107, 110–11, 113, 233,
246, 271
critical slowing down 8, 14
critical states 246–7
criticality 106, 246–7
cross-correlations 48–9
cross-modal interactions 184

dance 265
decentring distortion 164
decision making 31, 34–5, 47, 120, 160,
182, 190, 230, 271
degeneracy 117, 182, 230, 241–2, 244,

255–6, 262, 277, 282–3, 294, 306,
310–11, 314–16, 322
degrees of freedom: biomechanical 27, 47,
56; motor system 311, 316;
performance 328; spectral 68, 70–1, 77
deterministic models 145
detrended fluctuation analysis (dfa) 86,
92–3, 101, 134, 279
dimension reduction tool 151
direct linear transformation 164
direct perception 184
displacement trajectories 233
distal cues 321
dorsal visual system 321
dyadic system 107, 109–10, 116, 120,
233–4, 237
dynamics: cognition 19; intrinsic 55, 75,
243–4, 253, 255–7, 316, 325; overlap
266–70; pattern analysis 191, 205;
pattern forming 160, 161, 232; systems
3, 13, 87, 91, 100, 249

early specialization 255
ecological dynamics model 160, 229–32,
236–7, 262, 313–14, 323
ecological psychology 181, 251, 308, 311,
319, 320
ecological validity 322
effort tolerance 62
egocentric viewpoint 178–9
embedding theorem 89
emergence 3, 9, 18, 23, 25, 31, 75–7, 105,
112–14, 117, 120–1, 150, 167, 169,
171, 232, 245, 251, 253, 256, 265, 272,
281, 284, 296, 307, 313, 315, 316, 320,
326
emotions 327–30
entropy 85, 91–4, 97, 100, 138–9, 143,
265, 308; approximate entropy (ApEn)
92–4, 138; definition 91–2; geometric
entropy index 308; Kolmogorov-Sinai
entropy (KS) 92–3; sample entropy
(SampEn) 85, 94–5, 97–101
epigenetics 254
ergodicity 15, 264, 269–70, 294; breaking
264, 270
equilibrium 160, 209, 232, 284, 300, 308,
312, 316
experimental design 45, 180–1, 323, 325,
329
environment-agent systems 175
expertise 54, 149, 178, 180, 241–78, 306,
310, 313–16; acquisition of 241–3, 246,
250–1, 255–6; in climbing 308–12,

315; in kayaking 312, 314–15
expert performance 180, 241–4, 250, 255, 257, 278, 313–14, 330
exploratory 57, 307, 310; behaviour 57, 310; practice 307
exploration 14–15, 147, 175, 253, 261, 264–5, 267, 269, 272, 289, 301, 313, 329
exploratory breadth 264–5, 270
exponential function 299

fatigue-induced spontaneous termination point (FISTP) 66–8, 71, 73
fidelity 165, 178, 184, 324–6
field hockey 51, 136, 195, 287–8
finger waggling 208, 296–8
fluency 270, 308–9
fluctuations 3, 14–15, 26, 31, 46, 67–8, 70, 75, 77, 85–6, 92–3, 133–4, 165, 203–4, 213, 232–3, 246, 266, 272, 279–80; fluctuation process 203
functional behaviour 175, 184, 245, 261
functional synergies 105, 112–13, 120–1
fractal 75, 91–2, 99, 279
futsal 56, 114–15, 138, 141, 216, 231, 233–6

gait 46, 48, 50–1, 53–4, 99, 146, 279–80
genetic 241–5, 254–6, 295
goal-directed adaptive behaviour 180
goal orientation 327–8
goal-scoring opportunities 163, 167, 171–2

head-mounted display 176–7
hierarchically soft-assembled 261, 263, 270
Hilbert transform 52, 212, 215
HKB model 47, 296–8
homogeneity assumptions 293, 294
Hubert-Gamma method 151
Hysteresis 13, 31, 79, 149, 279

ice-climbing 282, 307–12
identification parameters 150
immersion 176, 178
individual-constraint coupling 277
individual differences in learning 293–4, 297, 299–303, 306–7, 309–10
individual environment coupling 283, 308, 311
in-phase 48, 50–2, 113–16, 208–9, 212–16, 223, 280, 283, 286, 311; attraction 114–16, 214, 216; behaviour

210, 212; coordination 208, 214, 280, 283, 286, 311
information 18–21, 25–8, 33–5; action coupling 175; detection 308, 323–4; movement coupling 55, 322, 325
in situ 111, 176, 182, 323
instability *see also* loss of stability 19, 22–3, 26–7, 137, 169–71, 209, 232, 245, 252, 288, 213–16
intentions 21, 25, 27, 32, 35, 67, 73, 76, 78, 106, 210, 230, 264, 278, 280, 282–4, 307, 309, 321, 323, 328
inter-centroid distance 167, 169, 171
internal validity 321
interpersonal distances 105–7, 110–13, 121, 161, 183–4
intra-individual analysis 294
intra-individual variability 310–11
intra-technical error of measurement 166

Judo 328

Karhunen-Loève transformation 154
Kayaking 307, 314–15
Kohonen maps 151

learning 19–20, 25–34, 92; design 56, 321, 323–7, 329, 330; motor 14, 26, 254, 293–304; process 204, 250, 288, 299; task 28–30, 299, 324–5, 328–9; timescales of 293, 295–6, 299–301, 303, 306; rate 299; supervised 151
level of description 19, 20–4, 29
limbic system 321, 327
limitations in averaging 293, 294, 295, 299, 303
locomotion 53, 278–9, 301, 308
long-range correlations 91, 99, 133–5, 279
loss of stability *see also* instability 8, 31, 47, 67, 72–3, 76–8, 169, 171, 314

memory recall 309
mesoscopic protectorate 24
metastability 14, 26–7, 46–7, 244, 245, 250, 254, 256, 262, 306, 312, 316; performance region 47, 313; region
movement form 262, 264–5, 272, 309, 313
movement output 309, 313
multifunctionality 6, 31
multi-layer-perceptrons 151
multistability 15, 27, 31, 65, 282, 284, 306, 310–11, 312, 315–16

naturalistic 22, 45, 179
neighbourhood preservation 152
networks 5, 11, 117, 121,152, 190, 194–7, 199–202, 205, 211, 217, 223; artificial neural 152, 190, 194–7, 199–202, 205, 211, 217, 223; social 117, 121
neurobiological system 11, 54, 56, 230, 242, 244, 254–5, 262, 264, 277, 278, 282–3, 285, 306, 308, 310, 323, 324
nodes 152, 154, 156–7
noise 92, 134, 128–9, 131, 134; brown 92; pink 92, 134; white 92, 128–9, 131, 134
nonlinearity 10, 15, 18, 78, 85, 87–90, 98, 101, 110, 113–14, 250, 254, 262
nonlinear dynamical systems 4–6, 87, 172
nonlinear pedagogy 253, 263, 323, 327, 329–30
non-stationarity 92, 98–9, 127–8, 134, 229–30, 236–7

optic array 181
optic flow 180–1
optical distortion 164
optimization 44, 261
order parameter *see also* collective variable 7, 11, 65–7, 69, 73, 79, 151, 160–1, 167–71, 211, 263–6, 270
order-order transition 167, 169
overlap order parameter 264, 266

parametric stabilization 21, 27
pattern formation 22, 282
pattern recognition 191, 194, 201–2, 205, 222–3
pedalo riding 300–1
perception-action coupling 180–2, 327
perceptual work-space 301
performance curves 295, 299
performance indicators 229–30, 237
performance variability 171, 245, 278
perception-action landscape 265, 270, 272
persistence 74–5, 77, 133
phase space 88–9, 211–12
phase relation 11, 29, 48, 51, 113–15, 171, 208, 213, 216, 223, 233, 279, 287, 296–7, 301, 311
phase transition *see also* transition 3, 8, 11, 13–14, 23, 30–2, 46–7, 52, 70, 107, 109, 111–12, 116, 150, 160–1, 212–13, 233, 297, 327, 329
pleiotropy 242, 255, 262
position data 195, 199–200, 214, 218, 221

postural stability 93, 301, 308, 310, 312, 315
power function 295
power law 295
practice 109, 117, 183, 241, 251, 256; deliberate 241, 256; design 109, 117, 321; organization 183; representative 117, 251
principal components analysis 52–3, 266, 300
process analysis 194–5
proximal cues 321–2
psychobiological integration 62, 66, 76–7, 79
psychobiological model 64, 72–3

qualitative analysis 201–3, 221
quantitative analysis 201–2, 221, 223, 229

race walking 279
racket sport 205, 210
reciprocity 46, 182
recurrence quantification analysis (RQA) 89–91, 98
redundancy 97, 314, 316
rehabilitation 34, 44, 56–7
relative phase 26, 28, 30, 46, 48, 51, 55, 113–14, 116–17, 208–10, 212–16, 223, 233–4, 264, 279, 281, 296–7, 301
relative stretch index 167, 170–1
relative velocity 107–8, 110, 112–13, 161, 183
relaxation time 8–9, 15, 28, 68, 269–70
repeller 5–7, 14, 19, 25
replica symmetry breaking 263
representative design 180, 251, 319–23; experimental task 161; functional interaction 181; learning design 323, 326–27, 329–30
residual analysis technique 166
rock climbing 307–9, 315
rollerball 301–3
rugby union 110–13, 161, 181–3, 321, 325–6
rugged potential landscape *see also* rugged energy landscape 14–15
rugged energy landscape *see also* rugged potential landscape 68
running correlations 110–12, 114

sampling rate 89–90, 94, 99
scale invariance 75
1/f scaling 86
selection via instability 26

self-determination theory 327
self-efficacy 327–8
self-implemented network 155
self-interaction 5, 10
self-organization 3, 10, 24–5, 35, 46, 71, 114, 122, 160, 230, 250, 256, 271, 288, 299–301, 323
self-organizing maps 54–5, 152–4, 190–2, 205
sequential analysis 229, 236
sequential dependence 85–7, 89, 92
signal processing 165, 171
signature movements 155
simulation 190, 193–5, 201, 204
simulation of constraints 323–5, 327
skill acquisition 28–30, 45, 244–54, 262, 316, 323, 326
soccer *see* association football 55–7, 87, 135–7, 149, 155–6, 179, 191–9, 202–4, 219, 286–7, 295, 320, 323, 325–6
soft-assembled 77–8, 262–3, 265–70
spatial awareness 308
spatial feedback 301
spatial randomness 141
spectral density function 125, 129–31, 134
squash 194–8, 209–10, 213, 223
stability 7, 11, 19, 24–5, 27–8, 31–4, 55–6, 63, 72, 77–8, 107, 111–12, 114, 126, 296–7, 306, 311, 313–14, 316, 329
stability analysis 279
stationary 90, 92, 94, 98–9
stationarity 90
stochastic processes 126–8
surface area 214, 216
symmetry 12–13
symmetry breaking *see also* decision making 12–13
synergies 46

tactical pattern 195–7, 201, 221–2, 230
talent development 250, 252–4, 256
talent identification 250, 252–4, 256
task-specific device 56
team dynamics 149, 155
team centroid 55, 167, 214, 215, 286
team sports 105–7, 109–10, 112–14, 117, 120, 125, 134, 136, 141, 190, 195, 201–2, 205, 208, 210, 214, 230–2, 236–7
temporal feedback 301
tennis 52, 114, 155, 157, 179, 194–6, 209–13, 223, 322
time-discrete variables 145–6
time series 125–35, 138, 142, 294, 301
time series analysis 89–90, 134, 294, 301
topological control parameter 32
track and field 294
tracking operator 166

variability 56, 150, 155, 241, 263, 278–8, 293, 306–7, 310–11, 313–16; adaptive 306, 310–11; compensatory 284; functional 279–80; movement 56, 155, 241, 263, 278–88, 293; movement pattern 56, 150, 306–7, 311, 314–16; movement system 56, 278, 313
vectors 94–6, 99 coding 49–51
ventral visual system 321
vicarious functioning 321
video-tracking 161
virtual positional coordinates 163
volition states 66, 71–2
volleyball 61, 149, 157, 194–5, 197, 199
two-landscape model 299, 301, 303

Waddington's landscape model 295
weight lifting 294

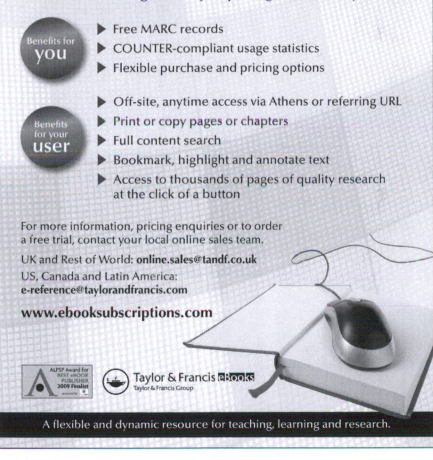